Contemporary Issues in Mental Health: Concepts, Policy, and Practice

CONTEMPORARY ISSUES IN MENTAL HEALTH:
CONCEPTS, POLICY, AND PRACTICE

edited by

James A. LeClair and Leslie T. Foster

Canadian Western Geographical Series

Volume 41

Copyright 2007

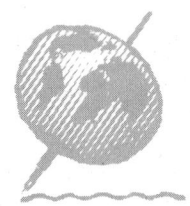

Western Geographical Press

DEPARTMENT OF GEOGRAPHY, UNIVERSITY OF VICTORIA
P.O. BOX 3050, VICTORIA, BC, CANADA V8W 3P5
PHONE: (250)721-7331   FAX: (250)721-6216
EMAIL: HFOSTER@OFFICE.GEOG.UVIC.CA

Canadian Western Geographical Series

editorial address
Harold D. Foster, Ph.D.
Department of Geography
University of Victoria
Victoria, British Columbia
Canada

Since publication began in 1970 the Western Geographical Series (now the Canadian and the International Western Geographical Series) has been generously supported by the Leon and Thea Koerner Foundation, the Social Science Federation of Canada, the National Centre for Atmospheric Research, the International Geographical Union Congress, the University of Victoria, the Natural Sciences Engineering Research Council of Canada, the Institute of the North American West, the University of Regina, the Potash and Phosphate Institute of Canada, and the Saskatchewan Agriculture and Food Department. Generous support has also been received from the BC Ministry of Children and Family Development. This volume has received grants from the BC Ministry of Health and from Nipissing University.

CONTEMPORARY ISSUES IN MENTAL HEALTH:
CONCEPTS, POLICY, AND PRACTICE

(Canadian western geographical series 1203-1178; v. 41)
Includes bibliographical references.
ISBN 978-0-919838-31-4

1. Mental health--Canada. 2. Mental illness--Canada. 3. Mental health services--Canada. 4. Mental health policy--Canada. I. LeClair, James A. (James André), 1969- II. Foster, Leslie T., 1947- III. Series.

RA790.7.C3C657 2007   362.20971   C2007-902518-8

Copyright 2007 Western Geographical Press

ALL RIGHTS RESERVED

This book is protected by copyright.
No part of it may be duplicated or reproduced
in any manner without written permission.

Printed in Canada

Series Editor's Acknowledgements

Several members of the Department of Geography, University of Victoria co-operated to ensure the successful publication of this volume of the Canadian Western Geographical Series. Special thanks are due to the Technical Services Division. Diane Braithwaite undertook the very demanding tasks of copy editing, typesetting, and layout, while cartography and cover design were in the expert hands of Ole Heggen and Ken Josephson respectively. Their dedication and hard work is greatly appreciated.

University of Victoria
Victoria, British Columbia
April, 2007

Harold D. Foster
Series Editor

Acknowledgements

Over the course of the development of this volume many individuals have provided assistance and encouragement along its somewhat winding road to completion. We would like to express our appreciation to the numerous authors who developed their chapters and patiently incorporated not only our editorial comments, but also those of the external peer reviewers. At the same time, we owe a great thanks to the many individuals who acted as peer reviewers. Their comments have not only improved the quality of individual chapters, but that of the volume as a whole. To both of these groups we are indebted.

We would also like to thank the British Columbia Ministry of Health and Nipissing University, both of which provided grants to enable this volume to be prepared and published, and the British Columbia Ministry of Children and Family Development for allowing one of the editors the time to work on the early planning of this volume. Without their support this volume would not have been possible.

We are indebted as well to Ferruccio Sardella, who graciously allowed us to reproduce his work for three of the volume's plates. For more information about his work, please get in touch with him at *contact@ferrucciosardella.com*.

Finally, we gratefully acknowledge the staff of the Western Geographical Press for their hard work throughout the production of this volume: Harry Foster, as overall editor for the series, provided continuing encouragement and advice; Diane Braithwaite did a superb job in assisting in final copy editorial work and catching and fixing many points which we missed; and Ken Josephson and Ole Heggen, who undertook the final development of figures, maps, and the design of the cover for the volume. Thanks to each of you.

James A. LeClair, *Associate Professor*
Nipissing University

Leslie T. Foster, *Adjunct Professor*
University of Victoria

Contents

Series Editor's Acknowledgements v
Editors' Acknowledgements v
List of Figures xi
List of Tables xii
List of Plates xiii

1   Introduction 1
     James A. LeClair and Leslie T. Foster

2   Mental Health Status in Northern Ontario 5
     Mary Ward

Introduction 5
The Region 5
Health Status in Northern Ontario 8
Implications 15
References 16

3   Youth in British Columbia: Their Mental Health 17
     Roger S. Tonkin

Introduction 17
Background 17
Prevalence 21
The BC Example 23
Issues and Challenges 30
Conclusion 34
Acknowledgements 35
References 36

4   Youth Leaving Care: Mental Health Issues 39
     Deborah Rutman, Carol Hubberstey, April Feduniw, and Erinn Brown

Introduction 39
Youth in Transition From State Care and Mental Health 39
Research Process 43
Findings 44
Physical and Mental Health 45

Physical and Mental Health Conditions 46
Homelessness 48
Marijuana Use 49
Family Relations, Social Supports, and Community Involvement 49
Summary and Conclusions 51
Endnotes 52
References 52

5   MENTAL HEALTH ISSUES AMONG CANADA'S HOMELESS YOUTH 55
Elizabeth Votta and Susan Farrell

Prevalence of Youth Homelessness in Canada 55
A Case Study of Canadian Homeless Youth 57
Mental Health Issues Among Canada's Homeless Youth 58
Risk Factors for Poor Mental Health Outcomes 62
Summary and Conclusions 69
References 70

6   CROSS-DISCIPLINARY PERSPECTIVES ON CHILDREN'S MENTAL HEALTH 77
James A. LeClair

Introduction 77
Data Collection and Behavioural Assessment 80
Ecological Analysis 82
Individual- and Family-level Analyses 85
Contextual Analyses 89
Multivariate Analysis 91
Discussion 92
Limitations of the Data 94
Conclusion 96
Acknowledgements 98
References 98

7   PSYCHOSOCIAL INFLUENCES OF SCHOOL CULTURE 103
Gord Miller

Introduction 103
Definitions of Key Terms and Concepts 105
Psychosocial Factors Influencing School Culture 106
Approaches, Programs, and Strategies That Impact School Culture 112
Examples of Program Innovations and a Data Measuring Tool 120
Summary 124
Recommendations for Future Research 124
References 127

8 Elder Abuse: A Consequence of Risk and Anxiety in Everyday Life 137
Kari Brozowski

Introduction 137
Overview of the Research on Elder Abuse 138
The Risk of Ageing in an Ageist Society 141
Interpersonal Risk and Elder Abuse 144
The Role of Public Policy and
    Institutional Support in an Ageing Society 147
Conclusion 149
Acknowledgement 150
References 150

9 Some Psychosocial Implications of Mass Pollutant Release Events 153
Lisa Kadonaga

Introduction 153
Types of Pollutant Release Situations 154
Complexity and Uncertainty 155
Physiological Impacts of Pollution 155
Psychological and Psychosocial Symptoms 157
Perceptions of Pollution 157
Stress as an Additional Complication 158
Mitigating Factors 159
Perception and the Media 161
Conclusion 162
References 163

10 Under the Weather: The Biometeorology of Mental Health Status 167
Lisa Kadonaga and James A. LeClair

Introduction 167
Sunlight and Seasonal Affective Disorder 168
Temperature Effects 170
The Role of Relative Humidity and Weather Variability 171
Wind and Air Pressure Changes 173
Air Quality Issues 173
Seasonality and Cyclical Effects 174
Climate Change 175
Conclusion 177
References 178

11 DEVELOPING A RESEARCH-POLICY PARTNERSHIP TO IMPROVE CHILDREN'S MENTAL HEALTH IN BRITISH COLUMBIA 183

Charlotte Waddell, Cody A. Shepherd, and Jayne Barker

Introduction 183
Motivation for the Partnership 184
Developing the Partnership 187
Challenges for the Partnership 190
Sustaining the Partnership 194
Conclusion 196
Acknowledgements 196
References 196

12 AN EDUCATIONAL RESPONSE TO MENTAL HEALTH ISSUES IN THE CLASSROOM 199

Darlene Brackenreed, Ron Common, Lorraine Frost, Warnie Richardson, and Paula Barber

Introduction 199
The Study 200
Results of the Study: Phase One 201
Results of the Study: Phase Two 202
Discussion 203
Outcome of the Study 203
References 205
Appendix A: Mental Health Issues Questionnaire 206

13 TEACHER STRESS AND STIGMA IN NORTHERN ONTARIO 211

Kristen Ferguson, Lorraine Frost, Kristian Kirkwood, and David Hall

Introduction 211
Method 213
Results 215
Discussion 219
Limitations of the Study 221
Suggestions for Future Research 222
Conclusion 223
References 224

14 Dangerous Medicine: Social Control of the Mentally Ill and the Police Role 227
Gregory P. Brown and Ron Hoffman

Introduction 227
The Epidemiology of Police Contact with
    Mentally Ill Persons in Canada 229
Historical Notes on the Social Control of the Mentally Ill 231
Deinstitutionalization and Growth of
    Community Mental Health 232
The Role of the Police in the Social Control of the Mentally Ill 232
Police Responses to Dealing with Persons with a Mental Illness 234
Rethinking the Police Role in Responding to
    Mentally Ill Persons in Crisis 235
Epilogue 237
References 237

15 Integration of Mind: How Superstition Amplifies Discrimination and Blocks Empowerment 243
Tim King

Introduction 243
The Mind as Myth 243
Philosophy of the Mind 244
Rational Enquiry Makes For Less Stigma 245
The Brief History of Mental Illness: Our Prejudices Show 245
The Negative Cycle 246
The Positive Cycle 247
Conclusion 248
References 249

List of Figures

2.1	Mental health hospitalizations by geographic area and sex, 2003	13
2.2	Mental health diagnoses by geographic area and sex, 2003	13
2.3	Suicide hospitalization by geographic area, 2003	14
2.4	Suicide mortality by geographic area, 2000 and 2001	14
3.1	Percentage of BC students who attempted suicide in the past year	24
3.2	Proposed public health strategy (adapted from Waddell et al., 2005)	25
3.3	Percentage of BC students who expect to live to be at least 25 years old	29
3.4	Percentage of school youth with emotional distress	30
3.5	Positive mental health by gender and age	34
6.1	Schools in the study area	80
6.2	The study area	81
6.3	Distribution of problem behaviour	85
11.1	Public health strategy to improve children's mental health	188
11.2	Framework of the *Child and Youth Mental Health Plan for BC*	189

LIST OF TABLES

2.1	Physical and mental health indicators by geographical area and sex (%)	9
2.2	Health indicators by geographical area, both sexes combined (%)	10
3.1	Prevalence of child/adolescent mental disorders: Canada versus British Columbia	22
3.2	Emotional health problems in special populations (%)	26
3.3	Emotional health problems in at-risk youth populations (%)	26
3.4	Emotional health problems in other youth populations (%)	27
3.5	Emotional health problems and engagement in multiple risk behaviours (%)	27
3.6	Positive mental health by health service delivery area (%)	28
3.7	Attempted suicide in the past year by Health Service Delivery Area (%)	33
4.1	Time 1 & 2 – Participants by gender	43
4.2	Time 1 – Youth rating their health as 'excellent' or 'good'	46
4.3	Time 1 – Past or current health condition	47
4.4	Time 1 – Current mental health concerns	47
6.1	Census tract prevalence of problem behaviour	84
6.2	Ecological correlations	86
6.3	Chi-Square analysis results	88
6.4	Hierarchical logistic regression analysis results	90
6.5	Multivariate analysis: Final model	91
7.1	Schematic framework for examining factors which influence school culture	126
11.1	Prevalence of children's mental disorders and population affected in British Columbia and Canada	185
13.1	Binary logistic regression models of teacher stress: Ontario, 2005 (exponentiated beta coefficients)	217
13.2	Binary logistic regression models of teacher stigma associated with stress: Ontario, 2005 (exponentiated beta coefficients)	217

List of Plates

1	Path Less Travelled	xiv
2	Counting Pebbles	38
3	No Vacancy	54
4	Chrysallis	76
5	Involvement	102
6	Genome	136
7	Electric Storm	182
8	Sitting, Waiting	210
9	Jailhouse Perspective	226
10	Meaning	242
11	Labyrinth	250

Plate 1 "Path Less Travelled" (J. LeClair) ▸

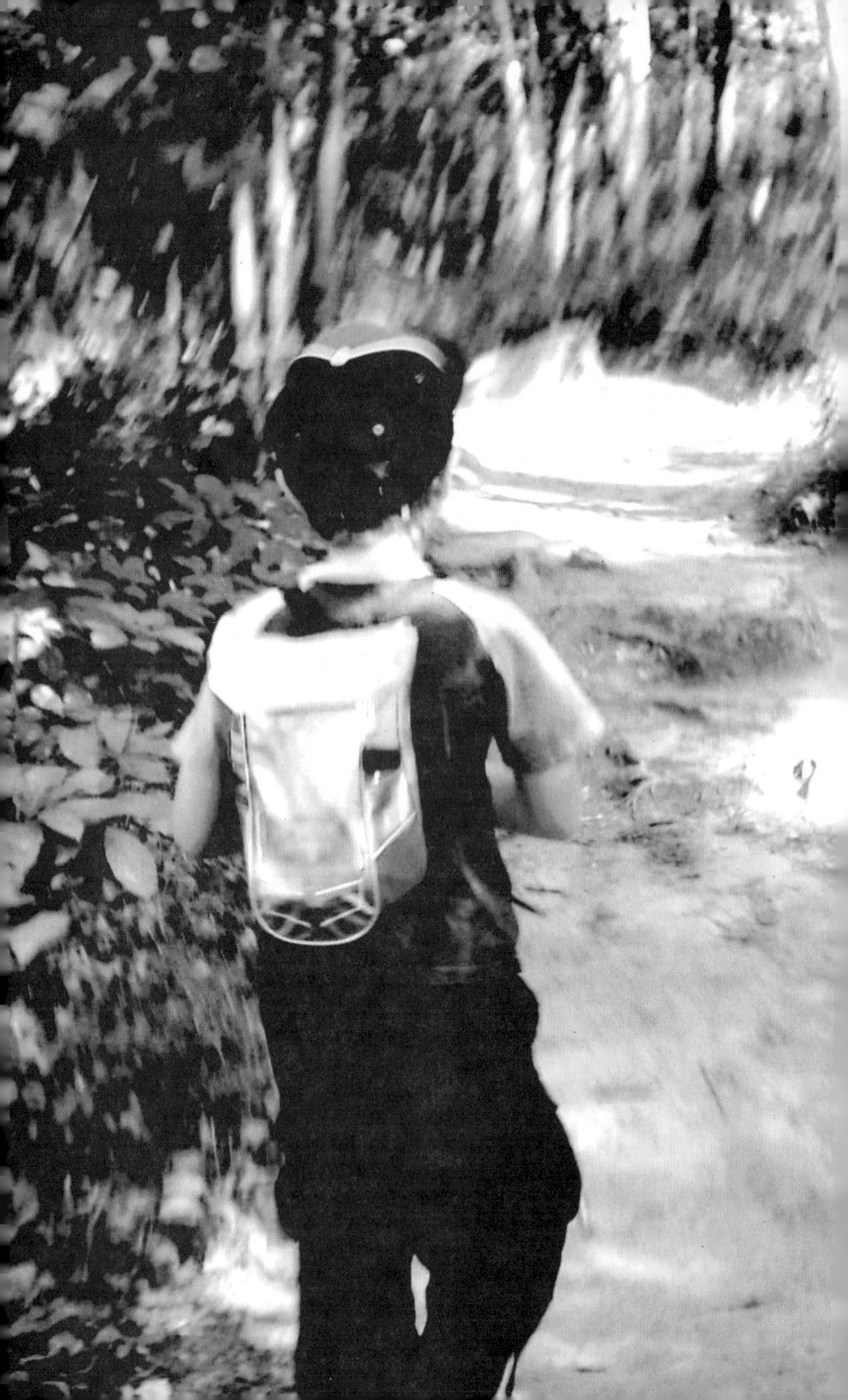

Introduction

James A. LeClair
Department of Geography, Nipissing University

Leslie T. Foster
School of Child and Youth Care and Department of Geography, University of Victoria

In any single year, approximately 20% of the population of Canada will suffer from a mental illness (Health Canada, 2002): 3% will experience a serious disorder, and an additional 17% will experience a mild to moderate illness (Standing Senate Committee on Social Affairs, Science and Technology, 2006). Recent data from the Canadian Community Health Survey (2005) indicate that about 4.8% of the population (not including those in institutions or on Indian reserves) aged 12 and over report fair to poor mental health when responding to the question, "In general, would you say your mental health is excellent, very good, fair, or poor." Females have a higher percentage of fair to poor mental health (5.1%) when compared to males (4.4%). Geographically, Newfoundland and Labrador, at 3.5%, has the lowest percentage reporting only fair or poor mental health status, while British Columbia and Nunavut, at 5.8%, have the highest percentage reporting compromised mental health (Statistics Canada, 2006).

The economic burden associated with mental health problems is also substantial; Stephens and Joubert (2001) identify it as among the costliest ill-health conditions in Canada, with an estimated total cost of $14.4 billion in 1998 alone. Mental illness is the leading cause for disability claims in Canada, accounting for up to one third of claims, and up to 70% of the costs associated with them (Standing Senate Committee on Social Affairs, Science and Technology, 2006). Depression alone accounted for productivity losses totalling $2.6 billion in 1998, and is a leading cause of disability worldwide (Gilmour and Patten, 2007).

In spite of the obvious importance of this health problem, further illustrated by the fact that 192,562 hospital stays in 2003-2004 were due primarily to mental health diagnoses (Canadian Institute for Health Information, 2006), almost 22% of those seeking treatment report that they cannot get help (Government of Canada, 2006).

Within a Canadian public-policy context, then, the problem of mental illness does not appear to be the "invisible plague" of which Torrey and Miller (2001) wrote. Since 2002, no less than four major reports on mental illness in Canada have been released, each of them cited herein.

The content of this volume reflects a large diversity of perspectives on mental health and illness, from both within and outside the academy. Attention is paid to the prevalence of mental health problems in specific populations, selected determinants of mental health, and to policy- and practice-related challenges faced in the provision of mental health services. Given the breadth of perspectives and issues related to mental health—consider the potential for multiple volumes concerning the determinants of mental health alone—the material covered is deliberately selective rather than exhaustive. Our focus is on vulnerable populations—most notably children and youth, the "1.2 million young Canadians who live with anxiety, attention deficit, depression, addiction, and other disorders" (Standing Senate Committee on Social Affairs, Science and Technology, 2006, p.135), and on what might be deemed 'alternative' perspectives on factors influencing mental health outcomes. The result is a wide-ranging and somewhat eclectic collection of readings intended to enhance and expand upon the recently-increasing volume of reports on mental health and illness that serve to raise awareness of this important health issue.

In Chapter 2, Ward examines the burden of mental health problems in Northern Ontario, a region 'at risk' and, in the three chapters that follow, attention is paid to mental health issues among youth. Specifically, Tonkin (Chapter 3) offers insight into the mental health status of British Columbia's youth, Ruttman and colleagues (Chapter 4) consider mental health issues in youth leaving care in the Province of British Columbia, and Votta and Farrell examine mental health issues among homeless youth in Canada.

Although the importance of mental health problems is now widely acknowledged, the causes underlying mental illness are still poorly understood. In Chapter 6, LeClair examines the wide range of potential determinants of children's mental health identified across disciplines and, in the four chapters that follow, consideration is given to what might seem rather unexpected determinants of mental health. In Chapter 7, Miller offers insight into the impacts of school culture, while Brozowski (Chapter 8) considers the complex (and potentially dangerous) interplay of low-level mental health problems and inter-generational relationships in a late-modern context. In Chapter 9, Kadonaga examines the psychosocial symptomatology—most notably tension and anxiety—that can follow exposure to major toxic release events, and the importance of information and official transparency in mitigating these effects. Finally, in Chapter 10, Kadonaga and LeClair consider some of the ways in which weather- and climate-related factors might influence our psychosocial and behavioural well-being.

Given the seriousness of mental health problems in Canadian society, and particularly the central (and quite costly) role played by both general and psychiatric hospitals in service provision, the development of responsive public policy seems critical. To this end, Waddell and colleagues (Chapter 11) consider the development of British Columbia's child and youth mental health plan. In Chapter 12, Brackenreed and colleagues characterize teachers as being on the 'front line' of mental health services provision for children, and discuss the development of university-level mental health-oriented curriculum that will better prepare classroom teachers for this role. And what of the state of mental health of these front-line teachers-cum-therapists? Ferguson and co-workers (Chapter 13) identify some of the factors linked to high levels of occupational stress, and the perception of stigma around such stress among classroom teachers.

The degree of integration into broader society of those with mental illness has clearly changed over time. The most notable development in this trajectory is undoubtedly the move toward deinstitutionalization, a trend that Torrey and Miller (2001) liken to confusing "civil liberty with the right to remain insane" (p. 4). While it is difficult to advocate for the involuntary incarceration of those with severe mental health problems, have things really changed? Between 1967 and 2004, there has been a 61% increase in the percentage of criminal offenders with mental disorders identified upon admission to Correctional Services, and fully 12% of offenders require immediate treatment for a serious disorder (Standing Senate Committee on Social Affairs, Science, and Technology, 2006). In British Columbia, 43% of inmates entering prison meet the criteria for one or more current or lifetime diagnoses for a mental disorder—a figure that soars to 84% when substance abuse problems are included (Government of Canada, 2006). In Chapter 14, Brown and Hoffman consider some of the troubling implications of increasing rates of interaction between police and the mentally ill, a seemingly inevitable consequence of the disjointed and oft-dwindling resources available to those in need of mental health services.

While belief in the clinical reality of mental health problems is implicit in the content of this volume, we recognize that the very notion of mental illness is contested. Szasz (1970), for example, suggests that the "ethical convictions and social arrangements" based upon this (ostensibly erroneous) belief in mental illness "constitute an immoral ideology of intolerance" (p. xv) which he likens to the Inquisition. Is mental illness merely a social construction reflective of the hegemony of the psychosocial-neurocognitive majority? In Chapter 15, the last in this volume, King examines some of the barriers to acknowledging and accepting mental illnesses as we do physical illnesses. This transition is an important one, for if it is achieved, those who suffer the burdens of mental illness may no longer be "other," but simply one of "us."

In today's fast changing world of globalized societies, it is increasingly evident that the mental health of the population is being compromised. As the opening sentence of this chapter reveals, fully one-fifth of the population suffers from a mental health issue in any given year. Along with this statistic comes a continuing tendency for sufferers to self-medicate through the use of drugs and alcohol, often because of the stigma associated with the term 'mental illness,' and the ensuing reluctance to seek professional help. This only serves to increase the burden of mental illness and its negative consequences for societal well-being.

Even as we write this introduction, the latest Ipsos-Reid survey of 1,000 Canadians and 1,000 Americans concerning depression in the workplace suggests that depression has major career ramifications, and 24% of those surveyed think that those suffering from depression could "just snap out of it if they really wanted to" (as quoted in the *Victoria Times Colonist*, February 15, p. A6). Highlighting the stigma associated with mental health problems, nearly 80% of those surveyed indicate that a worker suffering from depression should keep it secret to avoid damaging future career opportunities.

With an aging society, this burden will only increase, as older people indicate poorer mental health than younger age groups in the population. It is hoped that, in some small way, the variety of perspectives presented in this volume can help to focus more attention on specific dimensions of mental health, thus helping to improve the overall health of the country.

REFERENCES

Canadian Institute for Health Information (2006). *Hospital Mental Health Services in Canada, 2003-2004*. Ottawa: CIHI.

Gilmour, H., and Patten, S.B. (2007). Depression and work impairment. *Health Reports*, 18, 9-22.

Government of Canada (2006). *The Human Face of Mental Health and Mental Illness in Canada. 2006*. Ottawa: Minister of Public Works and Government Services Canada.

Health Canada (2002). *A Report on Mental Illnesses in Canada*. Ottawa, Canada.

Standing Senate Committee on Social Affairs, Science and Technology (2006). *Out of the Shadows at Last: Transforming Mental Health, Mental Illness and Addiction Services in Canada*. Ottawa: Standing Senate Committee on Social Affairs, Science and Technology.

Statistics Canada (2006). Statistics Canada Website. Accessed January 2006 from http://www.statcan.ca/english/freepub/82-221-XIE/2006001/tindex.htm#f.

Szasz, T.S. (1970). *The manufacture of madness: A comparative study of the Inquisition and the mental health movement*. New York: Harper Colophon Books.

Stephens, T., and Joubert, N. (2001). The economic burden of mental health problems in Canada. *Chronic Diseases in Canada*, 22, 18-23.

Torrey, E.F., and Miller, J. (2001). *The invisible plague: The rise of mental illness from 1750 to the present*. Piscataway, NJ: Rutgers University Press.

Mental Health Status in Northern Ontario

Mary Ward
*Northern Health Information Partnership &
Northern Ontario School of Medicine (East Campus)*

Introduction

As noted elsewhere in this volume, mental health problems exert a significant toll on the well-being of the population, with as many as 20% of all Canadians experiencing a mental health problem during any given year (Health Canada, 2002). While significant, even this number may well underestimate the magnitude of the problem, as mental health-related events are often poorly documented by traditional data sources. For example, it has been suggested that suicide attempts are under-reported by as much as 63% (Rhodes, Links, Dawe, Cass, and Janes, 2002). Other examples of poorly-captured mental health-related data include those pertaining to mental well-being, the use of medications for mental health problems, the prevalence of untreated depression, and perceptions of social support and isolation.

As is the case with health status in general, there seems to be considerable geographical variation in mental health; some regions have a greater burden of mental health problems in their populations than others. This chapter examines selected mental health indices as well as rates of hospitalization and death resulting from mental health-related diagnoses for Northern Ontario, a region of unique geographical character and significant overall health status issues. Within-region comparisons, in addition to comparisons with the Province of Ontario, are drawn in order to examine the significance of mental health problems within this region 'at-risk.'

The Region

Northern Ontario, which accounts for approximately 80% of Ontario's landmass, is home to only about 7% of its population (866,087 of 12,238,300 people). This vast region—approximately equivalent to the combined area of France, Germany, Switzerland, Belgium, and the Netherlands (Vainio, Ward, and the Northern Health Issues Strategy Steering Committee, 2004)—has a population density of about one person per square kilometre, a figure that is strikingly lower than that for the considerably smaller but more populous southern region of the province, which has a density of 192 people per square kilometre.

With respect to the demographic structure of Northern Ontario, census data show that, although the provincial population is increasing overall, the North is in a state of decline. For example, the population of the province in 1990 was 10,341,433, rising to 10,964,925 in 1995, and 11,685,380 in 2000. While the population of Northern Ontario grew between 1990 and 1995 (increasing from 899,519 to 908,756 residents in that period), the population has fallen steadily since, with a 2000 population of 881,437, and an estimate for 2003 of 866,087 (Statistics Canada, 2003). Two mechanisms that have been cited to explain this population decline are the aging of the population, and youth out-migration (Northern Health Issues Strategy Steering Committee, 2004).

The overall demographic decline of the North is coupled with its diminished socio-economic position relative to the growing southern region. Northern Ontario is disadvantaged with respect to both income–average incomes were about $6,000 lower than the provincial average in 2001–and educational attainment. Not surprisingly, unemployment is significantly higher in the North than it is in the South (Northern Health Information Partnership, 2004)

Northern Ontario Health Status: An Overview

The region in question has a number of unique health status issues. In general, the prevalence of health risk factors is higher than for the province as a whole. For example, rates of smoking and levels of alcohol consumption are higher in the North, as is the proportion of those with high blood pressure. As well, the overall mortality rate is higher in the North than for the province in general, a trend which is also apparent for specific causes of mortality, including those for circulatory disease, cancer, respiratory disease, and injuries and poisonings. As a consequence, hospitalization rates are significantly elevated in the region (Northern Health Information Partnership, 2004)

Sources of Data and Limitations

In general, little comprehensive information concerning the mental health status of the population of Northern Ontario has been available. As a result, the release of the Canadian Community Health Survey Mental Health Supplement from Statistics Canada has been an important addition to the small body of population-based databases on the subject. Hospitalization and mortality data, while long available, show only the tip of the mental health 'iceberg,' in that they typically reveal only the most serious mental health-related illnesses and events (most notably suicide and parasuicide). The stigma of mental illness—and the consequent reluctance of some to seek medical assistance—further limits such utilization data. To illustrate, an analysis of the 1994-1995 National Population Health Survey examined the care-seeking behaviour of those who had experienced a Major Depressive Episode (MDE). Despite the widespread availability of treatments for depression, just 43% of Canadians who met the criteria for having an MDE in the past year (approximately 487,000 individuals) report seeking the advice of a health professional, and only one in four of those who experienced an MDE report four or more consultations (Diverty and Beaudet, 1997). In addition, hospitalization data do not include admissions to provincial psychiatric hospitals. As a result, it seems likely that patients with chronic mental illnesses are under-represented in the data.

One final issue which compromises the utility of hospitalization data for analyses of mental health-related issues is the method employed in the coding of data. Mental health diagnoses are often under-represented because they are not coded as the 'most responsible diagnosis.' For example, if a patient presents to the emergency department with a serious injury and is subsequently admitted to hospital, the visit will often be coded with the injury being the most responsible diagnosis, even when the injury was caused by the patient's mental state. Consequently, data sources on mental health issues are inevitably not as inclusive as other databases, such as the Cancer Registries maintained by Cancer Care Ontario.

While hospitalization and mortality data need to be considered in light of their limitations, the national surveys produced by Statistics Canada are widely considered the 'gold standard' for population-based survey data. Accordingly, such data sources are highly useful, particularly when paired with data from Vital Statistics and Hospitalization records.

For the purposes of this chapter, population health data were derived from the Canadian Community Health Survey (CCHS) Mental Health Supplement [Cycle 1.2] (Statistics Canada, 2002), while mortality and hospitalization data were obtained from the Provincial Health Planning Database (Queen's Printer for Ontario, 2003) from Mental Health in Northern Ontario (Northern Health Information Partnership, 2005). Although the CCHS provides excellent information about the mental health status of the population in question, it should be noted that it does not include homeless individuals, those living in institutions, or on-reserves—populations which are generally known to have an increased risk for mental health issues (Scott, 1993; MacMillan, MacMillan, Offord, and Dingle, 1996). In contrast, Vital Statistics and Hospitalization records are considered inclusive of the population.

ICD-9 and ICD-10 Data Coding

For the purposes of this discussion, mental health diagnoses were coded using the International Classification of Diseases, 10th revision (ICD-10, F00 to F99). Due to small numbers in the Northern Ontario region, suicide mortality typically shows increased variability in comparison with the province. Often, when small numbers are present, several years of data are used to show suicide mortality trends in the North. The advent of the ICD-10 classification system in 2000 mortality data limits comparisons with older, ICD-9-based data. Therefore, as the classification differs between the two systems of coding, it is considered unwise to perform trend analyses using both coding systems. Accordingly, only 2 years of data are presented herein, and no attempt to ascertain trends from these data is made.

Northern Ontario Defined: Geographical Issues

In order to allow a comparative assessment of mental health status in Northern Ontario, data are presented for the Province of Ontario as a whole, for Northern Ontario in general, and for the three former Northern Ontario District Health Councils: Northern Shores (which includes the census divisions of Nipissing, Timiskaming, Parry Sound, and Muskoka); Algoma, Cochrane, Manitoulin, and Sudbury (which includes the census divisions of Algoma, Cochrane, Manitoulin, Sudbury District, and Sudbury Regional Municipality); Northwestern Ontario (which includes the Kenora, Thunder Bay, and Rainy River census divisions).

HEALTH STATUS IN NORTHERN ONTARIO

A number of physical and mental health status-related variables, as discussed in the paragraphs which follow, are summarized in Tables 2.1 and 2.2.

Physical Health Status and Related Lifestyle Factors

In general terms, the population of Northern Ontario has lower overall physical and mental health status than the population living elsewhere in the province. When comparing measures of overall health, Northern Ontario has a significantly lower proportion of individuals reporting very good or excellent physical well-being for both sexes combined and for males alone (both sexes: 54.3% vs. 48.1%; males: 57.1% vs. 49.3%). On the other hand, physical activity levels are significantly higher for Northerners than for the provincial population as a whole (27.1% vs. 33.4%). This can be attributed in part to the increased availability of outdoor recreation in the region. Unfortunately, the proportion of those with normal body weight is lower (for both sexes) in the North (35.3% vs. 41.4%). Clearly, physical activity is not synonymous with physical fitness.

With respect to chronic ill-health conditions, they are more prevalent in the North than in the province as a whole. In the case of females, the between-regions difference is statistically significant (Ontario: males 66.4%, females 74.8%; North: males 71.3%, females 80.9%).

Several measures of ease or difficulty with daily living are also captured in the data. This is reflective of those who may have chronic conditions that

Table 2.1 Physical and mental health indicators by geographical area and sex (%)

	Ontario Males	Ontario Females	North Males	North Females	ACMS Males	ACMS Females	Northern Shores Males	Northern Shores Females	Northwest Males	Northwest Females
Physical activity (active)	31.1	23.4	37.0*	29.9*	34.3	29.2	40.3	**27.5**	37.8	33.9*
BMI (normal)	38.0	46.0	32.3	39.4	36.3	39.0	33.4	36.3	**25.8***	44.1
Mental well-being (very good/excellent)	70.7	65.3	66.5	61.7	62.7	64.6	71.8	58.5	67.3	59.8
Physical well-being (very good/excellent)	57.1	51.6	49.3*	46.9	47.0*	50.2	47.3	40.3*	54.8	47.6
Mental health resource use	6.0	11.4	8.1	13.3	**9.4**	12.6	**7.3**	14.0	**7.1**	**13.8**
Depression	3.7	6.4	4.9	8.5	**6.9**	**8.3**	**	**	**	**7.3**
Medication use***	13.1	20.4	17.8	26.8*	20.5*	24.7	**16.0**	32.0*	**15.3**	25.3
Disability days-0 †	89.2	84.0	86.8	83.1	88.7	84.0	85.8	79.2	84.8	85.3
Emotional social support	92.1	92.8	93.3	93.8	95.8*	94.0	93.8	92.8	89.3	94.4
Tangible social support	92.6	92.5	94.7	92.3	90.5	87.2	97.6*	95.2	98.3	97.0*
Workstress (high)	29.1	30.2	25.1	34.1	28.1	32.7	**19.3***	**34.3**	**25.8**	36.1
Stress (high)	23.1	24.3	17.6*	23.6	17.5	25.1	**17.2**	22.7	**18.2**	21.5
Difficulty with tasks	22.8	26.1	30.2*	34.4*	29.4	33.1	37.1*	41.7*	24.7	29.1
Help with tasks	9.0	18.2	12.4	22.3	**13.3**	19.1	**13.1**	28.9*	**10.4**	21.4
Chronic conditions	66.4	74.8	71.3	80.9*	71.6	79.3	77.1*	80.8	65.4	84.2*
Panic disorders	6.0	8.5	8.12	9.3	**10.6**	**9.1**	**7.1**	**	**	**7.4**

* Statistically significant as compared to Ontario; ** Suppressed due to small sample size; *** In past 12 mo, includes medications for sleep, diet, anxiety, mood, depression, psychosis, stimulants; **Bold - High sample variability, use estimate with caution**
† Total number of days spent in bed because of illness or injury in previous two weeks
Source: This analysis is based on Statistics Canada, Canadian Community Health Survey, Mental Health Supplement, Cycle 1.2. 2002. All computations, use and interpretation of these data are entirely that of the author.

Table 2.2 Health indicators by geographical area, both sexes combined (%)

	Ontario	North	ACMS	North Shores	Northwest
Physical activity (active)	27.1	33.4*	31.6	33.9	35.9*
BMI (normal)	41.4	35.3*	37.5	34.7	32.3
Mental well-being (very good/excellent)	67.9	64.1	63.7	65.2	63.7
Physical well-being (very good/excellent)	54.3	48.1*	48.7	43.8*	51.4*
Mental health resource use	8.7	10.7	11.1	10.6	**10.2**
Depression	5.1	6.7	7.6	**	**4.9**
Medication use***	16.8	22.3*	22.7*	23.9*	20.0
Disability days-0 †	86.5	84.9	86.2	82.5	85.1
Emotional social support	92.5	93.6	94.8	93.3	91.7
Tangible social support	92.6	93.3	88.6	96.2	97.5*
Workstress (high)	29.6	29.3	30.4	26.1	30.4
Stress (high)	23.7	20.6	21.5	19.9	19.7
Difficulty with tasks	24.5	32.3	31.4*	39.4*	26.8
Help with tasks	13.7	17.4*	16.4	21.0*	15.6
Chronic conditions	70.7	76.2	75.6	78.9*	74.3
Panic disorders	7.3	8.7	9.8	**9.3**	6.3

* Statistically significant as compared to Ontario; ** Suppressed due to small sample size; *** In past 12 mo., includes medications for sleep, diet, anxiety, mood, depression, psychosis, stimulants; **Bold - High sample variability, use estimate with caution**
† Total number of days spent in bed because of illness or injury in previous two weeks
Source: This analysis is based on Statistics Canada, Canadian Community Health Survey, Mental Health Supplement, Cycle 1.2. 2002. All computations, use and interpretation of these data are entirely that of the author.

lead to activity limitations and other difficulties. In Northern Ontario, there is an increased prevalence of individuals who have difficulty with day-to-day tasks (for both sexes, and for males and females separately). There is also a higher proportion of individuals requiring help with their daily tasks in Northern Ontario (both sexes, 13.7% vs. 17.4%).

When comparing data for the DHC areas, a number of differences are apparent. Physical well-being is significantly lower among Algoma, Cochrane, Manitoulin, and Sudbury DHC males in relation to the province as a whole (57.1% vs. 47.0%), and in the Northern Shores DHC, physical well-being is likewise significantly lower for both sexes combined (54.3% vs. 43.8%) and for females (51.6% vs. 40.3%). This area also reports a significantly higher prevalence for difficulty with daily tasks (24.5% vs. 39.4% overall; 22.8% vs. 37.1% for males; 26.1% vs. 41.7% for females). Females in the Northern Shores DHC also report a significantly elevated need for help with tasks (18.2% vs. 28.9%), and there was a significantly higher prevalence of chronic conditions in both sexes (70.7% vs. 78.9%) and for males (66.4% vs. 77.1%).

The Northwestern Ontario DHC has the highest proportion of physically active individuals within the North (35.9%). In contrast, levels of physical well-being for both sexes are significantly lower (54.3% vs. 51.4%). As with other Northern DHCs, the prevalence of chronic conditions in females is significantly higher than for the province as a whole (74.8% vs. 84.2%).

Mental Health Status: Medication Use

'Medication use' includes all use of prescription stimulants or medications intended to address problems with sleep, diet, anxiety, mood, depression, or psychosis. The most commonly used are those to help with sleep, anti-depressants, and anti-anxiety medications.

Medication use is higher in Northern Ontario than in the province as a whole for both sexes combined, and for females (both sexes: 16.8% vs. 22.3%; females: 20.4% vs. 26.8%); the observed difference is significant for females. Consideration of intra-regional variations in medication use reveal significantly elevated uptake for both sexes combined (16.8% vs. 22.7%) and for males (13.1% vs. 20.5%) in the Algoma, Cochrane, Manitoulin, and Sudbury DHC. Medication use was likewise elevated in the Northern Shores DHC for females (20.4% vs. 32.0%), and for both sexes combined (16.8% vs. 23.9%).

Mental Health Status: Stress and Social Support

While males in Northern Ontario report significantly lower levels of high stress (23.1% vs. 17.6%), other stress indices, such as work stress (high), do not show significant differences. The leading reported sources of stress differ between males and females. For Ontario males, they are (in order of importance) work situation (selected by 24%), time (14%), and finances (12%). For Ontario females, they are time (16%), work situation (14%), and finances (10%). Northern Ontario males are very similar to those in the Ontario-wide data (work situation, 21%; finances, 12%; time, 11%), but Northern females show an interesting difference in that the leading stressors are work (14%), their own physical problems (12%), and time (11%) (Statistics Canada, 2002).

Information for two measures of social support is available: emotional support and tangible social support. Emotional support includes support from individuals in various facets of social life, whereas tangible social support deals with support for tasks such as meal preparation or errands.

Although reported social support does not differ significantly between the province as a whole and the North, there are some notable variations between the observation for the province and for specific DHCs. In the Algoma, Cochrane, Manitoulin, and Sudbury DHC, males have significantly higher levels of emotional support in comparison with the province (92.1% vs. 95.8%). Likewise, men in the Northern Shores DHC report significantly higher tangible social support than men in Ontario as a whole (92.6% vs. 97.6%), while in Northwestern Ontario, tangible social support is significantly higher for females (92.5% vs. 97.0%).

Mental Health Hospitalizations

Sex-specific mental health hospitalization rates are presented in Figure 2.1 for Ontario as a whole, for Northern Ontario, and for each of the Northern DHC areas. While there are no significant differences between mental health hospitalizations between males and females overall, there are for specific geographical areas. Northern Ontario has a significantly higher hospitalization rate than for the province as a whole (males: 91.0 per 100,000 vs. 149.6 per 10,000; females: 90.1 per 100,000 vs. 154.2 per 10,000). This finding is consistent with the increased rate of hospitalizations for all causes noted for the region. For Ontario, 11.5% of all in-patients also received a mental health diagnosis; the North is similar with 13.7% of in-patients likewise diagnosed.

A recent analysis of child mental health also reveals a high proportion of in-patients with mental health diagnoses. In children aged 6 or less, it is uncommon to have a mental health diagnosis. However, for 7- to 13-year-olds from Ontario, 8.2% of boys had a diagnosis related to mental health problems and 8.9% of girls had such a diagnosis. For Northern Ontario, mental health problems are slightly more common with 8.7% of boys and 10% of girls receiving a related diagnosis. When examining the data for 14- to 19-year-olds, the prevalence increases greatly: in Ontario males, 21.7% had a mental health diagnosis, and 20.8% of females had a mental health diagnosis. For Northern Ontario, the data are similar (23.7% of males; 19.1% of females) (Northern Health Information Partnership, 2003).

Regional variations in rates of hospitalization are notable. The Algoma, Cochrane, Manitoulin, and Sudbury DHC has the highest hospitalization rate in the North (males: 149.6 vs. 162.2 per 10,000; females: 154.2 vs. 168.2 per 10,000). By comparison, the Northern Shores DHC has a significantly lower hospitalization rate than the North as a whole (males: 120.0/10,000; females: 130.1/10,000), although it remains higher than the rate observed for the province.

Not surprisingly, mental health diagnoses follow a similar trend (Figure 2.2). Specifically, Northern Ontario has a significantly higher rate of mental health diagnoses than Ontario as a whole, while the Algoma, Cochrane, Manitoulin, and Sudbury DHC is significantly higher than the Northern rate, and the Northern Shores DHC rate is significantly lower than for the North, but still higher than for the Province of Ontario as a whole.

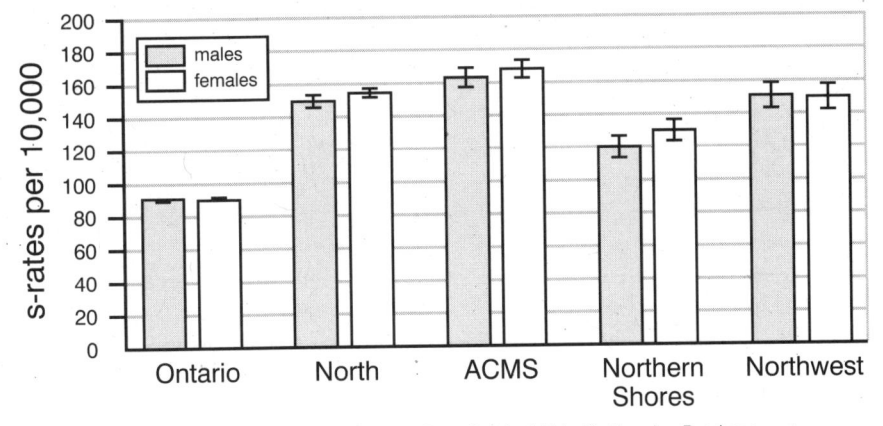

Mental Health Status in Northern Ontario 13

Figure 2.1 Mental health hospitalizations by geographic area and sex, 2003

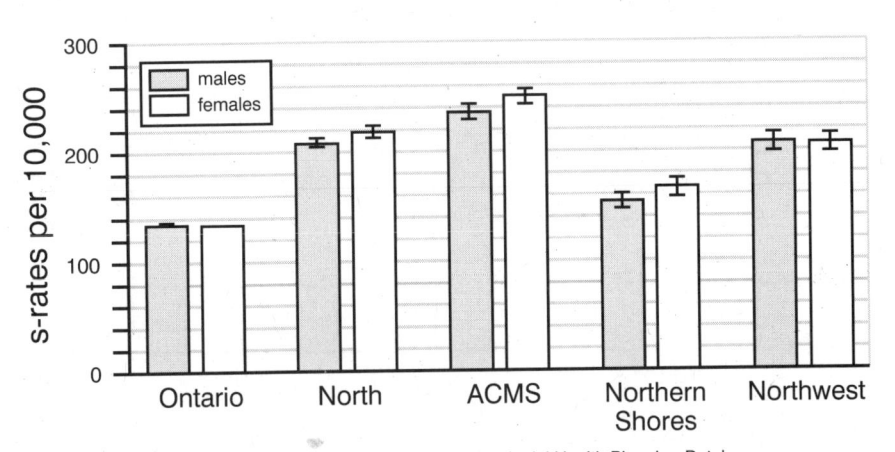

Source: Ontario Ministry of Health and Long-Term Care, Provincial Health Planning Database

Figure 2.2 Mental health diagnoses by geographic area and sex, 2003

Source: Ontario Ministry of Health and Long-Term Care, Provincial Health Planning Database

Suicide Hospitalizations and Mortality

Suicide data reveal a troubling trend in the Northern region (Figures 2.3 and 2.4). Northern Ontario suicide-related hospitalizations occur at more than double the provincial rate (8.3 per 10,000 vs. 19.2 per 10,000). There are no significant differences between Northern DHC areas, but clearly this is an area of serious concern for the region as a whole. Suicide mortality data further support this trend. It is worth noting that the Northern Shores DHC, which has the lowest mental health diagnosis and hospitalization rate, also has the lowest suicide mortality rate.

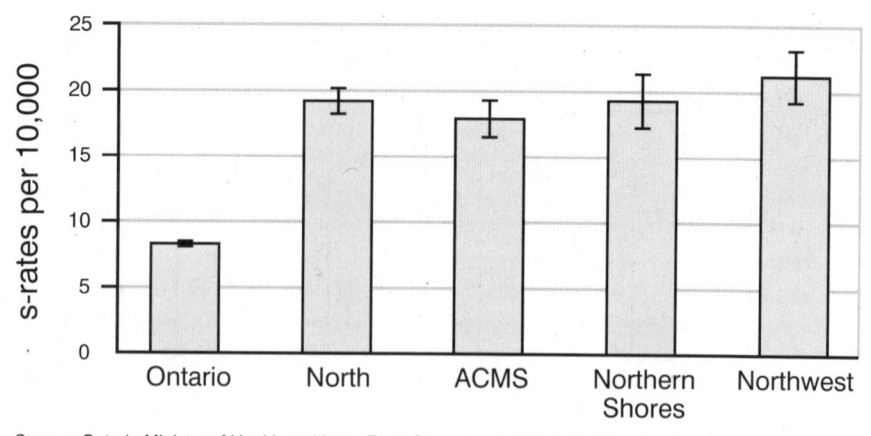

Figure 2.3 Suicide hospitalization by geographic area, 2003

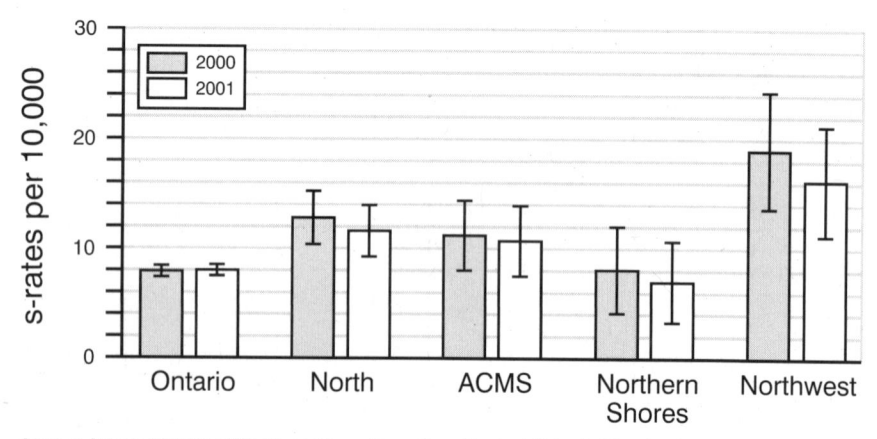

Source: Ontario Ministry of Health and Long-Term Care, Provincial Health Planning Database

Figure 2.4 Suicide mortality by geographic area, 2000 and 2001

Source: Ontario Ministry of Health and Long-Term Care, Provincial Health Planning Database

Recent injury data reveal that suicide is the leading cause of premature death in Northern Ontario (as measured by Potential Years of Life Lost [PYLL]), outranking motor vehicle incidents, accidental poisonings, intentional injury, and falls. It is particularly troubling that the rate of premature death from suicide in Northwestern Ontario is nearly three times the provincial rate: the rate of PYLL in Ontario in 1999 was 2.7 per 1,000, while in Northern Ontario as a whole it was 5.2 per 1,000, and for Northwestern Ontario the rate was 7.8 per 1,000. The lowest rates in the North are observed for the Algoma, Cochrane, Manitoulin, and Sudbury DHC and the Northern Shores DHC, at 3.8 per 1,000 and 4.9 per 1,000 respectively. When looking at the data for mortality, a similar trend emerges. In Ontario, in 2000, the leading cause of death for 10- to 19-year-olds was transportation accidents. For Northern Ontario, it was suicide. In 20- to 34-year-olds, the leading cause of death for the province and the North were transportation accidents. For 35- to 54-year-olds, however, the leading cause of death in the North was, once again, suicide (Northern Health Information Partnership, 2004).

A recent report cites some important sex differences to consider: young women (aged 15 to 19) appear more likely to contemplate suicide than do young men (82% vs. 92% having never contemplated suicide). As well, there is typically a higher rate of attempted suicide among women, although men are more likely to succeed in their suicide attempt (Northern Health Information Partnership, 2003). In addition, an analysis of suicide attempts and mortality by age suggests that the decrease in suicide attempt-related hospitalizations in the 20- to 35-year-old group may be related to the noted increase in suicide mortality between the ages of 20 and 40. It would seem that individuals in the 20- to 40-year-old age cohort are typically more successful when they attempt suicide.

One last piece of evidence highlights the importance of suicide as a cause of mortality in Northern Ontario. Suicide data collected for the Province of Ontario as a whole show that suicide mortality decreased during the years 1986 through 1999. Unfortunately, data for the same time period reveal that suicide mortality in Northern Ontario is increasing.

IMPLICATIONS

There are a number of positive findings in the overall health data. Physical activity levels, for example, are high in the North, particularly in Northwestern Ontario. Levels of social support are also generally very high, which is an important means of psychological support.

Less encouraging are the relatively high rates of both mental health problems and medication use. In general terms, women are at greater risk in the region than are men, for both physical and mental well-being. Most troubling of all is the high rate of suicide mortality in the region.

Despite the obvious importance of mental health-related morbidity and mortality in the North, utilization of mental health resources remains low: only 1 out of 10 in the region has sought professional help for mental health-related issues. This could be the result of many factors, including suppressed need, or the stigmatization associated with seeking help from mental health professionals. Other issues impacting negatively upon service uptake may include geographical or income-related barriers to access, or lack of knowledge or availability of services in this generally underserviced region.

While some aspects of life in Northern Ontario undoubtedly promote positive physical and mental well-being—observe the high rates of physical activity and social support, for example—the area is characterized by relatively high rates of negative health determinants, including low income, low educational attainment, prevalent smoking, and unhealthy body weights. While it goes beyond the intended scope of this chapter to investigate what causal mechanisms are at work in increasing the burden of mental health-related morbidity and mortality in Northern Ontario, it is perhaps not surprising that relatively poor socio-economic conditions and higher rates of negative health behaviours are echoed by poor population health status. Indeed, the higher prevalence of mental health issues in Northern Ontario accompanies much of the well-established evidence of poor health status in the region overall.

In general, one can see that the population of Northern Ontario is at higher risk for a number of physical and mental health issues. The most vital implication to consider overall is that, even for indicators that are similar to the province as a whole, there is still a need to increase attention and services for mental health issues in the Northern region of Ontario.

REFERENCES

Diverty, B., and Beaudet, M.P. (1997). Depression: An undertreated disorder? *Health Reports*, 8, 9-18.

Health Canada (2002). *A report on mental illnesses in Canada*. Catalogue H39-643/2002E. Ottawa: Health Canada.

MacMillan, H.L., MacMillan, A.B., Offord, D.R., and Dingle, J.L. (1996). Aboriginal health. *Canadian Medical Association Journal*, 155, 1569-1578.

Northern Health Information Partnership (2004). *Injuries and poisonings in Northern Ontario*. Sudbury: Northern Health Information Partnership.

Northern Health Issues Strategy Steering Committee (2004). *An overview of health status and the health care system in Northern Ontario*. Sudbury: Northern Health Information Partnership.

Queen's Printer for Ontario (2003). *Ontario Ministry of Health and Long-Term Care Provincial Health Planning Database*. Toronto: Health Planning Branch, Ontario Ministry of Health and Long Term Care.

Rhodes, A.E., Links, P., Dawe, I., Cass, D., and Janes, S. (2002). Do hospital Ecodes consistently capture suicidal behaviour? *Chronic Diseases in Canada*, 23, 139-145.

Scott, J. (1993). Homelessness and mental health. *British Journal of Psychiatry*, 162, 314-324.

Statistics Canada (2002). *Canadian Community Health Survey, Mental Health Supplement. Cycle 1.2*. Ottawa: Statistics Canada.

Statistics Canada (2003). Statistics Canada 2001 Community Profiles. *http://www.statscan.ca*, Accessed October 21, 2003.

Vainio, E., Ward, M., and the Northern Health Issues Strategy Steering Committee (2004). *The northern health strategy: Northern solutions for northern issues*. Sudbury: Northern Health Information Partnership.

Youth in British Columbia: Their Mental Health

Roger S. Tonkin
The McCreary Centre Society, Burnaby, BC

INTRODUCTION

Youth Mental Health is a term with many meanings and even more challenges. In British Columbia's health system, youth mental health is like a foster child; it lacks a clear identity, has been moved from home to home, and no discipline seems prepared to adopt it. Moreover, as with foster children, we have little hard evidence upon which to base our understanding of how best to promote it, monitor it, and provide services for it.

In this chapter the author will draw upon 40 years of clinical and research experience with youth issues in Canada to demonstrate the evolution of our mental health system of "foster care." The available evidence base, conceptual frameworks, and seminal writings by authoritative Canadians will be briefly reviewed in order to set the author's approach in context. In addition, the experience and rich data base relevant to youth mental health in BC will be outlined. Finally, the chapter will address some of the emerging contemporary issues and challenges that today's youth confront and the youth mental health system will need to address.

BACKGROUND

There is neither a clear chronologic definition of the term youth nor a clear definition of youth mental health. Also, there are no clear indicators of what constitutes mental health in our youth. For the purposes of this chapter, youth are considered to be adolescents entering puberty, in the secondary school age range, or emerging into adulthood. In this more functional approach to a definition of youth, offering a specific age grouping is deliberately avoided. In their paper "The Structure of Psychological Well-Being Revisited," Ryff and Keyes analysed six distinct dimensions of wellness in adults and provided the provisional conclusion that there is more to being well than feeling happy and satisfied with life (Ryff and Keyes, 1995). Perhaps the same multitask agenda of their research will need to be directed towards furthering our understanding of youth mental health.

The World Health Organization (WHO) offers a working definition of mental health: "Mental health is a state of well-being in which the individual realizes his or her own abilities, can cope with the stresses of life, can work productively and fruitfully, and is able to make a contribution to his or her community" (source: www.who.int/mentalhealth/resources). However, its language, while intended to cover all ages, is adult-oriented and not developmentally appropriate. Also, it addresses two functions: namely, preventing and treating all forms of mental and neurological disorders and mental retardation, not just promoting mental health and well-being. This author prefers the Health Education Authority definition as outlined below by Dwivedi and Harper (2004).

While many jurisdictions have struggled to define it, most resort to discussing the prevalence of mental health problems or disorders. Some outline the attributes or characteristics of mentally healthy youth. For example, Dwivedi and Harper's 2004 handbook explores the issue of definition and quotes the Health Education Authority in the UK as defining mental health as "... the emotional and spiritual resilience which enables us to enjoy life and to survive pain, disappointment and sadness. It is a positive sense of well-being and an underlying belief in our own and other's worth" (p. 17). In Australia, focus groups were brought together to define youth mental health but proved unsuccessful in doing so (Keys Young, 1997). They knew what mental health meant to them but could not be any clearer about defining it.

Williams and Kerfoot co-edited an impressive book on child and adolescent mental health services in the UK (2005). It is both current and comprehensive, but they failed to enunciate a simple definition. Peter Hill, a chapter author, tackles the definitional issue and concludes:

> ...mental health in children and adolescents is indicated by: a capacity to enter into, and sustain, mutually satisfying relationships; continuing progression of development; an ability to play and learn, so that attainments are appropriate for age and intellectual level; a developing sense of right and wrong; the degree of psychological distress and maladaptive behaviour being within normal limits for the child's age and behaviour (2005, p. 178).

In their Preface, Williams and Kerfoot concluded that "Hitherto, children's mental health has been a neglected topic in the domains of healthcare, social care, and education policy and investment" (2005, p. viii).

The 2002 federal document *A Canada Fit for Children* is a 122 page declaration of Canada's actions and intentions in response to the UN Convention of the Rights of the Child. However, it devotes only one page to mental health and fails to offer any definition. Two other earlier documents, the report of the Commission on Emotional and Learning Disorders in Children (CELDIC) (1970) and the third Canadian Institute for Child Health's *The Health of Canada's Children* (Kidder, Stein, Fraser, and Canadian Institute for Child Health, 2000) are more specific in their focus on mental health issues. However, neither offers a definition of mental health that can be used as a positive quantitative measure of youth mental health.

Waddell, McEwen, Shepherd, Offord, and Hua, in their excellent review paper "A public health strategy to improve the mental health of Canadian children" (2005), provide a thorough and up to date overview, but focus on "policy-relevant research in children's mental health and development" (p. 226). Waddell and co-authors have taken a broad population-based, determinants of health approach, and the application of this approach to depression in adolescence is further explored by Fuks-Geddes, Fielden, and Frankish (2005). Their chapter outlines the determinants of depression in youth, discusses the difficulty in defining youth depression, and concludes that "Adolescent mental health can be one barometer used to gauge future patterning of the socio-economic gradient and population health" (p. 80), but it is left to Willms, using National Longitudinal Study of Children and Youth (NLSCY) data, to attempt to demonstrate how to portray social gradients (2002).

These few references are reflective of the poorly developed "state of the art" in youth mental health in Canada and elsewhere. While our country has excellent scholars and clinicians in the mental health field, their focuses have largely been upon children's mental health and/or the identification and treatment of mental disorders in children or adolescents. Canadians such as Offord (2000 and 2005) and Steinhauer (2001) are representative of excellence in leadership, while studies such as the CELDIC, the Ontario Child Health Study (Offord, Boyle, Fleming, Monroe Blum, and Rae Grant, 1989), and the NLSCY (Willms, 2002) exemplify excellence in scholarship. As with *A Canada Fit for Children*, their work places its emphasis on children and pays little attention to the community mental health system. Youth seem to be included, but as an afterthought, and clearly are a secondary focus.

This situation is a logical outcome of the fragmented, discipline-bound approaches taken to preparing our professionals to deal with contemporary youth issues. As identified in the proposal for the National Training Initiative in Adolescent Health (*www.cps.ca/english/prodev/ntiah*), no one professional discipline provides a secure home for youth issues. Few training and research programs in Canada provide specialist training in adolescent problems. For example, the field of psychiatry, while linked to mental health, does not offer adolescent-specific training or licensure and remains largely concerned with diagnosis and treatment of children. Similarly, child-oriented disciplines such as developmental psychology, pediatrics, and social work only offer elective training and research opportunities. Canada has nothing comparable to the multidisciplinary Society for Adolescent Medicine in the United States (*www.adolescenthealth.org*).

This situation is also a function of the changing fiscal and social context experienced by today's youth and by youth serving agencies. It is also a reflection of the low priority given to the interdisciplinary Child and Youth Mental

Health Services by most provincial governments. In the last decade an emphasis on Early Child Development and Child Care has driven policy and program development. The flow of federal and provincial dollars has reinforced these priorities and the federal government has a less than impressive track record in promoting youth mental health as a priority. More recently, the recognition of the importance of securing youth input and engaging/empowering youth that is reflected in *A Canada Fit For Children* is embodied in such federal programs as the Centre of Excellence in Children's Well-Being – Youth Engagement (CoE-YE) (*www.tgmag.ca/centres*). The work of the CoE-YE is a move toward the principles and frameworks for promoting youth health outlined by Powelson and Tonkin in their chapter on Positive Youth Development (2005). This has fostered a shift in emphasis in youth mental health away from classical mental health frameworks to it being a function of empowerment. The context for our understanding of youth mental health is also likely to be further changed by three evolving research streams: the neuroscience of brain development in puberty (Dahl, 2004); the study of emerging adulthood (18-34 years) (Settersten, Furstenberg, and Rumbaut, 2005), and the evaluation of the treatment and psychopharmacology of adolescent depression (Brent, 2005).

This situation has also been shaped by changes in intervention approaches in mental health. The well established interdisciplinary networks of Child Guidance/Community Mental Health Services have seemed to operate in parallel with primary care physicians and psychiatrists (perhaps a result of the fee for service system). In the early days, provinces such as Saskatchewan and Ontario introduced a system of community-based Child Guidance Clinics and BC has built upon those experiences. These programs focused on the learning and emotional development of school-aged children. Later on, tertiary care teaching hospitals, especially those dedicated to children, developed psychiatric diagnostic services and in-patient assessment and treatment units. In the 1970s, hospitals like the BC Children's Hospital (then called Children's Hospital) introduced multidisciplinary diagnostic clinics and in-patient units dedicated to adolescents. Specialized adolescent in-patient psychiatric services were a later addition, but have since grown rapidly and focused on the excellence of the academic and clinical programs that they offer. However, as Waddell and co-authors (2005) point out, a renewed emphasis upon prevention and early intervention seems to be in order. They advocated for a clearer understanding of the differences between prevention and early intervention.

Some mental health services are age specific or have other restrictive mandates such as Child Protection or juvenile justice. For example, Child and Adolescent Forensic Psychiatric programs, an important adjunct to the classical psychiatric medical model, have age limits defined by the court orders of the juvenile justice system. Similarly, community-based individual clinical consultative and intervention services may limit accessibility by virtue of location, hours of operation, or fee schedules. Universal programs such as crisis intervention and counselling services (Kids Help Line: info@kidshelp.sympatico.ca) also serve an adolescent clientele. They are much more accessible to teens, but often face limitations in the availability of referral to follow-up resources. School-based counselling services, innovative community approaches such as Youth Net (www.youthnet.on.ca), specialized summer or boot camp programs, and internet-based mental health information sites or the Canadian Health Network (www.canadian-health-network.ca) round out the panoply of interventions. However, as Waddell and co-authors (2005) point out, less than 25% of children and youth with mental health problems ever receive any specialized services. We have yet to properly address the "intolerable" (p. 470) findings outlined in the 1970 CELDIC report.

Prevalence

Waddell and co-authors (2005) report that "At any given time, 14 percent of children aged 4 to 17 years (over 800,000 in Canada) experience mental disorders that cause significant distress and impairment at home, at school, and in the community" (p. 226). Their paper also provides a useful table (see Table 3.1) of the prevalence of children's mental disorders (p. 228). It is important to note that these estimates do not include older adolescents or children and adolescents who have not been identified as having a specific, diagnosable mental disorder. This distinction is important to parents and teachers of symptomatic children or adolescents who are never "picked up" and to primary health care providers who feel ill equipped to intervene. I describe such youth as "the worried mentally unwell."

The four most prevalent diagnosed mental disorders are those relating to anxiety, hyperactivity, conduct, and depression. The prevalence estimate for the latter is 3.5% (Waddell et al., 2005), whereas the self-reported prevalence of suicide attempts by BC students in grades 7-12 is 7% (Tonkin, Murphy, Chittenden, Jackson, and McCreary Centre Society, 2004). It is important to understand the basis for this discrepancy as it reflects the magnitude of the unreported mental health burden in the general adolescent population. Later in this chapter these reported prevalences of the key mental disorders will be contrasted with the population-based data for mainstream students and special populations of out of school youth in BC. BC data on some of the determinant factors (such as place of residence, ethnicity, and abuse history) that affect prevalence rates will also be presented.

The prevalence of youth mental health problems in individual adolescents is often masked by our focus on youth as issues or behaviour problems. Their engagement in problem behaviours not seen as manifestations of youth mental health problems obscures the mental health dimension. Examples of these problem behaviours include their participation in various risky or criminal behaviours or having dropped out of school and/or become street-involved. Conversely, all risky or experimental behaviours should not be explained as

Table 3.1   Prevalence of child/adolescent mental disorders: Canada versus British Columbia

Disorder	Estimated prevalence in Canada [1]	Age range for Canadian estimates	Estimated prevalence in BC [2]
Anxiety disorder	6.4	5-17	15%
ADHD/hyperactivity	4.8	4-17	n/a
Conduct disorder	4.2	4-17	n/a
Depressive	3.5	5-17	7% [3]
Substance abuse	0.8	9-17	8% [4]
Obsessive compulsive disorder	0.2	5-15	n/a
Eating disorder	0.1	5-15	3% [5]
Schizophrenia	0.1	9-13	n/a
Bipolar disorder	<0.1	9-13	n/a

[1] From Waddell, C., McEwen, K., Shepherd, C. A., Offord, D. R., and Hua, J. M. (2005, March). A public health strategy to improve mental health of Canadian Children. *Canadian Journal of Psychiatry*, 50(4), 226-2332

[2] From Adolescent Health Survey III, McCreary Centre Society (2003) – BC students in grades 7-12 (approx. 12-18 yrs)

[3] Percent of BC students who attempted suicide in the past year

[4] Percent of BC students who used marijuana on 20+ days in the past month and/or used alcohol on 20+ days in past month and/or binge drank on 6+ days in past month

[5] Percent of BC students who vomited on purpose after eating 2-3 times a month and/or their activities are limited due to being overweight or underweight ("keeps you from doing things other kids your age do")

being due to mental health problems. In fact, for the majority of adolescents, testing limits and experimentation is a sign of healthy adolescent development. However, studies of BC youth who engage in multiple risky behaviours or become street-involved indicate that a greater proportion of them also report experiencing significant emotional distress (McCreary Centre Society, 1999, 2001, 2002; Tonkin et al., 2004; and Murphy, Chittenden, and McCreary Centre Society, 2005).

The occurrence of significant negative life events may influence the prevalence of youth mental health problems among affected youth. These occurrences include bullying, discrimination, abuse, family dysfunction, neglect, and exploitation. However, as the BC data demonstrate, the impact of these occurrences upon youth mental health may be ameliorated by the youth's resilience and personal assets and by their degree of connectedness to family and school (Tonkin et al., 2004). Finally, prevalence estimates for mental disorder in adolescents may be low because the affected adolescents and their families are resistant (for social or cultural reasons) to the perceived stigmatization of being labelled as having a mental disorder.

The federal government and its various policies and programs could have an important influence on our understanding of the prevalence of youth mental problems. Research funding priorities, monitoring and evaluation of programs, and sharing of data between jurisdictions remains an unresolved challenge. In the absence of a unifying National Youth Agenda (Kidder and Rodgers, 2004), the approach to youth policy and programs is scattered among many departments. While Canada once had a Minister of State for youth, no one in the current federal or provincial ministries champions youth issues. The mental health problems of children and youth are not yet a federal priority.

Provision of mental health services is a provincial responsibility. The Mental Health Act in each province should, but does not necessarily, determine the cut-offs between child and adult programs. For this reason, approaches and priorities often differ. The model used in BC allows communities and their mental health teams to set referral priorities under the Act. This is particularly true with respect to youth mental health. Only recently has there been any impact from the efforts of mental health advocates on youth mental health concerns at either the federal or provincial levels.

THE BC EXAMPLE

The responsibility for youth mental health in BC is nominally with the Ministry of Child and Family Development (MCFD). However, other ministries such as Health, Education, Solicitor General, and Attorney General each have defined roles that have a direct impact on youth mental health and the provision of services to them. Various aboriginal branches of government, the Representative for Children and Youth, and the municipalities and their local services (e.g., recreation, police, various non-profits) join the list of agencies who could or should have the mental health needs of youth on their agenda.

BC is a "young" province with a frontier mentality. Due to its geography, the concentration of population in its lower mainland area, its ethnic diversity, and the special needs of the aboriginal community, the unmet mental health needs of BC's youth population are a source of community concern. However, things are improving. Beginning in 2004 the MCFD spearheaded a long term approach to child and youth mental health and now has a youth mental health policy (www.mcf.gov.bc.ca/mental_health/mh_publications/cymh_plan). The Child Mental Health Unit at the University of BC (www.childmentalhealth.ubc.ca) worked in concert with government but has relocated to the Children's Health Policy Centre at Simon Fraser University. Its major focus is on the health and mental health of children and adolescents (0 to 19 years). Excellent tertiary care mental health diagnostic and treatment services and academic leadership are available via the programs at BC Children's Hospital (BCCH). Outreach mental health teaching and consultation is becoming more widely available, and highly specialized services for adolescents with conditions such as autism, ADHD, FASD, and eating disorders are now in place.

Despite these many advances over the past decade, the suicide attempt rate among BC students has not changed (Figure 3.1). One can only speculate as to why this is so. The most obvious explanation is that youth who attempt suicide generally do not seek professional help (a finding confirmed by Waddell et al., 2005). It may also be that suicide attempts are a reflection of the endemic levels of depression, anxiety, and situational crises that are interpreted as part of the normal challenges of adolescence. Indeed, 3% of BC students reported having a "mental or emotional condition" that kept them from "doing some things other kids your age do."

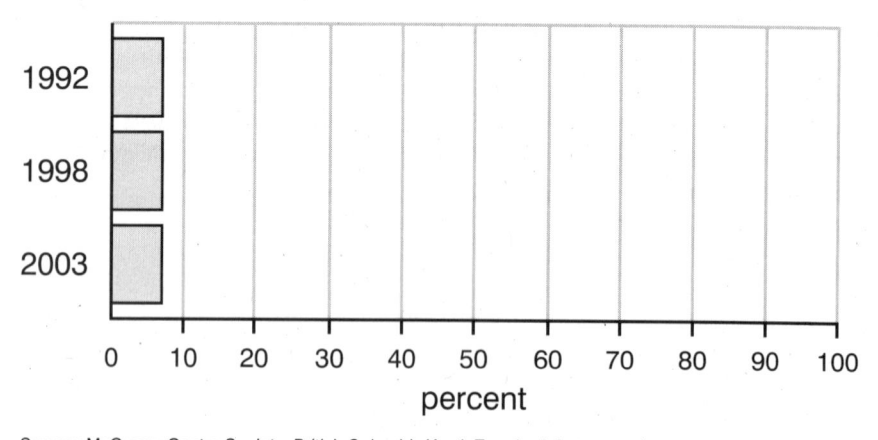

Source: McCreary Centre Society. *British Columbia Youth Trends: A Retrospective, 1992-2003*, 2005.

Figure 3.1 Percentage of BC students who attempted suicide in the past year

Another explanation, partially supported by the data, is that the seriousness of the majority of these attempts is underestimated. More adolescents (16%) report considering and planning a suicide than actually attempting, and much fewer (2%) report needing professional help to deal with the outcome (Tonkin et al., 2004). In addition, the trend in adolescent suicide mortality rates among BC adolescents has declined over the past two decades (Tonkin, Murphy, and McCreary Centre Society, 2002). These comments and explanations may well apply to most youth in BC, but for some, especially Aboriginal youth, the scenario is much bleaker (van der Woerd, Dixon, McDiarmid, Chittenden, Murphy, and McCreary Centre Society, 2005). For example, the suicide attempt rate for on-reserve aboriginal students is 18%, while the rate for off-reserve aboriginal students is 11%.

Mental health during adolescence is a stepping stone to mental health in adulthood. Adolescence is also the time when lifelong afflictions such as alcoholism and addiction, psychosis, obsessive compulsive disorder, and bipolar disorder make their appearance. These DSM IV classified disorders are of much lower prevalence than the sub-clinical mental health problems of the mainstream student population (Table 3.1). The demands that these disorders or clinical conditions place on the mental health care system are much higher. The improvements noted earlier in the BC example are largely devoted to addressing these more specialized needs and, as Waddell and co-authors (2005) symbolize in their Venn diagram (Figure 3.2), these needs become the smallest element within their proposed public health strategy.

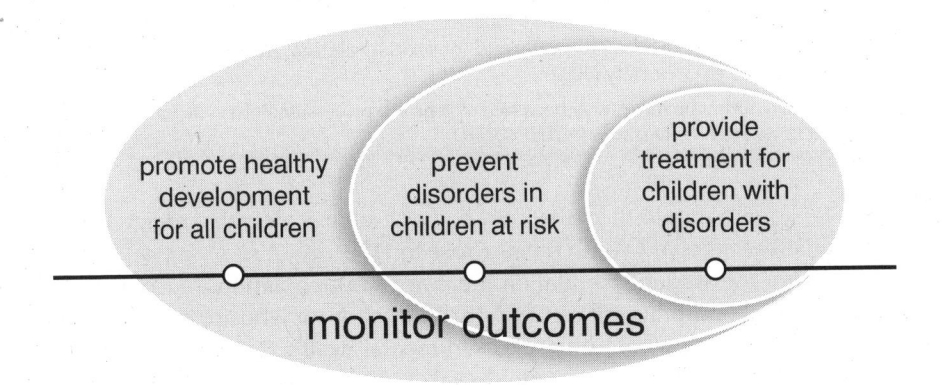

promote healthy development for all children

prevent disorders in children at risk

provide treatment for children with disorders

monitor outcomes

Adapted from Waddell et al. (2005)

Figure 3.2 Proposed public health strategy

The crossover between mental disorders and milder mental health problems is sometimes murky. One of the goals of this chapter is to examine and illuminate that crossover. The data are soft and the scales contrived, but there are important differences in self-reported anxiety, depression, hyperactivity, and conduct disorder between mainstream and special adolescent populations. However important and useful these comparisons are, they must be viewed with caution as the data are derived from surveys that used slightly different sampling methodologies and time frames (see *www.mcs.bc.ca*). Nevertheless, for these special populations (e.g., aboriginal, street-involved, youth in custody, previously abused, or sexually exploited) the rates are much higher than for mainstream students (Table 3.2). For example, 18% of aboriginal students can be defined as anxious, while out-of-school street-involved youth report the higher levels of anxiety (29%), emotional distress (21%), and suicide attempts (27%). Youth in custody report the highest rates of professionally diagnosed ADHD/hyperactivity. Four percent of youth in custody report that

Table 3.2 Emotional health problems in special populations (%)

	Aboriginal[1]	In custody[2]	Street[3]	Abused[4]
Anxiety	18	22	29	31
Emotional distress	10	13	21	19
Attempted suicide in past year	12	13	27	18
ADHD/Hyperactivity[5]	n/a	33	27	n/a

[1] BC Aboriginal students, Adolescent Health Survey III, McCreary Centre Society (2003)
[2] BC Youth in custody, McCreary Centre Society (2004)
[3] Street involved youth in five BC communities, McCreary Centre Society (2000)
[4] BC students who have been physically and/or sexually abused, Adolescent Health Survey III, McCreary Centre Society (2003)
[5] Percent of youth who have "ever been told by a health professional that you have Attention Deficit Hyperactivity Disorder (ADHD/ADD)"

a professional had told them that they had a chronic anxiety disorder, whereas among street-involved youth the rate rose to 11%.

Within the student population there are sub-populations, such as those with chronic conditions, issues of sexual orientation, or who appear older than they really are, for whom differences in mental health status are also noted. With the exception of students with sexual orientation concerns, these rates are less marked than for street-involved or out-of-school youth. However, the extent of the mental health burden among these student sub-groups may come as a surprise (Table 3.3).

Table 3.3 Emotional health problems in at-risk youth populations (%)

	Chronic health condition or disability[1]	Lesbian, gay or bisexual[2]	Look older than same age peers[3]
Anxiety	22	36	20
Emotional distress	12	22	11
Attempted suicide in past year	10	25	10

[1] BC students who reported having a physical disability or long-term illness that limits their activities. Adolescent Health Survey III, McCreary Centre Society (2003)
[2] BC students who identified themselves as lesbian, gay or bisexual. Adolescent Health Survey III, McCreary Centre Society (2003)
[3] BC students who reported looking older than their same-aged peers. Adolescent Health Survey III, McCreary Centre Society (2003)

Students who seem to be coping with their adolescence still may report more anxiety, emotional distress, and suicide behaviour than the majority of their peers. For example, obese and overweight adolescents, those who are bullied or discriminated against, or live in rural regions of BC also reported elevated rates (Table 3.4). Of particular interest are the much higher rates among students who have tried marijuana before the age of 13 years and the even higher rates among those students who report engaging in three or more risk behaviours (Tables 3.4 and 3.5).

Table 3.4 Emotional health problems in other youth populations (%)

	Obese[1]	Bullied[2]	Rural[3]	Early marijuana use[4]
Anxiety	19	22	14	24
Emotional distress	10	13	8	15
Attempted suicide in past year	9	10	8	16

[1] BC students with a Body Mass Index that is classified as obese for their age and gender, Adolescent Health Survey III, McCreary Centre Society (2003)

[2] BC students who were verbally harassed, purposely excluded or physically assaulted at school in the past year. Adolescent Health Survey III, McCreary Centre Society (2003)

[3] BC students who live in the Kootenay-Boundary, East Kootenay, Northwest, Northern Interior, or North Vancouver Island Health Service Delivery Areas. Adolescent Health Survey III, McCreary Centre Society (2003)

[4] BC students who tried marijuana before the age of 13 years. Adolescent Health Survey III, McCreary Centre Society (2003)

Table 3.5 Emotional health problems and engagement in multiple risk behaviours (%)

	0 risk behaviours	1-2 risk behaviours	3+ risk behaviours
Anxiety	8	17	36
Emotional distress in past month	3	9	24
Suicide attempt in past year	<1	7	32

Source: Adolescent Health Survey III, McCreary Centre Society (2003)

The following four risk behaviours were counted:
- 1+ physical fights in past year
- skipped school in past month
- ever tried illegal drugs (not including marijuana)
- considered suicide in past year

The data are not robust enough to enable conclusions on cause and effect. However the relationship between mental health concerns and issues such as sexual orientation, early use of marijuana, or engaging in three or more risky behaviours gives cause to pause and rethink our ideas about who, among adolescents, are at risk for a mental health problem. We might wonder to what extent the 14% overall prevalence estimate of Waddell and co-authors (2005) represents the proverbial tip of the youth mental health iceberg.

These data might discourage some, but after 40 years of clinical experience I confess to a more hopeful and positive outlook. The McCreary Centre Society's Adolescent Health Survey (AHS) data sets reveal an impressive degree of stability in the indicators commonly used to monitor youth health (Tonkin, Murphy, Lee, Saewyc, and McCreary Centre Society, 2005). It is reassuring that 97% of students expect to be alive at age 25 years (Tonkin et al., 2004). Overall, the attitudes and behaviours of BC youth have been consistently positive and, in fact, in many areas have shown improvement (Table 3.6).

Table 3.6 Positive mental health by health service delivery area (%)

Health Service Delivery Area	Positive mental health
Northwest	50
Northern Interior	49
Thompson Cariboo Shuswap	49
Okanagan	49
Kootenay Boundary	47
East Kootenay	48
North Vancouver Island	43
Central Vancouver Island	50
South Vancouver Island	50
Coastal	50
Vancouver	39
Richmond	45
Fraser North	50

Source: Adolescent Health Survey III, McCreary Centre Society (2003)

Note: Data not available for the Fraser South, Fraser East, and Northeast Health Service Delivery Areas.

Positive mental health is defined as BC students who:
- feel cared about "a lot" by one or both parents
- are very satisfied with their relationship with one or both parents
- like school
- report good or excellent heath status
- can think of some things that they are really good at

Of concern is the 10-12% of BC students who engage in a multiplicity of high risk behaviours (Tonkin, Poon, Murphy, and McCreary Centre Society, 2002). While this percentage is relatively low, the mental health burden of these students is more marked. Among students with no reported risk behaviours 8% are anxious, whereas 36% of students engaging in three or more risky behaviours report being anxious (Table 3.5). Also, an important percentage of them do not expect to reach age 25 (Figure 3.3). The presence of some self-protective behaviours, such as reported condom use and safety belt use, is quite high and has shown recent improvement (Tonkin et al., 2004). Other, more complex protective factors such as connectedness to family and school are part of most students' lives and, where present, may prevent more serious mental health issues from arising. For example, emotional distress in those traumatized by sexual abuse is less prevalent in students with medium to high levels of family connectedness (Figure 3.4) (Tonkin et al., 2002).

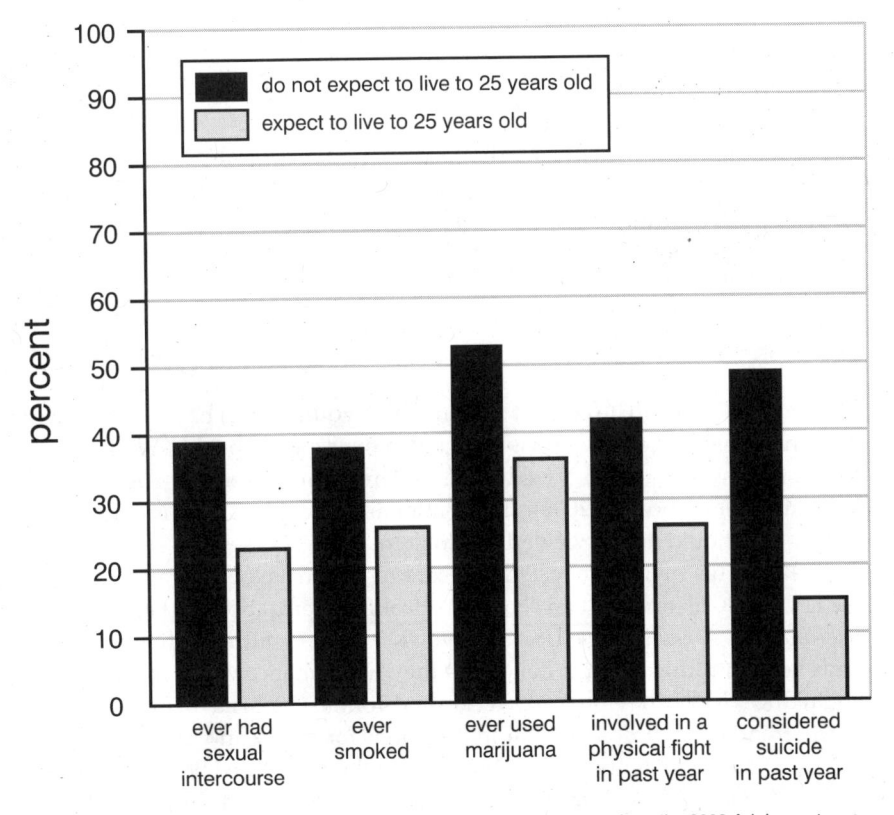

Source: McCreary Centre Society. Healthy Youth Development: Highlights from the 2003 Adolescent Health Survey. (2004)

Figure 3.3 Percentage of BC students who expect to live to be at least 25 years old

[Bar chart showing percentage of school youth with emotional distress by family connectedness and sexual abuse status. Low family connectedness: sexual abuse ~35%, no sexual abuse ~16%. Medium-high family connectedness: sexual abuse ~15%, no sexual abuse ~5%.]

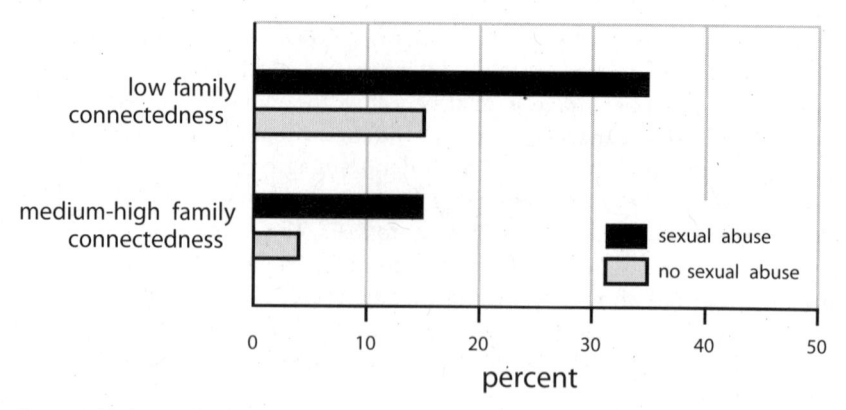

Source: McCreary Centre Society. *Healthy connections: Connectedness and BC youth.* 2000.

Figure 3.4 Percentage of school youth with emotional distress

ISSUES AND CHALLENGES

The author is aware of many international, national, federal-provincial-territorial, provincial, and non-governmental reports that have already addressed issues of mental health or, more specifically, youth mental health, but they are either outdated, in the grey literature, or have had little impact. Therefore, the author has chosen not to present an exhaustive review of the literature. Rather, this section will focus on some of the more contemporary issues and challenges. The list is selective and will only offer highlights for the reader to focus upon.

Societal Context: The context within which youth issues have been viewed influences their behaviour and is reflected in their mental health. Williams and Kerfoot stress the need to consider the contemporary context in our approach to youth mental health (2005). Internationally, there is a growing sentiment that youth should not be viewed as problems but as possessing strengths and resilience. This trend is reflected in recent reports from organizations such as the UN, UNICEF, and the Pan American Health Organization (PAHO). In countries such as Australia, the US, and the UK various youth positive initiatives have been introduced in the belief that they will enhance youth mental health and reduce risky behaviours. Powelson and Tonkin (2005) have reviewed these recent trends and discussed their implications for policy and programs in BC.

Settersten, Furstenberg, and Rumbaut, in their co-edited book *On the Frontier of Adulthood* (2005), introduce the notion of emerging adulthood and make the case that adolescence, as a distinct developmental period, has undergone important changes and now extends well into the mid-thirties. This recent phenomenon has important implications for youth mental health and youth's connections to family. For example, the emerging adult remains dependent on family support (financial and social) longer and delays attainment of the traditional markers of adulthood (marriage, mortgage, and maternity). At the same time, certain mental disorders such as early psychosis, autism, and bipolar disorder continue to emerge and be diagnosed in youth, thus requiring integration of the family into the treatment team.

The new millennium includes an explosion of technology, and youth have rushed to adapt to it. In health promotion the primary function of the internet and web-based information sites has been to provide information and improve access to reliable, confidential, knowledge-based health information. However, this has not proven to be its primary use among youth. Adolescents do not turn to the internet for their mental health information. Peers remain their principal source of information, and support. Parents and mental health professionals continue to be a source of help, but not as a frontline resource. The youth mental health folklore stigmatizes mental health services. Youth are not averse to using the internet to engage in socialization (e.g., chat lines) or even less positive behaviours such as cruising sites that promote hate, pornography, gambling, and violence. This misuse of technology by youth, and the opportunity it creates for their exploitation by predators, is a contemporary version of an old issue and must adversely affect youth mental health. Unfortunately, we have no population-based measures of the pluses and minuses of the new information technology (IT).

The new brand of social conservatism could have an important impact on youth mental health. This conservatism, largely religion-based, offers youth opportunities to become engaged in meaningful ways. Their sense of closeness to their god empowers them, but it should also promote mental health in many. However, it is too early to conclude that religion fosters tolerance or understanding of mental disorders or that religion alone is enough to change youth risky behaviours for the better. For example, in the US, faith-based abstinence programs do not necessarily prevent early pregnancy or prolong virginity (Bruckner and Bearman, 2005).

Primary Care: There is general public recognition that Canada has insufficient medical manpower. This is particularly true of adolescent-oriented family physicians and psychiatrists. However, the very nature of the common mental health problems in adolescence calls for early identification and developmentally appropriate intervention by these physicians. To complicate matters, an adolescent's first call for help is not made to a counsellor, school nurse, or priest, but to family and peers, and as Waddell and co-authors also point out, only a fraction of these are self-referrals and few ever receive specialized care for their mental health problems (2005). The primary care provider in the youth's own community or school may be the adolescent's most logical resource, but competing demands for their services, fee schedules and referral restrictions, and provider discomforts with consent and confidentiality concerns conspire to make the logical impractical.

Early Intervention: Early adolescent mental health issues are amenable to both prevention programs and early intervention strategies (Canadian Institute for Health Information, 2005). The challenge is how to identify the issues and how best to respond. The goal is to prevent negative outcomes and not perpetuate/exacerbate the presenting issue. The prime consideration is how best to convert a behavioural challenge into an opportunity for positive growth. For example, adolescent girls who appear to be older than they really are, are at risk for sexual abuse, early first intercourse, and related risky behaviours. Would raising the legal age of consent for intercourse solve this problem? Would earlier sex education be better than more accessible emergency contraception? Would the morning after pill reduce suicide attempts by early teens? Obviously there is no one right or even simple answer. Nor is there solid enough evidence to base an answer upon. However, it is encouraging to note more recent efforts to address the challenge of primary prevention in child and youth mental health programs. Complex issues like mental health will demand more comprehensive solutions, and the voices of youth themselves will need a place in their formulation.

Evidence Base: Public perception is that youth are the root of society's problems. They are seen as violent, criminal, apathetic, and self destructive. Nothing could be further from the truth. The evidence or the clinical reality tell us that yes, some youth do engage in too risky stuff too often, but most are full of positive energy and hope. The importance of this more positive message is underpinned by the data reported by the Canadian Institute for Health Information publication *Improving the Health of Young Canadians* (2005). Mental disorders do exist among youth, but most clinicians will confirm that these afflicted youth try to overcome their mental disorders and want to get on with their lives. However, we lack the evidence to demonstrate how or how well they do this. We are just beginning to evaluate the impact of our interventions upon the course of their disorder. This lack of an evidence base on the effectiveness of treatment is appalling, but more disturbing is the failure of policy makers and program planners to heed the evidence that is available. For example, while crystal methamphetamine is a mental health scourge among street-involved youth, the political hyperbole concerning crystal methamphetamine use in our schools is contrary to the low prevalence of its self-reported use by students (Tonkin et al., 2004) or the trend towards its declining use.

Targeted Interventions: In BC, our evidence base in regard to adolescent health is fairly robust. In fact, it enables us to confidently state that the majority of students do quite well and, aside from universal interventions such as immunization, injury prevention and treatment, and reproductive health services, they have little need of special mental health services. However, we can also identify special sub-populations within schools and in the community who confront mental health problems. It is reasonable to assume that they would benefit from a balanced mix of universal programs to promote their mental health and targeted programs designed to identify specific mental health problems and intervene at their earliest stages. The evidence shows that difficult to reach, elusive adolescent populations, such as those who are street-involved, carry more than the normal burden of adolescent mental health problems and require targeted interventions. For example, the profile of suicide attempts among street youth reflects their burden of mental health problems. Similarly, important regional differences in suicide attempt rates exist (Table 3.7).

Table 3.7 Attempted suicide in the past year by Health Service Delivery Area (%)

Health Service Delivery Area	Attempted suicide in the past year
Northwest	7
Northern Interior	9
Thompson Cariboo Shuswap	7
Okanagan	8
Kootenay Boundary	8
East Kootenay	9
North Vancouver Island	5
Central Vancouver Island	7
South Vancouver Island	5
Coastal	6
Vancouver	6
Richmond	6
Fraser North	6

Source: Adolescent Health Survey III, McCreary Centre Society (2003)
Note: Data not available for the Fraser South, Fraser East, and Northeast Health Service Delivery Areas.

Differences in the indicators of student mental health vary according to age and gender. Younger students and male students exhibit healthier profiles (Figure 3.5). For example, 65% of 12 year old girls have positive mental health, but by 18 years of age the percentage drops to 39, while for 18 year old males it is 43%.

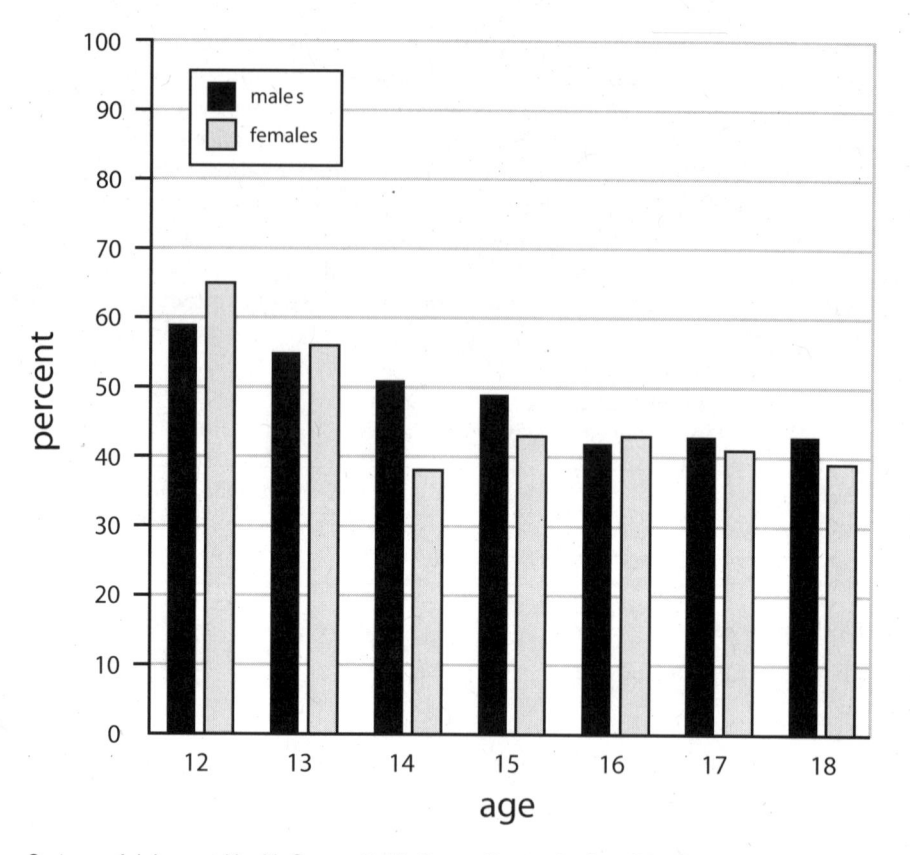

Source: Adolescent Health Survey III, McCreary Centre Society (2003)

Figure 3.5 Positive mental health by gender and age

Conclusion

In the absence of a clear definition of youth mental health, the discussion in this chapter has had to rely on showing the presence or absence of mental health problems among different populations of BC youth. It is clear that we have a long way to go before we can feel comfortable with the way we measure mental health, the extent to which we successfully apply the determinants of health approach (Fuks Geddes, Fielden, and Frankish, 2005), or the adequacy of the services intended to serve them. While progress has been made in areas such as provision of specialized services for mental disorders, the more general burden of mental health suffering, as reflected by the static nature of the suicide attempt rate among BC students, remains worrisome.

It is important to recognize that suicide is not the most common mental health problem among youth, but it is an example of how the emphasis tends to shift away from "health" and become placed on "risk." Issues of access to mental health services and mal-distribution of crisis intervention programs within regions of our province continue. Some regions report higher levels of suicide attempts and lower levels of overall self-reported mental health among their students (Table 3.7). Using Vancouver as the example, the percent of students with a history of a suicide attempt is among the lowest (6%), but the percentage with positive mental health is also the lowest (39%). Similarly, 48% of BC students reported having all five of the indicators of positive mental health but still 3% of that group reported severe emotional distress and 3% had attempted suicide in the past year. However, the data does not help us explain these apparent contradictions.

Coupling clinical and population-based approaches to identifying and understanding problems should stimulate newer thinking about youth mental health, while youth positive development intervention strategies hold out promise for the easement of the mental health burden that youth and their families bear. We have a long road ahead!

ACKNOWLEDGEMENTS

The Ministry of Children and Family Development, Government of British Columbia provides financial support for the Adolescent Health Survey, and the McCreary Centre Society conducts the surveys and publishes reports based on that data. The assistance of Aileen Murphy and Minda Chittenden in preparing the special tables for this chapter is much appreciated. Angela Ahn and Kathy Powelson of the McCreary Youth Foundation provided invaluable assistance with the assembly of the references and editing of the text. Dr. Terry Russell critiqued the draft chapter and offered several excellent references from the "grey literature." Dr. Charlotte Waddell carefully reviewed the text and tables and provided helpful comments.

Definitions used in Tables 3.1-3.5:

Anxiety: Percent of youth who during the past 30 days felt under strain, stress, or pressure "almost more than I could take" and/or were bothered by nervousness "extremely so to the point I couldn't do my work or deal with things."

Emotional Distress: Five items were used as an indicator of emotional distress. These included the frequency in the past 30 days of: feeling like being by oneself; feeling under strain, stress, or pressure; being bothered by any illness, physical problems, or fears about your health; being bothered by nervousness; and feeling sad, discouraged, hopeless, or had so many problems that you wondered if anything was worthwhile. The percent of youth who responded "all the time" or "extremely so" to two or more items were considered to be emotionally distressed. (Note: 8% of BC students in grades 7-12 were emotionally distressed in 2003.)

REFERENCES

Brent, D.A. (2005). Is the medication bottle for pediatric and adolescent depression half-full or half-empty? [Editorial]. *Journal of Adolescent Health*, 37(6), 431-433.

Bruckner, H., and Bearman, P.S. (2005). After the promise: The STD consequences of adolescent virginity pledges. *Journal of Adolescent Health*, 36(3), 271-278.

Canada (2004). *A Canada fit for children: Canada's plan of action in response to the May 2002 United Nations Special Session on Children*. Ottawa, ON: Government of Canada.

Canadian Institute for Health Information (2005). *Improving the health of young Canadians: Patterns of health and disease are largely a consequence of how we learn, live and work*. Toronto, ON: Canadian Institute for Health Information.

Commission on Emotional and Learning Disorders in Children (1970). *One million children: The CELDIC report*. Toronto, ON: Leonard Crainford for the Commssion on Emotional and Learning Disorders in Children.

Dahl, R.E. (2004). Adolescent brain development: A period of vulnerabilities and opportunities. *Annals of the New York Academy of Sciences*, 1021, 1-21

Dwivedi, K.N., and Harper, P.B. (2004). Introduction. In K.N. Dwivedi and P.B. Harper (Eds.), *Promoting the emotional well-being of children and adolescents and preventing their mental ill health: A handbook* (pp. 15- 28). London: Jessica Kingsley Publishers.

Fuks Geddes, C., Fielden, S., and Frankish, J. (2005). Determinants of health in special sub-populations of youth. In R.S. Tonkin and L.T. Foster (Eds.), *The youth of British Columbia: Their past and their future*. Canadian Western Geographical Series, Vol. 39 (pp. 63-102). Victoria, BC: University of Victoria, Department of Geography.

Hill, P. (2005). Mental health promotion, prevention, and early interventions in childhood and adolescence. In R. Williams and M. Kerfoot (Eds.), *Child and adolescent mental health services: Strategy, planning, delivery and evaluation* (pp. 177-185). New York: Oxford University Press.

Keys Young (1997). *Final report: Research and consultation among young people on mental health issues*. Canberra, Australia: Mental Health Branch, Department of Health and Family Services, Commonwealth of Australia.

Kidder, K., Stein, J. Fraser, J., and Canadian Institute of Child Health (2000). *The health of Canada's children* (3rd ed.). Ottawa, ON: Canadian Institute of Child Health.

Kidder, K., and Rogers, D. (2004). *Why Canada needs a national youth policy agenda*. Retrieved January 15, 2006 from the National Children's Alliance website: *http://www.national childrensalliance.com/nca/pubs/2004/youthpolicypaper.htm*

McCreary Centre Society (1999). *Our kids too: Sexually exploited youth in British Columbia: An Adolescent Health Survey*. Burnaby, BC: The McCreary Centre Society.

McCreary Centre Society (2001). *No place to call home: A profile of street youth in British Columbia*. Burnaby, BC: The McCreary Centre Society.

McCreary Centre Society (2002). *Between the cracks: Homeless youth in Vancouver*. Burnaby, BC: The McCreary Centre Society.

McCreary Centre Society (2003). *Healthy youth development: Highlights from the 2003 Adolescent Health Survey*. Burnaby, BC: The McCreary Centre Society.

Murphy, A., Chittenden, M., and The McCreary Centre Society (2005). *Time Out II: A profile of BC youth in custody*. Vancouver, BC: The McCreary Centre Society.

Offord, D.R. (2000). The mental health of children and youth [commentary on Chapter 8]. In K. Kidder, J. Stein, J. Fraser, and Canadian Institute of Child Health, *The health of Canada's children* (3rd ed., pp. 225-226). Ottawa, ON: Canadian Institute of Child Health.

Offord, D.R. (2005). Comparative analyses: Challenges facing CAMHS in North America. In R. Williams and M. Kerfoot (Eds.), *Child and adolescent mental health services: Strategy, planning, delivery and evaluation* (pp. 373-388). New York: Oxford University Press.

Offord, D.R., Boyle, M.H., Fleming, J.E., Monroe Blum, H, and Rae Grant, N. (1989). Ontario child health study: Summary of selected results. *Canadian Journal of Psychiatry*, 34, 483-491.

Powelson, K., and Tonkin, R.S. (2005). Definitions of positive youth development. In R.S. Tonkin and L.T. Foster (Eds.), *The youth of British Columbia: Their past and their future.* Canadian Western Geographical Series, Vol. 39 (pp. 123-144). Victoria, BC: University of Victoria, Department of Geography.

Ryff, C.D., and Keyes, C.L.M. (1995). The structure of psychological well-being revisited. *Journal of Personality and Social Psychology*, 69(4), 719-727.

Settersten, R.A. Jr., Furstenberg, F.F. Jr., and Rumbaut, R.G. (Eds.) (2005). *On the frontier of adulthood: Theory, research and public policy.* Chicago: University of Chicago Press.

Steinhauer, P.D. (2001). Clinical and service applications of the theory of resiliency with particular reference to adolescents. *International Journal of Adolescent Medicine and Health*, 13, 53-73.

Tonkin, R.S., Murphy, A., and McCreary Centre Society (2002). *Violence in adolescence: Injury, suicide, and criminal violence in the lives of BC youth.* Burnaby, BC: The McCreary Centre Society.

Tonkin, R.S., Poon, C., Murphy, A., and McCreary Centre Society (2002). *Accenting the positive: A developmental framework for reducing risk and promoting positive outcomes among BC youth.* Vancouver, BC: The McCreary Centre Society.

Tonkin, R.S., Murphy, A., Chittenden, M., Jackson, P., and McCreary Centre Society (2004). *Healthy youth development: Highlights from the 2003 Adolescent Health Survey III.* Vancouver, BC: The McCreary Centre Society.

Tonkin, R.S., Murphy, A., Lee, Z., Saewyc, E., and McCreary Centre Society (2005). *British Columbia youth health trends: A retrospective, 1992-2003.* Vancouver, BC: The McCreary Centre Society.

van der Woerd, K.A., Dixon, B.L., McDiarmid, T., Chittenden, M., Murphy, A., and McCreary Centre Society (2005). *Raven's Children II: Aboriginal youth health in BC.* Vancouver, BC: The McCreary Centre Society.

Waddell, C., McEwen, K., Shepherd, C.A., Offord, D.R., and Hua, J.M. (2005). A public health strategy to improve mental health of Canadian Children. *Canadian Journal of Psychiatry*, 50(4), 226-233.

Williams, R., and Kerfoot, M. (Eds.) (2005). *Child and adolescent mental health services: Strategy, planning, delivery and evaluation.* New York: Oxford University Press.

Willms, J.D. (Ed.) (2002). *Vulnerable children: Findings from Canada's National Longitudinal Survey of Children and Youth.* Edmonton, AB: University of Alberta Press.

Plate 2 "Counting Pebbles" (J. LeClair)

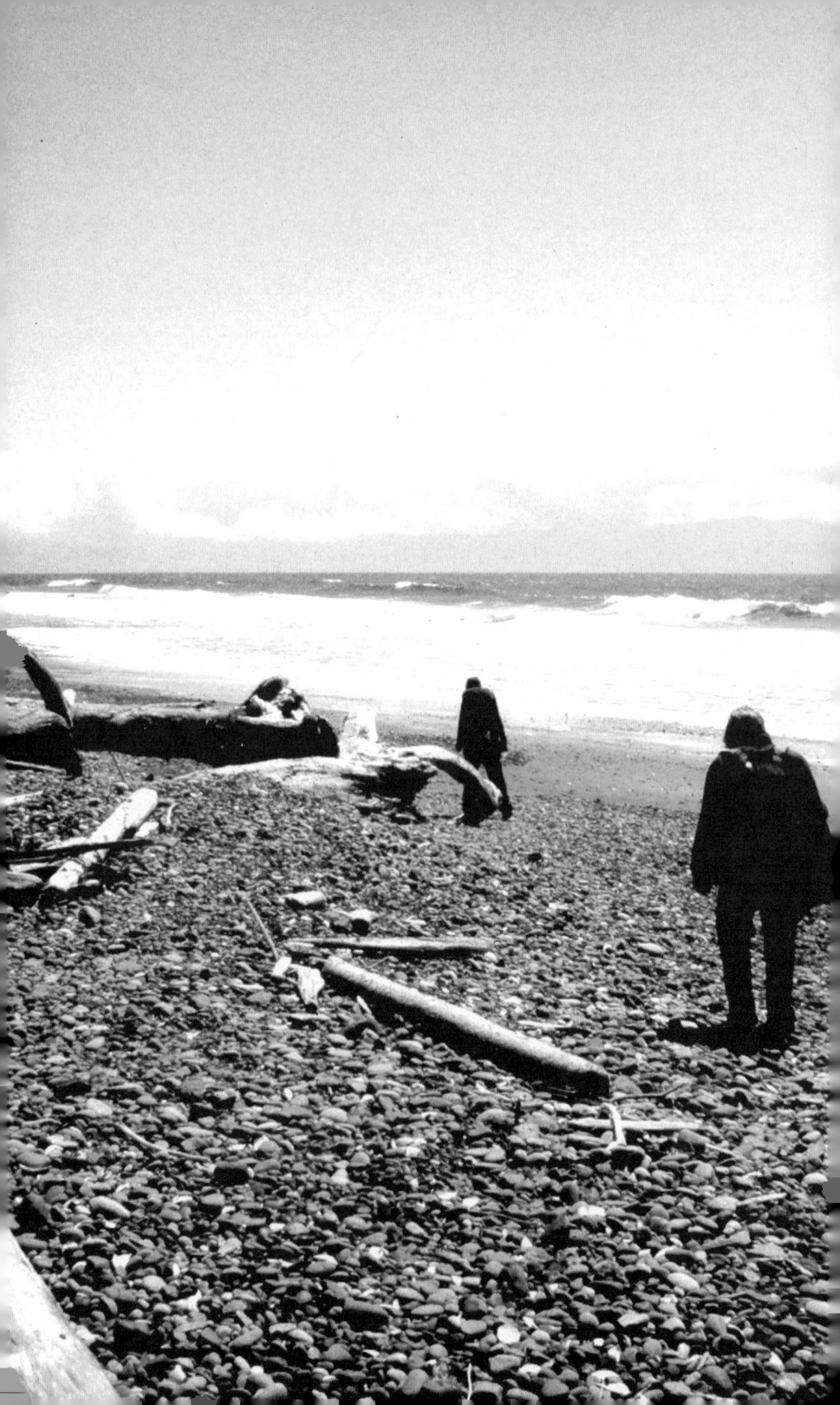

Youth Leaving Care: Mental Health Issues

Deborah Rutman, Carol Hubberstey,
April Feduniw, and Erinn Brown
School of Social Work, University of Victoria

Introduction

The *Promoting Positive Outcomes for Youth From Care* project is a prospective, 3-year study designed to examine what happens to youth living in two communities in British Columbia following their exit from government care. The overall goal of the project was to better understand the processes, supports, and resources that make a positive difference to youth and that help to lead to successful transitions from care.[1] Additional project objectives were to examine strategies to provide youth with peer support during the process of exiting care, and to provide opportunities for youth to voice their perspective on how successful transitions are defined. The project received funding from 2003-2006 from the Crime Prevention Partnership Program of the National Crime Prevention Centre (NCPC).

In other reports we have provided a snapshot of the experiences and life circumstances of youth in transition from care (Time 1 Report) and then approximately 9 months later (Time 2 Report) (Rutman, Hubberstey, Barlow, and Brown, 2005; Rutman, Hubberstey, Feduniw, and Brown, 2006). In this chapter, we focus on the mental health issues and concerns of youth in transition from state care, based on our findings from the first two waves of interviews with youth.

Youth in Transition From State Care and Mental Health

The concept of developmental transitions suggests that the life cycle consists of a series of important transitional periods that can be distinguished from the day to day changes and transformations experienced by infants, children, and youth. A transitional period can be defined as a "process or period in which change occurs, either from one state, stage, form, or activity, to another" (*Encarta*, no date).

The transition from adolescence to adulthood is widely regarded to be a critical transitional period (*www.growinghealthykids.com*) that takes places between the ages of 17 and 22 (Mech 1994). Key facets of the transitions are the development of social competence, self-direction, self-esteem, the acquisition of values, standards of conduct, and preparation in life-skills (Mech, 1994). Canadian research suggests that young people who make a successful transition to adulthood actually make four transitions (*www.growinghealthykids.com*):

- from school to work
- from their family home to creating their own family
- from being responsible members of a nuclear family to being responsible, contributing members of the community
- *from the care of others to managing their own health and well-being* (emphasis added)

Children and youth who enter the care of the state under the auspices of the child protection system bring with them experiences that result in significant histories of developmental delays and emotional adjustment problems (Foster and Wright, 2002). In BC, the *Child, Family and Community Service Act* is the legislative authority for Child Protection Services. Under the Act, anyone who has reason to believe that a child may be abused, neglected, or is for any other reason in need of protection, must report this information to the Ministry of Children and Family Development. If a report is substantiated, then a range of actions may be available, including: providing or arranging the provision of support services to the family; supervising the child's care in the home; or, protecting the child through removal from the family and placement with relatives, a foster family, or specialized residential resources

The pre-care experiences of children and youth entering foster care typically mean that they are "at risk for behavioural problems at home, in school, and in the community" (Trocmé et al., 1999, p. 2). In a review of the literature that was conducted as part of the evaluation of the "Looking After Children Project" in Canada, Kufeldt and co-authors (2000) noted that children taken into care displayed higher incidents of emotional and physical health problems than did children in the general population. The authors also found that the research literature regarding children in care indicated that one-third to one-half of children in care had mental health concerns. When age was taken into consideration, children over age 12 had higher rates of emotional health problems, whereas younger children had higher rates of physical health problems (Kufeldt et al., 2000, pp. 15-17).

It is evident, then, that children who enter the care system potentially have a range of pre-existing health problems that need to be addressed. While children and youth may receive care and treatment during their time in care, once they reach the age of majority, which in BC is age 19, they must exit the child welfare system, regardless of their abilities, skills, needs, or readiness. Furthermore, as Christopher (2005) poignantly describes, in as much as the parental role of government comes to an end, this occurs with finality and without further formal involvement of the 'parent,' regardless of the young person's financial, emotional, or practical support needs. Thus, it may be argued that youth leaving foster care at the age of majority enter the transition towards adulthood in a more "depersonalized and irreversible way" (Leslie and Hare, 2000, p. 20) than do other youth leaving home. Their leaving care experience may be more akin to an "expulsion" than a transition.

According to Flynn (2003), a significant proportion of youth who leave care at the age of majority need emotional support, along with practical assistance to locate suitable housing, educational programs, and employment, and to establish rewarding personal relationships. Silva-Wayne (1994) has also proposed that youth from care may need more support and assistance than others with more enduring support systems, in order to effectively manage the health and emotional residue of their pre-care and in-care experiences, along with their abrupt exit from care and accelerated transition to adulthood.

Canadian longitudinal research on outcomes for youth from care is essentially non-existent and has been recognized as a major knowledge gap by researchers, practitioners, and policy makers alike. Nevertheless, Tweddle's (2005, p. 7) review of findings from what does exist in the Canadian literature revealed that, compared to their peers, youth aging out of care were more likely to:

- leave school before completing their secondary education
- become a parent at a young age
- be dependent on social assistance
- be unemployed or underemployed
- be incarcerated/involved with the criminal justice system
- experience homelessness
- be at higher risk for substance abuse problems
- *have mental health problems* (emphasis added)

In the US, where outcomes for youth who have exited foster care are similarly troubling, several studies found that mental illness was more prevalent among youth who have lived in care than it was among youth who had not lived in care. Moreover, youth from care were also more likely to report difficulties maintaining behavioural and emotional control (Shin et al., no date).

Cook (1990, 1991), for example, reported that 38% of youth from care were diagnosed as emotionally disturbed. An extensive study of outcomes for youth at age 19 who had lived in care found that one-third of the participants in the study had at least one mental health diagnosis, the most prevalent being "PTSD, alcohol abuse, substance abuse, and major depression" (Courtney et al., 2005, p. 41). The study further noted that youth still living in care reported fewer mental health diagnoses than those who had already left care. The study's authors suggested that experiences of isolation and other environmental stressors, such as threats of conflict and violence and uncertainty about one's safety and well-being, may have been contributing factors to the higher rate of mental illness among those who had aged out of care.

Having a positive relationship with a stable, caring adult is an important asset and protective factor for young people as they navigate the transition from adolescence to young adulthood (Kurtz et al., 2000; Loman and Siegel, 2000; Mann-Feder and White, 2003). A review of best practices in the provision of youth services cited a 10 year study by Cook (1991) that found that high-risk youth experienced better outcomes post-care if they had strong support networks, including the presence of family members. Inglehart (1994), also cited in the best practices review, similarly found that contact with fathers enabled youth to find help and resources on their own. An earlier study by Courtney (1998) found that emotional and physical well-being was linked to the presence of a healthy and positive social support network. Youth exiting care with no obvious connections to biological family members, foster parents, social workers, teachers, or other positive adult role models were found to be especially vulnerable. Moreover, as noted by Courtenay's (1998) study, too many youth go through the transition experience without adequate support or direction with respect to accessing adult services such as mental health, income assistance, housing, and education programs. Without this support and advocacy, youth have to fend for themselves with complex systems.

Similar results have been reported in the UK. In one study of 101 young people leaving care, those with mental health or emotional or behavioural difficulties were vulnerable to poor outcomes (Dixon et al., 2004). As with other studies, these youth were more likely to report post-care instability, homelessness, poor employment outcomes, and weaker life skills.

A qualitative study of the experiences of youth leaving care in Australia likewise concluded that "when young people who have been in care leave care, they are more likely to experience homelessness, unemployment, early parenthood, *loneliness and despair*" [emphasis added] (Maunders et al., 1999, p. vii). Youth in the study recounted suicidal ideation, alcohol abuse, psychiatric breakdowns, and feelings of depression, along with their struggles to cope with the pressure and stress of managing on their own with few, if any, supports.

In all likelihood, the strong presence of mental health problems and concerns in youth who have exited care reflects a complex interplay of several factors, including pre-placement events, in-care experiences, as well as the leaving care process. Many young people living in care experience significant trauma, abuse, and neglect both prior to entering the care system and even during their time in care (Raychaba, 1988; Courtney et. al., 1998; Christopher, 2005), leaving them attempting to cope with unresolved internal conflicts. In view of the magnitude and degree of these risk factors, there is good reason to suspect that when the transition from foster care to independence is not well supported, youth are at greater risk for homelessness, sexual exploitation, victimization, involvement in the criminal justice and child welfare systems, and increased mental health issues.

Research Process

The project was a prospective, longitudinal (3-year) study following a cohort of youth in transition from care over a 2.5-year period. Two BC communities were involved: a metropolitan centre and a small city. The project team was comprised of two researchers with experience undertaking academic and community-based research, and two former 'youth in care' experienced in providing peer support.

The primary criteria for participation in the project were: (a) youth in care of the Ministry of Children and Family Development; (b) youth who either turned 19 in 2003 *or* would be doing so by December 2004. Although the project team did not have access to Ministry client information and thus could not directly contact eligible youth, the BC Ministry of Children and Family Development was the primary source of participant referral/recruitment; Ministry staff identified eligible youth and invited them to take part in the study.[2]

At Time 1, 37 youth participated in the study; 17 (46%) were under the age of majority and 54% were over age 19 and therefore had already aged out of care. As shown in Table 4.1, more than three-quarters of the study cohort at Time 1 were female (78%; n=29), and slightly less than one-quarter (22%; n=8) were male. At Time 2, 33 youth took part in interviews; the remaining 4 youths were lost through attrition. A total of 82% (n=27) of youth participants were female and 18% (n=6) were male.

Table 4.1 Time 1 & 2 – Participants by gender

Gender	Time 1 #	Time 1 %	Time 2 #	Time 2 %
Male	8	22	6	18
Female	29	78	27	82
Total	**37**	**100**	**33**	**100**

The research plan called for youth to take part in a total of four face-to-face interviews, scheduled 6 to 9 months apart. The Time 1 interview took about 90 minutes to complete and was used to establish baseline information for each youth. The Time 2 interview took about 60 minutes to complete. Interviews were conducted either in the participant's home, the project's research office, or another private setting of the participant's choice.

An interview guide was developed based on a review of the literature and consultations with national colleagues. Interview topics include: background information/demographics; in-care experiences; family relationships; parenting experiences; physical and mental health; substance use; educational experience; training and employment; source of income; social supports and community involvement; experiences of victimization and/or offending; self-care skills; and preparedness for leaving care. In addition, questions regarding homelessness were added to the Time 2 interview guide.

The interviews were not audio-taped; however, detailed notes were made by interviewers at the time of the interview, with every effort made to record participants' comments in their own words and terminology. Statistical analysis of the fixed choice interview questions was performed using SPSS; qualitative data analysis techniques were used on the open-ended interview data. The data and emerging themes were reviewed and discussed by all team members as a means of researcher triangulation.

While the number/percentage of youth participants lost to attrition from Time 1 to Time 2 was relatively small (11% of the sample), we anticipated at the outset of this study that participant attrition would likely be an issue given that this is a prospective study. We are also aware that this represents a limitation to the study, as we cannot ascertain how the absence of information from these missing participants affects our findings over time. Subsequent reports will focus on the various methodological issues and lessons associated with our study, including attrition and retention efforts.

FINDINGS

In this article we consider the experiences of study participants in relation to their self-reports of depression, anxiety, substance use, social supports/involvement in the community, and connection with family members. We begin by sharing the stories of two participants, Cassie and Nicola (not their real names; some personal information has been changed to protect privacy). Their stories speak to some of the experiences and related mental health issues faced by study participants upon exiting state care.

Cassie

At the time of the first interview, Cassie was within 8 weeks of turning 19 years old and "ageing out of care." She had been recently admitted into hospital for anxiety and panic attacks related to using cocaine. Cassie admitted to using cocaine, but explained that her feelings of panic and anxiety were more a result of feeling stressed and overwhelmed from living on her own. She said she was worried about losing the financial support of the Ministry for Children and Family Development's Independent Living program when she turned 19. Cassie wanted to find employment post-care, but had not completed high school and lacked adequate or reliable transportation as well as a plan for finding work. Transportation was a problem because Cassie lived away from easily accessed transportation links. If Cassie ended up on income assistance, her income would drop by about $200 per month.

Cassie did not feel prepared or ready to be totally on her own. She said:

> No, I don't want this yet. I have nothing to fall back on. There's more stuff I feel I need to know.

When Cassie was released from hospital, she started staying with a half-sister and the half-sister's 3-year-old son. The 3-year-old had behavioural issues and needed constant supervision, and Cassie's half-sister also struggled with mental health issues. Cassie stated that even though the household was not ideal for someone such as herself dealing with anxiety, she would rather be there than on her own at her apartment which was reportedly unsafe due to the easy accessibility of drugs and the presence of drug dealers and violence.

Nicola

At the time of the first interview, Nicola was a few days short of her 19th birthday and living in care on the Independent Living Program. Soon after leaving care, Nicola took up residence in a motel while searching for a permanent place to live. After a couple of months she was able to move into a group home.

Nicola said she suffered from high anxiety and other mental health concerns such as depression. She reported using marijuana on a daily basis to mitigate her anxiety. Getting appropriate support from health professionals was difficult for Nicola due to her suspicion of most people and her reported anxiety and inability to follow through on appointments. These behaviours also made it difficult for her to seek and retain employment.

At the time of the second interview, Nicola was aware that she needed to secure a regular source of income and was becoming increasingly anxious about this. Thus, with support, Nicola was trying to complete an application for income assistance under the Employment and Assistance for Persons with Disabilities Act, otherwise referred to as Persons with a Disability Designation (PWD). However, obtaining this designation requires completion of a 24 page application form along with supporting documentation from medical health professionals. Nicola, who also did not have a family physician, made several appointments with a doctor at a drop-in health clinic but at the last moment would refuse to go. Nicola's anxiety was such that she also was reluctant to apply for support through Adult Mental Health Services. She primarily spent her time in the house, with occasional forays to the store or Food Bank for food.

PHYSICAL AND MENTAL HEALTH

At Time 1, the majority of youth in our sample (65%) rated their health as good or excellent. While this is positive, our findings were striking in that substantially *fewer* participants reported themselves to be in good/excellent health relative to other recent surveys of BC youth. For example, the 2003 BC Adolescent

Health Survey, conducted by the McCreary Centre Society, reported that 86% of the youth in its sample stated that they were in good or excellent health (McCreary Centre, 2003). While the reasons for rating their health as 'fair' or 'poor' likely varied and youth were not specifically asked to explain their responses, one participant linked her self-perceived health rating to her former substance use:

> *I didn't rate my health as good right now because of past drug use. But I've quit drugs now.*

With only 65% of our sample reporting good or excellent health, our findings are more comparable to those of BC youth who had been abused or sexually exploited. As shown in Table 4.2, recent BC Adolescent Health Surveys found that 75% of female youth who had been abused and 55% of sexually exploited females rated their health as good or excellent (McCreary Centre, 2003).

Table 4.2 Time 1 – Youth rating their health as 'excellent' or 'good'

	% of sample
2003 Adolescent Health Survey (in school youth sample)	86
2002 Adolescent Health Survey of Youth who have been abused (female only sample)	75
"Promoting Positive Outcomes for Youth from care" study (1st Interview)	65
1999 Adolescent Health Survey of Sexually Exploited Youth (female only sample)	55

There was no difference between the males and females in our sample on self-reported health. This is in contrast to other research, including the BC Adolescent Health Survey (McCreary Centre, 2003), which found that girls assessed their health less favourably than did boys.

At Time 2, the proportion of youth who rated their health as good or excellent dropped to 55%—that is, participants' ratings of their health were comparable to youth in the general population who had been sexually exploited.

PHYSICAL AND MENTAL HEALTH CONDITIONS

We asked youth whether they had ever experienced or been diagnosed with a variety of health conditions. Overall, at Time 1 most participants reported that they had not experienced these conditions. The one exception to this was depression; more than one third of the youth (38%) reported that they had experienced or been diagnosed with depression. Indeed, of all the health problems included in the checklist, depression was the most frequently reported (Table 4.3).

As well, an additional 11% of our sample reported experiencing anxiety (which had not been listed separately, but emerged out of the "other" category of health conditions), and 14% reported having an eating disorder. These findings indicate that approximately two-thirds of young people in our study have experienced mental health problems or concerns.

Table 4.3 Time 1 – Past or current health condition

	Percent of sample (n=37)
Depression	38
Vision problem	30
Eating disorder	14
Hearing problem	8
Sexually transmitted disease	8
Anaemia	5
Herpes	3
Hepatitis	3
Other (includes anxiety)	41

Overall, relatively few youth in our study had concerns about their mental health at Time 1 (Table 4.4).

Table 4.4 Time 1 – Current mental health concerns

Have current mental health concerns?	% of sample(n=37)
Yes	14
No	84
Not sure	3

However, a number of participants did report concerns. For example, one participant stated:

> I had a psychiatric assessment just last week. I've been having really bad anxiety attacks and depression for a few years and have been on meds for a long time. I did see counsellors while in care and played

> with different meds but they didn't work. Now am seeing counsellor/psychiatrist on Mondays. I want to avoid meds and work through issues instead.

Moreover, all of the participants who indicated they had mental health concerns at Time 2 were females, a continuation of the pattern noted at Time 1 when all but one of the participants reporting a mental health concern or problem were females.

Direct comparisons between our findings and those of other surveys with BC youth cannot be made because of differences in interview/survey questions. Nevertheless, our findings with regard to self-reported experience/diagnosis of depression are generally consistent with the BC Adolescent Health Survey, which reported that 42% of female youth in school stated they had "emotional troubles" (McCreary Centre, 1999).

At Time 2, we asked participants whether, *in the previous 6 to 9 months*, they had experienced or been diagnosed with various health conditions. As at Time 1, the most frequently reported health condition was depression. A total of 48% (n=16) of participants either reported experiencing depression (n=10) or reported mental health concerns related to depression, or that they were currently being treated for depression (n=6). An additional participant reported a "drug-induced psychosis" that resulted in hospitalization. *Thus, at Time 2 a total of 51% (n=17) of participants reported depression-related symptoms, treatment and/or serious mental health concerns.* Participants described their experiences and symptoms in the following ways:

> I'm concerned about depression and post-partum depression.

> (I feel like I have) mild depression. I can't afford medication, so I just talk to people about it.

> I recently had to face issues that I left behind in my childhood. That's hard to deal with right now.

> I was admitted to (psychiatric unit of acute care hospital) for a drug-induced psychosis and continue to have the after effects.

> (I) agreed to go for a psychological assessment, by choice, and now I'm on anti-depressants.

HOMELESSNESS

At Time 2, participants were also asked whether they had ever been homeless, a question not posed at Time 1. Forty-five percent (n=15) of youth participants reported that they had experienced homelessness at some point in their life; analysis by gender revealed that 48% (n=13) of the females and 33% (n=2) of the males reported homelessness. In terms of when and for how long youth had been homeless, the data revealed that:

- Of all 'homeless' youth, 73% (n=11/15) were homeless from ages 13-16
- 53% (n=8/15) of homeless youth were homeless for more than 3 months

The circumstances under which youth became homeless varied considerably. For some, homelessness resulted after the young person got into conflict with a parent or caregiver or when a parent was no longer physically able to care for the youth; for others, involvement with drugs or alcohol led to homelessness; for still others, homelessness resulted from a break-up with a partner.

Nevertheless, further inspection of the data revealed that *80% (n=12) of the youth who reported experiencing homelessness also reported depression, depression-related symptoms or treatment, and/or another major mental health issue.*

Marijuana Use

Experimentation with alcohol and marijuana may be considered a common experience for teenagers, but some go beyond experimentation to the extent that their behaviours fall into the high risk category (Health Canada, no date). A high rate of substance use tends to be one of the poor outcomes associated with youth who have lived in care.

According to the 2003 BC Adolescent Health Survey, 55% of 17 year olds in BC reported that they used or had tried marijuana (McCreary Centre, 2003). By contrast, in our study, 81% (n=30) of youth at Time 1 reported that they currently used marijuana, had tried it, or had quit using it. Moreover, a sizeable percentage of all youth interviewed at Time 1 (41%) reported using marijuana daily or multiple times per week. Notably, 27% of our total sample at Time 1 reported using marijuana daily.

We were interested in knowing what the pattern of marijuana use was among youth who reported mental health concerns. Of the 17 youth who indicated a mental health problem or concern at Time 2, 70% (n=12) reported using marijuana and, of these, 41% (n=9) reported using it on a weekly or daily basis. Four youth who reported mental health issues said they did not use drugs at all.

Family Relations, Social Supports, and Community Involvement

As noted previously, having a positive relationship with a stable, caring adult is an important asset and protective factor for young people as they navigate the transition from adolescence to young adulthood (Kurtz et al., 2000; Loman and Siegel, 2000; Mann-Feder and White, unpublished). Drawing on Sarason's Social Support Questionnaire – Short Form (Sarason et al., 1987), youth participants were asked several questions related to their perceived support networks.

These questions included whether they had close and trustworthy friends, whether they had someone on whom they could depend for support, as well as the type of support they received (characterized as emotional, financial, and practical support), how involved they were in community activities, and how satisfied they were with the types and levels of support they experienced.

Overall, at Time 1 and Time 2, more than half the youth said that they were disconnected from one or both parents. At the same time, the majority reported having people whom they counted on for emotional and practical support. However, when we looked at these results more closely, it was evident that the support network was comprised of a mix of paid support people such as social workers, community agency staff, and mental health workers, as well as unpaid support people such as friends, boyfriends or girlfriends, (former) foster parents, and family members. For example, close to one-quarter of the 17 youth who reported mental health issues indicated at Time 1 that they received emotional support from a paid worker. Another one-quarter of this group reported that they did not have anyone they depended upon for emotional support. Yet another participant identified a youth who was part of the study (and also reported experiencing mental health problems) as someone she counted on for support. In subsequent interviews she reported that she had terminated this relationship due to the other youth's ongoing drug use. We provide this example to illustrate the tenuousness of the support networks upon which many youth purport to rely. Indeed, several of the youth who reported mental health problems indicated at Time 2 that one goal they had for their social relationships was to find healthier, more mature and reliable friends.

I want to find 'straight/clean' friends, goal oriented friends.

I want to meet more actual friends.

Finally, youth were asked what they perceived as being the best and worst aspects of leaving care. In terms of the worst or hardest aspects of leaving care, as at Time 1, the most frequently reported issue overall was *financial hardship*: participants discussed their difficulties in obtaining enough money to make ends meet, and their significant loss of income relative to that which they received in care:

A drop in income has been hard. I'm living on $200 less per month.

This theme was echoed by the 17 youth who reported mental health issues; half indicated they were worried about the financial implications and whether they were really ready to be on their own.

A second important theme was the *loss of supportive people* in participants' lives, and in particular, the loss of involvement by their social worker. One young person poignantly compared her situation to that of young people who grew up in their parents' homes:

> *I know 24 year-olds whose parents still make them lunch – I don't have that.*

Participants also spoke of the *difficulties in trying to access resources or programs via adult service systems* (e.g., income support or health/mental health care). Not having a support person or worker to help them navigate adult systems may have heightened their experience of distress.

> *Welfare workers aren't as involved or helpful. When you're on your own you are ON YOUR OWN. And they don't care.*

Lastly, some youth spoke conveying their loneliness and unease at being on their own at this point in their life.

> *Some nights I can't sleep because I'm not used to it yet.*

SUMMARY AND CONCLUSIONS

We began this chapter by noting the lack of longitudinal Canadian research on youth leaving care. The current study contributes to the emergence of a nascent body of Canadian literature on the subject. Sadly, the outcomes that the *Promoting Positive Outcomes for Youth From Care* project is beginning to document are in keeping with studies from other countries such as the US, Australia, and the UK. Relative to youth who have not lived in care, youth in transition from state care: had a lower level of education; were more likely to be on income assistance at age 19; engaged in higher levels of alcohol and drug use; and had a more fragile social support network, as well as tenuous ties to family. In our study, the single biggest concern was mental health and in particular, depression.

In terms of mental health issues, based on our Time 1 and Time 2 interviews, the picture emerging of these young people's experiences is highly disquieting. Among our sample of youth in transition from state care, depression has been the most frequently reported health issue. Depression and/or depressive symptoms/treatment were experienced by 48% of participants, a jump from 38% at Time 1. Moreover, 80% of the youth in our study who experienced homelessness also reported depression and/or major mental health issues. Our findings to date also suggest that many youth from care lack a strong support network and/or one comprised primarily of non-paid supports, and youth experience as a real loss the reduction in their network that occurs upon ageing out of care. Again, a tenuous social support system is particularly worrisome for youth who experience mental health problems.

In short, the leaving care experience neither facilitates nor allows for the full range of transitions described above that youth encounter as they enter adulthood, and puts former foster care youth under pressure to do more, sooner, and with fewer internal and external resources than their peers (Stein, 2002).

Endnotes

[1] A number of terms are used in the literature to refer to being in the care of the child welfare system, including being "in foster care," "in substitute care," "in government care," and simply "in care." In this report we use these terms interchangeably, and most often use the latter ("in care"), since that is the term most often used by youth themselves.

[2] A variety of other recruitment strategies were employed as well, including putting up posters in youth friendly organizations and alternative schools, talking with foster parents and school counsellors, and speaking with youth participants from a previous youth-based project that we had undertaken.

References

Boyd, M., and Norris, D. (1999). *The crowded nest: Young adults at home*. Canadian Social Trends. Statistics Canada, pp. 2-5.

Christopher, N. (2005). Youth from care, B.A. The barriers to university faced by a former youth in care. *Relational Child & Youth Care Practice*, 18(2), 19-28.

Cook, R. (1990). *A National Evaluation of Title IV-E Foster Care Independent Living Programs for Youth, Phase 1*. Rockville, MD: Westat.

Cook, R. (1991). *A National Evaluation of Title IV-E Foster Care Independent Living Programs for Youth: Phase 2 Final Report*. Rockville, MD: Westat.

Courtney, M., Dworsky, A., Ruth, G., Keller, T., Havlicek, J., and Bost, N. (2005). *Midwest evaluation of the adult functioning of former foster youth: Outcomes at age 19*. Chicago: Chapin Hall, Centre for Children, University of Chicago.

Courtney, M., Piliavin, I., Grogan-Kaylor, A., and Nesmith, A. (1998). *Foster youth transitions to adulthood: Outcomes 12 to 18 months after leaving out-of-home care: Notes and comments*. Madison, WI: School of Social Work and Institute for Research on Poverty, University of Wisconsin-Madison.

Dixon, J., Wade, J., Byford, S., Weatherly, H., and Lee, J. (2004). *Young people leaving care: A study of outcomes and costs. Research summary*. York: University of York.

Encarta (no date). *www.dictionary.msn.com*.

Farris-Manning, C., and Zandstra, M. (2003). *Children in care in Canada*. Child Welfare League of Canada (as retrieved from *www.cwlc.ca*).

Foster, L.T., and Wright, M. (2002). Patterns and trends in children in the care of the Province of British Columbia: Ecological, policy, and cultural perspectives. In M. Hayes and L.T. Foster (Eds.), *Too small to see, too big to ignore: Child health and well-being in British Columbia* (pp. 103-140). Victoria, BC: Western Geographical Press, University of Victoria.

Flynn, R. (2003). *Resilience in transitions from out-of-home care in Canada: A prospective longitudinal national study*. Unpublished Research Proposal.

Health Canada (no date). *Young people in Canada: Their health and well-being*. Ottawa: Health Canada, Publications.

Inglehart, A.P. (1994). Kinship Foster Care: Placement, services, and outcome issues. *Children and Youth Services Review*, 16, 107–22.

Kufeldt, K., and Stein, M. (2005). The voice of young people: Reflections on the process of leaving care and the care experience. In J. Scott and H. Ward (Eds.), *Safeguarding and promoting the well-being of children, families and communities* (pp. 134-148). London: Jessica Kingsley Publishers.

Kufeldt, K., Simard, M., and Vachon, J. (2000). *Looking after children in Canada – Final Report*. Ottawa: Social Development Partnerships of Human Development, Human Resources Development Canada.

Kurtz, D., Lindsey, E., Jarvis, S., and Nackerud, L. (2000). How runaway and homeless youth navigate troubled waters: The role of formal and informal helpers. *Child and Adolescent Social Work Journal*, 17(5), 115-140.

Leslie, B., and Hare, F. (2000). Improving the outcomes for youth in transition from care. *Ontario Association of Children's Aid Societies*, 44(3), 9-25.

Lindsey, D. (1994). *The welfare of children*. Oxford: Oxford University Press.

Loman, L., and Siegel, G. (2000). *A review of literature on independent living of youths in foster and residential care*. A Report of the Institute of Applied Research, St. Louis, Missouri.

Mann-Feder, V., and White, T. (2003). The transition to independent living: Preliminary findings on the experiences of youth in care. In K. Kufeldt and B. McKenzie (Eds.), *Child welfare: Connecting research, policy and practice* (pp. 217-225). Waterloo, ON: Wilfrid Laurier University Press.

Maunders, D., Liddell, M., Liddell, M., and Green, S. (1999). *Young people leaving care and protection: A report to the National Affairs Research Scheme*. Hobart, Tasmania: Australian Clearing House for Youth Studies.

McCreary Centre (1999). *Our kids too. Sexually exploited youth in BC: An adolescent health survey*. Burnaby, BC: McCreary Centre Society

McCreary Centre (2003). *Healthy youth development: Highlights from the 2003 Adolescent Health Survey III*. Burnaby, BC: McCreary Centre Society.

Mech, E. (1994). Preparing foster youth for adulthood: A knowledge building perspective. *Children and Youth Services Review*, 16, 141-145.

Raychaba, B. (1988). *To be on our own with no direction from home: A report on the special needs of youth leaving the care of the child welfare system*. Ottawa: National Youth in Care Network.

Rutman, D., Hubberstey, C., Feduniw, A., and Brown, E. (2006). *When youth age out of care: Bulletin of Time 2 Findings*. Victoria, BC: School of Social Work, University of Victoria.

Rutman, D., Hubberstey, C., Barlow, A., and Brown, E. (2005). *When youth age out of care: A Report on Baseline Findings*. Victoria, BC: School of Social Work, University of Victoria.

Rutman, D., Strega, S., Callahan, M., and Dominelli, L. (2002). Undeserving mothers? Practitioners' experiences working with young mothers in/from care. *Child and Family Social Work*, 7(3), 149-160.

Sarason, I., Shearin, P., and Sarason, B. (1987). Social Support Questionnaire. *Journal of Social and Personal Relationships*, 497-510.

Shin, H.S., and Poertner, J. (No date). *The well-being of older youth in out of home care who are headed to independence*. Urbana-Champaign, IL: Children and Family Research Centre, School of Social Work, University of Illinois.

Silva-Wayne, S. (1994). *Contributions to the resilience of foster care graduates*. DSW Thesis. Waterloo, ON: Sir Wilfred Laurier University.

Stein, M. (2002). Leaving care. In D. McNeish, T. Newman, and H. Roberts (Eds.), *What works? Effective social care services for children and families* (pp. 59-82). Oxford University Press.

Trocme, N., Nutter, B., MacLaurin, B., and Fallon, B. (1999). *Child Welfare Outcome Indicator Matrix*. Toronto: Bell Canada Child Welfare Research Unit, University of Toronto.

Tweddle, A. (2005). *Youth leaving care – How do they fare: A briefing paper*. Discussion paper for the Modernizing Income Security for Working Age Adults Project, Toronto, Ontario.

Plate 3 "No Vacancy" (Stefan Virtue)

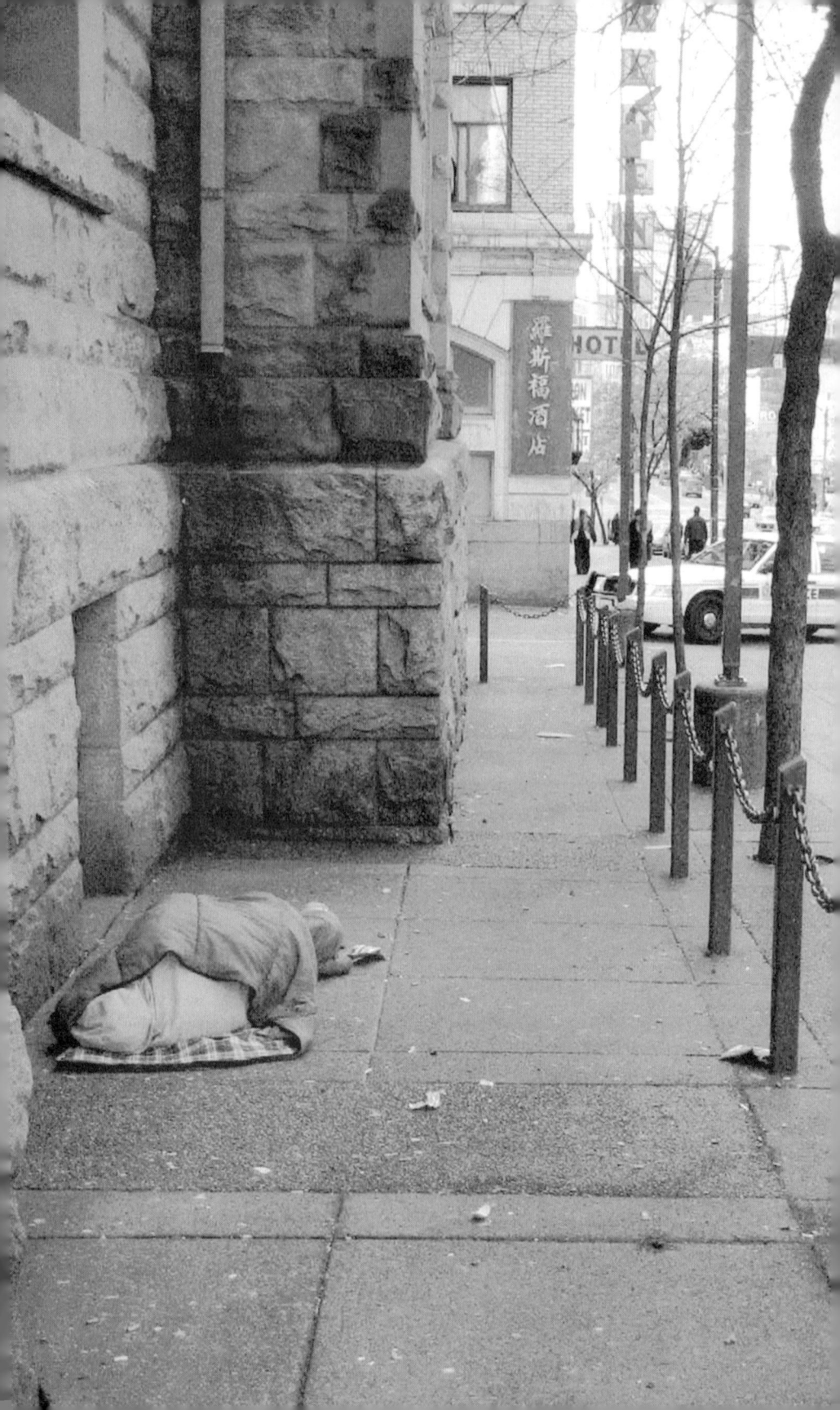

Mental Health Issues Among Canada's Homeless Youth

Elizabeth Votta
School of Nursing, University of Ottawa

Susan Farrell
Royal Ottawa Mental Health Centre, Institute of Mental Health Research, University of Ottawa

Homelessness is a significant social and public health issue, particularly among youth. Once on the street, homeless youth are at risk for victimization, lack of safe shelter, physical illness, HIV infection, involvement in criminal activity, mental health problems, injuries, and suicide (Greene and Ringwalt, 1996; Farrell, 2000; Farrell, Aubry, Klodawsky, and Pettey, 2000; Perkins, Tryssenaar, and Moland, 1998; Rotheram-Borus, 1993; Rotheram-Borus, Koopman, and Ehrhardt, 1991; Rotheram-Borus, Parra, Cantwell, Gwadz, and Murphy, 1996; Smart and Walsh, 1993; Unger et al., 1998; Votta and Manion, 2003, 2004). From a perspective that collectively considers individual, familial, and societal factors, researchers from various fields have increased their efforts to ascertain the prevalence of homelessness among Canada's youth, the antecedents of youth homelessness, and the mental and physical health outcomes of youth homelessness.

The purpose of this chapter is to provide an overview of the various mental health issues to which Canada's homeless youth are most vulnerable. It is not meant to be an exhaustive review of all possible research, programs, and literature, nor is it meant to be a comprehensive discussion of specific interventions or models. Rather, it will profile the various risk factors that Canada's male and female youth may be exposed to and experience and that may subsequently increase their risk of mental health problems. As an illustration, the chapter will present data obtained from a large sample of homeless male and female youth from a large urban centre in Ontario, Canada.

PREVALENCE OF YOUTH HOMELESSNESS IN CANADA

Homeless youth comprise a subgroup of adolescents that is increasing in number throughout Canada on a daily basis (National Secretariat on Homelessness, 2003). However, the exact prevalence of homelessness among

Canadian youth is difficult to determine. A 1989 study of the prevalence of HIV among Canada's street youth estimated that approximately 150,000 youth were runaways (Radford, King, and Warren, 1989). In 1992, Toronto's street youth population was estimated to be 5,000 to 12,000 (McCarthy and Hagan, 1992). More recently, federal statistics suggest that on any given night, 8,000 to 11,000 youth comprise the approximately 33,000 homeless Canadians (Edmonton Block Parent, 2006). Variability in and difficulties obtaining population estimates reflect the lack of an operational definition of 'homelessness' (Caputo, Weiler, and Anderson, 1997). Given this, critical questions such as the total number of homeless youth, their demographic profile, and their needs remain unanswered.

Definitional Problems

Defining youth homelessness is an issue with political, sociological, epidemiological, clinical, and practical implications. While there is no universally adopted definition of homelessness (Federation of Canadian Municipalities, 2004), most definitions encompass those who: are reliant on emergency shelters or transition houses on a temporary basis; spend nights in places such as the park or on the street; live with friends or relatives; live in an institution for lack of an appropriate alternative; and are at risk of homelessness because their accommodations are unsafe, insecure, or not affordable (City of Vancouver, 2005; Federation of Canadian Municipalities, 2004).

Consistent with this, homeless youth are now generally described as those who have left home with or without parental/guardian knowledge, have been thrown out of their homes, have left social service placements, and/or lack basic shelter provisions (Caputo et al., 1997; Rotheram-Borus et al., 1996; Unger et al., 1998; van der Ploeg and Scholte, 1997; Votta and Manion, 2004). Although all homelessness studies have identified youth as homeless by the location in which they were living at the time of study (e.g., street, shelter, abandoned building, park), only a few studies have used or specified a timeframe during which youth had been living in one of these locations in order to be considered homeless (e.g., living on the streets for two or more consecutive months, living in a makeshift street dwelling or emergency shelter service for 7 consecutive days) (Kipke, O'Connor, Palmer, and MacKenzie, 1995; Votta and Manion, 2003, 2004; Votta and Farrell, 2005). Some of these definitional issues have led to the etiology of classification systems.

Classification Systems

To better understand the homeless phenomenon, researchers have examined patterns of differentiating behaviours among homeless youth. Consequently, a number of studies report typologies based on primary motives for leaving, such as dysfunctional family dynamics or intolerable home situations, adolescent pregnancy, parental financial difficulties, school difficulties, criminal or delinquent acts, and physical and/or sexual abuse (Adams, Gullotta, and Clancy, 1985; Brennan, 1980; Hier, Karboot, and Schweitzer, 1990; Rotheram-Borus, Rosario, and Koopman, 1991; Shane, 1989). Classifying homeless youth by such demographic variables as gender or services accessed is relatively straightforward. However, problems may arise when more subjective characteristics or typologies are used for classification purposes. Youth may avoid answering direct questions or deliberately give incorrect answers, leading to inaccurate profiles of youth homelessness.

Although some previous studies classified youth according to their reasons for being on the street (e.g., 'running to,' 'running away,' 'throw away,' or 'forsaken') (Zide and Cherry, 1992), not all research uses typologies to classify homeless youth. Current researchers assert that the means by which a youth came to the street is only one aspect of their experience. Although a range of pre-homeless events may be reported, there are also many significant events and issues that face adolescents once they are homeless. This chapter does not distinguish between how youth came to the street; instead, it examines the range of issues related to their mental health that can affect them once homeless.

A Case Study of Canadian Homeless Youth

To illustrate the range of issues that affect Canadian homeless youth, this chapter will profile empirical findings from two recent Canadian studies that examined the impact of coping style, self-esteem, social support, and life events on male and female youths' psychological outcomes. The two studies will be presented to compare the experiences of homeless and housed youth (N = 494; 270 females and 224 males between 16 and 19 years of age) in a large urban centre in Ontario. Homeless and housed youth are used as comparison groups to understand how their experiences differ based on the experience of homelessness for some youth. In addition to illustrating the unique experiences of homeless youth, this research highlights differences in positive and negative life and health experiences between youth.

These studies used a definitional time-frame of 7 consecutive days (Votta and Manion, 2003, 2004; Votta and Farrell, 2005). Establishing a time-frame served the dual purpose of distinguishing between those youth truly in need of the shelter's emergency housing services, and those using the shelter for an isolated incident and who could return home (e.g., missed last bus home). Consequently, the research to be profiled throughout this chapter used the term 'homeless youth' to refer to male or female youth between the ages of 16 and 19, who were currently without a fixed address, and who, independent of their parent(s)/guardian, stayed in a shelter, service agency, makeshift street dwelling, or partner's/friend's dwelling, for at least 7 consecutive days.

Significant Life Events Prior to Life on the Street

There is no single pathway to the street for youth. If there were, methods for the prevention of homelessness would be much more clearly defined. Instead, each youth has a set of specific circumstances and life events that precipitated their street involvement. However, there also seem to be some commonalities in the stressful life events prior to being homeless reported by many youth. None of these reported events are assumed to cause homelessness; instead, they are recognized as contributing factors that can assist with understanding some of the antecedents to youths' experience of being homeless.

A 1995 study of street youth in Canada found that 74% of male youth and 90% of female youth reported experiencing at least one physically abusive event while living in their family home (Janus, Archambault, Brown, and Welsh, 1995). A Seattle sample found that 51% of youth had been physically abused before becoming homeless and 60% of girls had been sexually abused (Cauce et al., 2000). Kurtz, Kurtz, and Jarvis (1991) discovered that the problems arising from youths' experiences of physical and sexual abuse histories were additive, meaning that youth who experienced both physical and sexual abuse reported more problems than did those who were either physically or sexually abused. In addition, these youth experienced more problems with feelings of depression, low self-esteem, and suicide attempts/threats than non-abused homeless youth. Cauce and co-authors (2000) also found that over 50% of parents had substance abuse problems and over 70% had problems with the law.

A Case Study of Canadian Homeless Youth: Significant Life Events

Homeless youth cited various reasons for leaving home, including but not limited to: abuse; fights with parents; disagreement with family rules; family violence; parents' substance abuse; forced by parents; cultural conflict; and financial difficulties. Significantly more homeless male and female youth reported being in the care of child protection services and living in alternate care (foster home or group home) than their housed peers. Significantly more homeless youth reported parental substance abuse, having a deceased parent, or an unemployed parent.

MENTAL HEALTH ISSUES AMONG CANADA'S HOMELESS YOUTH

Although childhood events are not predictive of youth homelessness, they are important to understand as significant events that youth bring with them to the street, often placing them at greater risk of future negative events and poor health outcomes. Whatever their underlying reason for leaving home, once 'on the street,' homeless youth face numerous stressors, placing them at risk for mental health problems such as depression, physical health issues such as sexually transmitted infections, and increased risk factors for negative outcomes such as drug use, victimization, and injury. Studies conducted over the last 20 years to assess the association between mental health and homelessness indicate that depression, depressive symptoms, and other psychiatric problems are prevalent among homeless youth.

Depression and Depressive Symptoms

Recent estimates in the US suggest that over 35% of homeless youth have the symptoms of major depression (Nyamathi et al., 2005). However, these rates may be considered underestimates of the disorder. For example, more than 20 years ago, in their assessment of depression, mood, and conduct disorders in a sample of 118 New York homeless youth, Shaffer and Caton (1984) reported that depression was common in both males and females. A study of 45 homeless male youth in Ottawa indicated that, in the previous year, 27% reported experiencing mental health problems and 18% reported being diagnosed with a psychiatric illness (Farrell et al., 2000).

The link between depressive symptoms and substance use, social support, self-esteem, and parental substance abuse among homeless youth has also been examined. Smart and Walsh (1993) found that one-third of 145 youth reported feelings of depression often or always in the 3 months preceding their study. Self-esteem, perceived social support, length of time spent in a hostel, and parents' drug-use were the best predictors of depression. More recently, Litrownik and co-authors (1999) conducted a study in which they examined the prevalence of prior involvement with the mental health system in youth accessing an emergency shelter. Of the 295 youth interviewed, 11% reported a previous psychiatric hospital admission, 58% had been admitted to a psychiatric hospital in the year before their use of the shelter, and 43% had received counselling.

Few studies of youth homelessness have included comparison groups and/or differentiated between a diagnosis of major depressive episode (MDE) and depressive symptoms. A Canadian study reported that street youth had a higher mean level of depression than a sample of high school youth (Ayerst, 1999). In studies of homeless youth in California, 26% of homeless youth in Hollywood (Robertson, Koegel, and Ferguson, 1989) and 64% of homeless youth in Los Angeles (Unger et al., 1998) met criteria for MDE as per the American Psychiatric Association's Diagnostic and Statistical Manual (DSM). These rates were higher than incidence rates of 7% among community and high-school adolescents (Peterson et al., 1993).

Although the clinical implications of these findings are important in the study of youth homelessness, a discussion of depressive symptoms among homeless adolescents is complicated by several factors. First, few studies have included comparison groups or compared their results to those of standardized norms. Second, as no reported study has followed youth at risk longitudinally, or measured depression both before and after a homeless episode, it is difficult to determine if the reported levels of depression were precipitants or the result of youths' homelessness. Lastly, adolescents rarely experience depressed mood in the absence of other negative emotions (Compas and Hammen, 1994), and are often diagnosed with a depressive disorder and one or more co-morbid conditions (Rhode, Lewinsohn, and Seeley, 1991), which contributes to the complexity underlying studies of adolescent depression.

Internalizing and Externalizing Behaviour Problems

In addition to depression and depressive symptoms, research has looked at the overall categories of internalizing and externalizing behaviour problems among homeless youth as these categories are comprised of a number of mental health indicators. Internalizing behaviour problems are characterized as having somatic complaints, symptoms of anxiety or depression, and social withdrawal. Conversely, externalizing behaviour problems are characterized as delinquent and aggressive behaviour (Achenbach and Edelbrock, 1986, 1991). Using the Youth Self-Report Form (Achenbach and Edelbrock, 1986), homeless youth had higher total behaviour problem scores than housed youth. Homeless females also scored higher on the internalizing scale, while males scored higher on the externalizing scales (Cauce et al., 2000).

Use of Mental Health Services

Health service access and health status are consistently shown to be inversely related to one another among the homeless population. Although studies have consistently shown that homeless adults have high rates of health care utilization, it is primarily with the use of acute care services, such as emergency rooms, rather than consistent follow-up care with a treatment physician or health team (Kushel, Perry, Bangsberg, Clark, and Moss, 2002; Kushel, Vittinghoff, and Haas, 2001; Padgett, Stuening, Andrews, and Pittman, 1995). Comparable data for homeless youth are not readily available. Instead, rates of health service access are more often examined in terms of mental health services use. Research involving homeless youth suggests much lower patterns of use, for both physical and mental health services. Buckner and Bassuk (1997) found that, although rates of concurrent disorders (mental illness and substance use) were higher in a sample of American homeless youth, rates of utilization of mental health services were very low. In a recent study examining health utilization patterns pre- and during homelessness, Berdahl, Hoyt, and Whitbeck (2005) found that, unlike the adult population, homeless youth were accessing health care services not necessarily tied to acute services. They found that differences in utilization patterns were associated with family of origin, street experiences, timing of the first use of mental health services (pre- or during homelessness), race, and gender.

A Case Study of Canadian Homeless Youth: Mental Health Status and Use of Mental Health Services

Depressive Symptoms

Sixty-one percent (61%) of homeless female youth reported symptoms of depression in the clinical range as measured by responses to the Beck Depression Inventory. Among the male youth, 39% reported depressive symptoms in the clinical range. These rates were significantly higher than those reported by their housed peers.

Internalizing and Externalizing Behaviour Problems

Findings from the profiled studies differed slightly from those reported by Cauce and colleagues (2000). In the profiled studies of Canadian youth, which also used the Youth Self-Report Form, females were more likely to report higher levels of both internalizing and externalizing behaviour problem scores. Among the female homeless youth, 51% and 54% reported internalizing and externalizing behaviour scores in the clinical range, respectively. Among the male homeless youth, 44% and 48% reported internalizing and externalizing behaviour scores in the clinical range. Internalizing and externalizing scores for both males and females were higher than those for their housed peers.

High levels of depressive symptomatology and internalizing behaviour problems are of concern given previous findings associating depressive symptoms with lifetime suicide attempts, negative life-events, low self-esteem, and mental health problems among both male and female homeless youth. High prevalence of externalizing behaviour problems is also of concern given the high incidence of homeless youth's involvement with criminal activity, gangs, aggressive behaviour, and substance abuse.

Mental Health Service Use

Analyses of homeless youths' use of and access to health services indicated that approximately half of both male and female youth had used a variety of mental health services. Among male youth, 49% had consulted a psychologist or psychiatrist, 43% had sought help from a social worker, and 54% had received counselling from a therapist. Similar rates were evident among homeless female youth, with 49% having seen a psychologist or psychiatrist, 51% having consulted a social worker, and 51% having received counselling from a therapist.

RISK FACTORS FOR POOR MENTAL HEALTH OUTCOMES

There are many risk factors for poor mental health outcomes to which homeless youth are reported to be exposed that increase the likelihood of negative outcomes while homeless. Among the most prevalent risk factors in current literature that are subsequently discussed in this chapter are substance use, deviant subsistence strategies and victimization, unintentional and intentional injuries, risky physical health behaviours, membership in a sexual minority group, and maladaptive coping.

Substance Use

A 2005 review of the epidemiologic studies of the health of Canadian homeless youth found that substance use (both alcohol and drugs) was higher than that found among their housed peers (Boivin, Roy, Haley, and Galbaud du Fort, 2005). Substance use was also found to be related to higher rates of hepatitis and HIV infection, as well as a mortality rate that was 11 times the expected rate for youth. In a US study involving 226 homeless youth using an emergency shelter, Slesnick and Presopnik (2005) found that over 56% of the youth had a dual disorder – mental illness and substance use.

Previous national studies of substance use among the homeless in the US found that 70 to 90% of homeless youth abuse alcohol and/or drugs, with the risk of abuse increasing with age and the duration of homelessness (Nyamathi et al., 2005). In a study of Hollywood's homeless youth, Kipke and co-authors (1995) reported that 79% had used alcohol, 77% had used marijuana, 68% had used methamphetamine, 67% had used LSD, 54% had used cocaine, and 30% had injected drugs. These rates significantly exceeded those found in high school and community samples for all substances (Unger, Kipke, Simon, Montgomery, and Johnson, 1997).

In Canada, Roy and colleagues (2004) found that heavy substance use and homelessness were factors associated with mortality in a cohort of street youth in Montreal, Quebec. Over 90% reported use of cannabis and hallucinogens, 82% reported use of cocaine or crack, 46% reported injecting drugs, and 44% used drugs from two or more of the categories within the past month. These rates were higher than those of studies conducted in the 1990s. For example, McCarthy and Hagan (1992) reported that 80% of a sample of Toronto's homeless youth smoked marijuana, 42% reported cocaine use, 55% used hallucinogens, and 34% used amphetamines.

In another Toronto-based study, Smart and Adlaf (1991) discovered that alcohol and drug consumption were three times greater among Toronto's street youth, relative to a sample of non-homeless youth. They also reported a positive association between the amount of alcohol and drugs consumed by street youth 1 week before their study and increased time on the street; youth also self-identified alcohol consumption as a coping strategy. Findings obtained from a sample of 200 male street youth in Edmonton indicated that exposure to parental substance abuse increased street youths' risk of alcohol and hard-drug use (Baron, 1999). Histories of physical abuse and the presence of substance-using peers were related to the use of alcohol, marijuana, and psychedelic drugs, while long-term homelessness was positively associated with hard-drug use (Baron, 1999).

Typically, most youth homelessness studies have reported substance use patterns based on youths' responses to non-standardized measures. Farrell and colleagues (2000) reported that 36% and 57% of Ottawa's homeless youth self-reported problems due to current or past alcohol and drug use, respectively. Only a few studies have employed standardized criteria (from the DSM) to examine the prevalence of substance abuse disorders among homeless youth (Robertson et al., 1989; Kipke, Simon, Montgomery, Unger, and Iverson, 1997). In their assessment of the relationship between alcohol use and youth homelessness, Robertson and co-authors (1989) reported that 48% of youth met criteria for a diagnosis of either alcohol abuse or dependence; 24% met criteria for abuse only, 3% met criteria for dependence only, and 22% met criteria for both abuse and dependence. Although 66% of the youth reported alcohol consumption prior to their first homeless episode, only 15% perceived alcohol as a factor in their homelessness while 5% identified alcohol use as the precipitant to their homelessness (Robertson et al., 1989). Similar findings were reported by Kipke and colleagues (1997) in their assessment of drug and alcohol abuse disorders among homeless youth. Standardized criteria indicated that 43% of youth met criteria for both alcohol and drug abuse disorder, 32% met criteria for alcohol abuse and dependence, while 39% met criteria for drug abuse and dependence. Length of time homeless was positively associated with both the risk of "alcohol abuse" disorder and the risk of "drug abuse" disorder (Kipke et al., 1997).

**A Case Study of Canadian Homeless Youth:
Substance Use**

Sixty-eight percent (68%) of homeless females and 72% of homeless males reported drug use, which was significantly higher than rates reported by their housed peers. Daily drug use was reported by 37% of females and 35% of males.

Sixty percent (60%) of females and 69% of males reported alcohol use, again significantly higher rates than reported by their housed peers. Daily alcohol use was reported by 7% of females and 2% of males.

Forty-eight percent (48%) of females reported smoking more than half a pack of cigarettes per day; 32% smoked less than half a pack per day. Patterns were reversed for males with 27% smoking more than half a pack per day and 64% smoking less than half a pack per day.

Deviant Subsistence Strategies and Victimization

Numerous studies conducted in Canada and the US indicate that engagement in criminal acts (e.g., prostitution, robbery), delinquency (e.g., shoplifting, trespassing, loitering), and exposure to violence and violent victimization is widespread among homeless youth (Kipke et al., 1995; Kipke et al., 1997; Koopman, Rosario, and Rotheram-Borus, 1994; Smart and Walsh, 1993; Unger et al., 1997; Unger et al., 1998). Numerous studies also indicate that substance use/abuse and criminal acts related to drug use (e.g., drug possession and trafficking) are widespread among homeless youth (Baron, 1999; Farrell et al., 2000; McCarthy and Hagan, 1992; Smart and Adlaf, 1991; Unger et al., 1997; Unger et al., 1998). In much research, these activities are classified as deviant subsistence strategies, meaning activities that are criminal in nature done to promote survival while homeless. Engagement in such acts has been noted to increase with length of time homeless and to increase risk for other negative outcomes such as mental illness, substance use and poor physical health (Tyler and Cauce, 2002; Whitbeck, Hoyt, and Yoder, 1999).

Many homeless youth employ subsistence and survival strategies that increase the chances of victimization (Gaetz, 2004; Kipke et al., 1997; Tyler and Cauce, 2002; Whitbeck, Hoyt, and Bao, 2000; Whitbeck, Hoyt, Yoder, Cauce, and Paradise, 2001; Whitbeck, Chen, Hoyt, Tyler, and Johnson, 2004). In a study of Toronto's homeless youth, Janus and colleagues (1995) reported that 56% had been physically victimized while homeless and 51% had been threatened with a weapon. A recent study of victimization in Ottawa found that 61% of homeless female youth and 32% of homeless male youth had been sexually abused since becoming homeless; 44% and 39%, respectively, had been the victim of a violent crime (Farrell and MacDonald, 2006).

A Case Study of Canadian Homeless Youth: Deviant Subsistence Strategies

Forty percent (40%) of male youth reported current legal problems. In addition, 27% of males reported being on probation, 27% reported impending court dates, and 62% reported having been arrested in the past. Lower rates were reported among homeless females: 7% reported being on probation, 14% reported impending court dates, and 15% reported a prior arrest for criminal behaviours.

Unintentional and Intentional Injuries

Although different age groups experience different injuries at varying rates, injuries are nonetheless a leading cause of death among Canadians (SMART RISK, 1998). By virtue of their involvement with deviant subsistent strategies and substance use, homeless youth are at high risk for unintentional injuries.

Unfortunately, in some cases these situations may put them at risk for intentional injuries presenting in the form of victimization such as interpersonal violence. Homeless youth are also at risk for intentional injuries such as self-harm and suicidal behaviours.

In one of the first national studies of street youth from 10 Canadian cities, Radford and colleagues (1989) reported that, of its 712 respondents, 25% had suicidal thoughts. Later studies reported increasingly higher rates of suicidality. In Toronto, 27% of street and shelter youth (N = 390) reported at least one prior suicide attempt (McCarthy and Hagan, 1992). One year later, in another study involving Toronto's homeless youth (N = 145), this number had risen to 42% (Smart and Walsh, 1993). In a study of youth attending various substance-abuse treatment programs in Ontario (Smart and Ogborne, 1994), 53% of the youth identified as 'street youth' had attempted suicide (n = 261), compared to 30% of the youth identified as 'non-street youth' (n = 586).

A number of studies conducted in the US report findings consistent with data recorded for homeless youth in Canada and youth in the general population. In an epidemiological survey conducted over a 2 week period, Shaffer and Caton (1984) found that 16% and 33% of male and female runaways, respectively, had attempted suicide. In a series of interviews conducted with 576 runaway youth over a 2 year period, Rotheram-Borus (1993) reported that 37% of the youth had previously attempted suicide; 44% had made an attempt within the previous month. Other studies involving homeless youth also cited reports of prior suicide attempts ranging from 30 to 50% (Smart and Adlaf, 1991; Stiffman, 1989; Unger et al., 1997; Unger et al., 1998). These rates were higher than those reported from high school samples (3-13%) (Andrews and Lewinsohn, 1992; Garland and Zigler, 1993; Garrison, 1989; Smith and Crawford, 1986), community samples (2%) (Earls, 1989; Velez and Cohen, 1988), and adolescent clinic patients (12%) (Joffe, Offord, and Boyle, 1988).

Although homeless males tend to report fewer suicidal behaviours than females, rates of suicidal ideation among males and females tend to be similar (Shaffer and Caton, 1984; Rotheram-Borus, 1993; Unger et al., 1997; Unger et al., 1998). Among both male and female runaways and homeless adolescents, life-time suicide attempts have also been positively associated with substance abuse, negative life-events, running away, mental health and behaviour problems, low self-esteem, family instability, sexual and physical abuse, and having a friend who attempted suicide (Stiffman, 1989; Greene and Ringwalt, 1996; Yoder, 1999).

A 2003 study conducted in the US reported that homeless youth had very high rates of suicidal ideation and that almost 20% had attempted suicide (Desai, Liu-Mares, Dausey, and Rosenheck, 2003). Tyler and colleagues (2003) reported that widespread self-mutilation (up to 45% reporting an act of deliberate self-harm) in homeless youth was associated with symptoms of depression, and engagement in deviant subsistence strategies, which are reviewed in the subsequent section.

A Case Study of Canadian Homeless Youth: Unintentional and Intentional Injuries

Thirty-five percent (35%) of homeless males reported thoughts of suicide in their lifetime; 8% reported suicidal ideation in the 3 months prior to the study. Relative to their housed peers (4%), more homeless males reported past suicide attempts (21%). Higher rates of both suicidal ideation and past attempts were found among females. Whereas 41% reported lifetime suicidal ideation, 30% reported thoughts of suicide in the previous 3 months. Like their male counterparts, more homeless females (51%) reported past suicide attempts than did their housed peers (40%).

Among the females, high rates of injuries, both those requiring medical attention (37%) and those for which medical attention was not sought (39%), were also reported. Among the injuries requiring medical attention were broken bones (4%), sprains (28%), cuts (12%), head injuries (16%), and burns (12%). Among the injuries for which medical attention was not sought were dislocated joints (18%), sprains (29%), cuts (21%), head injuries (4%), and burns (7%). Data specific to unintentional injuries were not collected of the homeless male youth.

Health Status

Although the focus of this chapter is on mental health issues among homeless youth, given the transient lifestyle associated with homelessness, homeless youth's physical health is concurrently at risk and therefore warrants a brief discussion.

Findings from a study of Toronto's runaway and street youth indicate that in comparison to 2% of non-runaway youth, 16% of runaway and 38% of street youth rated their physical health as poor (Smart, Adlaf, Walsh, and Zdanowicz, 1994). Unger and colleagues (1998) reported that length of time from home was a factor in youths' subjective ratings of their physical health; youth who had been homeless for more than 1 year reported poorer physical health than did youth who had been homeless for less time.

Homeless youth are also at high risk for HIV infection, sexually transmitted diseases, pregnancy, and unsafe sexual behaviours. Compared to 7% of national samples in the US, 50% of homeless adolescent males have had more than 10 sexual partners in their life; homeless youth also have higher prevalence rates of sexually transmitted diseases (50-70%) and pregnancy than non-homeless youth (Booth, Zhang, and Kwiatkowski, 1999; Kipke et al., 1995; Robertson et al., 1989; Rotheram-Borus et al., 1991; Sweeney, Lindegren, Buehler,

Onorato, and Janssen, 1995). A Washington, DC study indicated that youth without social networks, consisting of strong, affective, and supportive bonds between a few friends, were more likely to report illicit drug use, multiple sex partners, and survival sex than youth with a social network (Ennett, Bailey, and Federman, 1999). Radford and co-authors (1989) reported similar findings for Canadian street youth. Of 712 youth interviewed, two-thirds reported having had five or more sexual partners in their lifetime, compared to 17% of college/university students; 32% of street youth also reported that they never used a condom when engaging in sexual intercourse.

**A Case Study of Canadian Homeless Youth:
Health Status**

Comparisons of physical health issues between homeless male and female youth indicated that females reported significantly more physical health problems (63%) than males (26%). However, both male and female homeless youth reported significantly more physical health problems than their housed peers. Most frequently cited physical problems were respiratory ailments (e.g., asthma), diabetes, allergies, and headaches.

Membership in a Sexual Minority Group

Limited research has examined the differences between the experiences of gay, lesbian, bisexual, and transgender (GLBT) homeless youths and their heterosexual peers in terms of augmented risk associated with membership in a sexual minority group. In a prevalence study in Portland, Oregon, GLBT youth were found to represent approximately 26% of the homeless population, but to be over-represented in the percentage of youth reporting high rates of depression and suicidal ideation (Noell and Ochs, 2001). Cochran and colleagues (2002) found that, based on self-reports, homeless youth who identified themselves as members of a sexual minority group were at increased risk for negative outcomes such as victimization, substance use, and mental health problems. Membership in a sexual minority group has also been linked to an increase in deviant subsistence strategies for survival (Whitbeck et al., 2004), thus increasing the risk for a myriad of negative physical and psychological outcomes as a result of being homeless.

Maladaptive Coping

The ability to effectively cope with stress is a skill that differentiates between adolescents at low and high risk for maladjustment (Jeffries McWhirter, McWhirter, McWhirter, and Hawley McWhirter, 1994). Elevated levels of stress among adolescents are associated with various physical and psychosocial problems, including low self-esteem, delinquent conduct, poor school performance, and depressive symptoms (Adams, Gullotta, and Clancy, 1994; Barnet, Joffe, Duggan, Wilson, and Repke, 1996; Compas, 1987a, 1987b; Compas, Orosan, and Grant, 1993).

Studies conducted to assess the impact of stress and manner of coping among street youth are limited to a few conducted in large urban North American cities. Unger and colleagues (1998) reported a positive association between stressful life events and depressive symptoms, substance use, and poor physical health. In another study, homeless male youth identified an inability to find work and housing, loss of contact with family and friends, and being the victim of violence as their most stressful life-events (Farrell et al., 2000). Relative to high school youth, Ayerst (1999) found that street youth reported a higher number of stressors and were more likely to engage in substance use and self-harm to cope; in contrast, high school youth were more apt to use productive problem-solving and talk to someone they trusted.

Disengagement coping is characterized by such strategies as problem avoidance, wishful thinking, social withdrawal, and avoidance of negative emotions and thoughts (Carver and Scheier, 1994). Current findings indicate that the disengaging coping style is associated with poor psychological and physical outcomes in adult cancer patients (Carver and Scheier, 1994). Among adolescents, the beneficial effects of engagement coping appear to be greatest in response to stressors which adolescents perceive as controllable (e.g., academic stressors) (Compas et al., 1988). In contrast, adolescents with a disengaging coping style, high levels of stress, and/or low social support are at greater risk for depression, poor physical health, and substance abuse (Compas et al., 1993).

To date, only one known study involving homeless male youth has examined coping style and its theoretical or clinical association with psychological adjustment (Votta and Manion, 2003, 2004). Homeless male youth were more likely to have a disengaging coping style than housed male youth. Analyses indicated that disengagement coping and self-worth were significant predictors of depressive symptoms, suicidality, and both internalizing and externalizing behaviour problems in homeless male youth. In its counterpart study with homeless female youth, unlike the male homeless youth, female youth did not report greater use of a disengaging coping style than non-homeless females (Votta and Farrell, 2005). Despite this, disengagement coping style was a significant predictor of externalizing behaviour problems among homeless females. For both groups of homeless youth, these findings indicate that their coping style may not be adaptive to deal with the stress in their lives.

SUMMARY AND CONCLUSIONS

Clinical and Research Implications

Homeless youth, males and females alike, are a vulnerable group of young people at high risk for a number of poor health outcomes, particularly mental health problems. The clinical and policy implications of the issues highlighted in this chapter are far-reaching.

Current research indicates a high prevalence of depressive symptomatology among homeless youth, as well as a tendency for maladaptive coping. There are two main implications to this finding. First, having a coping style that tends toward disengagement may contribute to the chronicity of existing mental health problems or exacerbate existing risk factors. Second, rather than serving as a contributing factor, the disengagement coping style may serve as a barrier to service use. This would suggest that shelter staff, outreach workers, and youth-services agencies be aware of youths' coping style and the potential value in providing services that are youth-friendly in nature. Greater knowledge regarding the stability of coping style could also speak to the feasibility and approach required for early intervention programs for at-risk youth.

Health care professionals should be trained to work with homeless youth. As the recipients of service and participants in research, youth should be included in the decision-making, planning, and implementing processes. In addition, researchers should be non-judgemental and caring (Canadian Pediatric Society, 1999; Virley O'Connor and MacDonald, 1999).

The vast array of mental, physical, and psychosocial problems common among homeless youth indicate that clinical, outreach, and research interventions must provide an equal complement of services that target specific problems such as substance abuse, suicidality, depression, violence, and involvement in criminal activity. Further, homeless youth would likely benefit from youth-specific services and interventions that are designed to decrease the incidence of risk-taking behaviours, reduce the prevalence of psychosocial difficulties, and foster adaptive coping patterns.

Despite the number of negative outcomes for which homeless youth are at risk, there are a few positive or protective factors that, if available or developed, may mitigate some of the consequences of homelessness. This is not to suggest that such factors reduce all risk associated with homelessness, but rather that the impact of these negative risk factors may be buffered by positive or protective factors. Youth homelessness studies have typically assessed negative traits and behaviours such as hostility, depression, substance use, criminality, poor self-concept, and lack of support. Further research is needed to determine if positive traits such as optimism, adaptability, and resiliency (which includes cohesive relationships, pro-social peer attachments, physical and mental attributes, social capital, ability to plan for the future, strong school attachment, and long-term participation in social and recreational activities)

(Totten and Quigley, 2003) can serve as protective factors against the risks for homelessness and poor health outcomes among youth facing the adversity of homelessness.

Future Directions

With continued homelessness, youths' vulnerability increases by known gender differences in street-related risk behaviour and patterns of victimization. Preventing chronic homelessness provides cost savings to social, health, and mental health systems. Two keys to preventing chronic homelessness for youth involve the early detection of risk factors and the identification of protective factors that promote resilience. In addition, the development of flexible social and housing policies that allow for ongoing opportunities for youth to access education, health services (including concurrent treatment), and supportive housing are required to meet the needs of homeless youth (Frankish, Hwang, and Quantz, 2003).

Currently there is no systematic way to assess and predict which at-risk youth will become homeless. Further, the complex interaction between predictive factors, risk factors, service system involvement, and psychosocial adjustment has not been systematically assessed as an effective way to prevent homelessness among both male and female youth. Given the increasing number of homeless youth in Canada, research of this nature is particularly important.

The goal of this chapter was to profile the myriad of issues affecting homeless youth, both before and while on the street. Unfortunately, while many of the negative psychological, social, and physical risk factors and outcomes have been well documented over time, the problems nonetheless persist. This suggests that previous policies and interventions have not been as uniformly effective as hoped, and that innovative solutions to address the negative sequelae of homelessness are still required.

REFERENCES

Achenbach, T., and Edelbrock, C. (1986). *Youth self-report profile*. Burlington: University of Vermont, Department of Psychiatry.

Achenbach, T., and Edelbrock, C. (1991). *Manual for the youth self-report and profile*. Burlington: University of Vermont, Department of Psychiatry.

Adams, G., Gullotta, T., and Clancy, M.A. (1985). Homeless adolescents: A descriptive study of similarities and differences between runaways and throwaways. *Adolescence, 10*, 715-724.

Andrews, J.A. and Lewinsohn, P.M. (1992). Suicidal attempts among older adolescents: Prevalence and co-occurrence with psychiatric disorders. *Journal of the American Academy of Child and Adolescent Psychiatry, 31*, 655-662.

Ayerst, S.L. (1999). Depression and stress in street youth. *Adolescence, 34*, 567-575.

Barnet, B., Joffe, A., Duggan, A.K., Wilson, M.D., and Repke, J.T. (1996). Depressive symptoms, stress, and social support in pregnant and postpartum adolescents. *Archives of Pediatric and Adolescent Medicine*, 150, 64-69.

Baron, S.W. (1999). Street youths and substance use: The role of background, street lifestyle, and economic factors. *Youth and Society*, 31, 3-26.

Beck, A., Steer, R., and Garbin, M. (1988). Psychometric properties of the Beck Depression Inventory: Twenty-five years of evaluation. *Clinical Psychology Review*, 8, 77-100.

Berdahl, T.A., Hoyt, D.R., and Whitbeck, L.B. (2005). Predictors of first mental health service utilization among homeless and runaway adolescents. *Journal of Adolescent Health*, 37, 145-154.

Boivin, J.F., Roy, E., Haley, N., and Galbaud du Fort, G. (2005). The health of street youth: A Canadian perspective. *Canadian Journal of Public Health*, 96, 432-437.

Booth, R.E., Zhang, Y., and Kwiatkowski, C.F. (1999). The challenge of changing drug and sex risk behaviors of runaway and homeless adolescents. *Child Abuse and Neglect*, 23, 1295-1306.

Brennan, T. (1980). Mapping the diversity among runaways. *Journal of Family Issues*, 1, 189-209.

Buckner, J.C., and Bassuk, E.L. (1997). Mental disorders and service utilization among youths from homeless and low-income housed families. *Journal of the American Academy of Child and Adolescent Psychiatry*, 36, 890-900.

Canadian Pediatric Society (1999). *Street Youth Health Care: Telephone Survey*. Ottawa, Canada: Health Promotions and Programs Branch, Health Canada.

Caputo, T., Weiler, R., and Anderson, J. (1997). *The Street Lifestyle Study*. Ottawa, Canada: Minister of Public Works and Government Services Canada.

Carver, C.S., and Scheier, M.F. (1994). Situational coping and coping dispositions in a stressful transaction. *Journal of Personality and Social Psychology*, 66, 184-195.

Cauce, A.M., Paradise, M., Ginzler, J.A., Embry, L., Morgan, C.J., Lohr, Y., and Theofelis, J. (2000). The characteristics and mental health of homeless adolescents: Age and gender differences. *Journal of Emotional and Behavioural Disorders*, 8, 230-239.

City of Vancouver (2005). Homeless Action Plan, http://vancouver.ca/commsvcs/housing/pdf/ HAP(June2005).pdf (accessed February 10, 2006).

Cochran, B.N., Stewart, A.J., Ginzler, J.A., and Cauce, A.M. (2002). Challenges faced by homeless sexual minorities: Comparison of gay, lesbian, bisexual and transgender homeless adolescents with their heterosexual counterparts. *American Journal of Public Health*, 92, 773-777.

Compas, B.E. (1987a). Stress and life events during childhood and adolescence. *Clinical Psychology Review*, 7, 275-302.

Compas, B.E. (1987b). Coping with stress during childhood and adolescence. *Psychological Bulletin*, 101, 393-403.

Compas, B.E., Malcarne, V.L., and Fondacaro, K.M. (1988). Coping with stressful events in older children and young adolescents. *Journal of Consulting and Clinical Psychology*, 56, 405-411.

Compas, B.E., Orosan, P.G., and Grant, K.E. (1993). Adolescent stress and coping: Implications for psychopathology during adolescence. *Journal of Adolescence*, 16, 331-349.

Compas, B.E., and Hammen, C.L. (1994). Child and adolescent depression: Covariation and comorbity in development. In R.J. Haggerty, L.R. Sherrod, N. Garmezy, and M. Rutter (Eds.), *Stress, risk, and resilience in children and adolescents: Processes, mechanisms, and interventions* (pp. 225-267): Cambridge University Press.

Desai, R.A., Liu-Mares, W., Dausey, D.J., and Rosenheck, R.A. (2003). Suicidal ideation and suicide attempts in a sample of homeless people with mental illness. *Journal of Nervous and Mental Disease*, 91, 365-371.

Earls, F. (1989). Studying adolescent suicidal ideation and behaviour in primary care settings. *Suicide and Life Threatening Behavior*, 19, 99-119.

Edmonton Block Parent (2006). Homeless Street Kids in Canada (numbers), *http://www.edmblockparent.com/newsletter/* (accessed February 23, 2006).

Ennett, S.T., Bailey, S.L., and Federman, E.B. (1999). Social network characteristics associated with risky behaviors among runaway and homeless youth. *Journal of Health and Social Behaviour*, 40, 63-78.

Farrell, S. (2000). *An examination of homelessness from a stress perspective*, Doctoral Dissertation, University of Ottawa.

Farrell, S., Aubry, T., Kladowsky, F., and Pettey, D. (2000). *Describing the homeless population of Ottawa-Carleton*. Centre for Research on Community Services, Faculty of Social Sciences, University of Ottawa, Ottawa, Canada: On-line Fact Sheet.

Farrell, S.J., and MacDonald, S-A. (2006, in preparation). *The relative association of victimization on the mental health of Canadian homeless youth*.

Federation of Canadian Municipalities (2004). *Quality of life in Canadian communities*. Vancouver, British Columbia.

Frankish, C.J., Hwang, S.W., and Quantz, D. (September, 2003). *Homelessness and health*. Canadian Institutes of Health Research. Ottawa, Ontario.

Gaetz, S. (2004). Safe streets for whom? Homeless youth, social exclusion and criminal victimization. *Canadian Journal of Criminology and Criminal Justice*, 46, 423-55.

Garland, A.F., and Zigler, E. (1993). Adolescent suicide prevention. *American Psychologist*, 48, 169-182.

Garrison, J. (1989). Studying suicidal behaviour in the schools. *Suicide and Life-Threatening Behaviour*, 19, 120-130.

Greene, J.M., and Ringwalt, C.L. (1996). Youth and familial substance use's association with suicide attempts among runaway and homeless youth. *Substance Use and Misuse*, 31, 1041-1058.

Hier, S.J., Korboot, P.J., and Schweitzer, R.D. (1990). Social adjustment and symptomatology in two types of homeless adolescents: Runaways and throwaways. *Adolescence*, 25, 761-771.

Janus, M.D., McCormack, A., Burgess, A., and Hartman, C. (1987). *Adolescent runaways: Causes and consequences*. Toronto: Lexington Books.

Janus, M.D., Archambault, F.X., Brown, S.W., and Welsh, L.A. (1995). Physical abuse in Canadian runaway adolescents. *Child Abuse and Neglect*, 19(4), 433-447.

Jeffries McWhirter, J., McWhirter, B.T., McWhirter, A.M., and Hawley McWhirter, E. (1994). High- and low-risk characteristics of youth: The five Cs of competency. *Elementary School Guidance and Counselling*, 28, 188-196.

Joffe, R.T., Offord, D.R., and Boyle, M.H. (1988). Ontario Child Health Study: Suicidal behaviour in youth ages 12 - 16 years. *American Journal of Psychiatry*, 145, 1420-1423.

Kipke, M.D., O'Connor, S., Palmer, R., and MacKenzie, R.G. (1995). Street youth in Los Angeles: Profile of a group at high risk for Human Immunodeficiency Virus infection. *Archives of Pediatrics and Adolescent Medicine*, 149, 513-519.

Kipke, M.D., Simon, T.R., Montgomery, S.B., Unger, J.B., and Iversen, E. (1997). Homeless youth and their exposure to and involvement in violence while living on the streets. *Journal of Adolescent Health*, 20, 360-367.

Koopman, C., Rosario, M., and Rotheram-Borus, M.J. (1994). Alcohol and drug use and sexual behaviours placing runaways at risk for HIV infection. *Addictive Behaviours*, 19, 95-103.

Kurtz, P.D., Kurtz, G.L., and Jarvis, S.V. (1991). Problems of maltreated runaway youth. *Adolescence*, 26, 543-555.

Kushel, M.B., Vittinghoff, E., and Haas, J.S. (2001). Factors associated with the health care utilization of homeless persons. *Journal of the American Medical Association*, 285, 200-206.

Kushel, M.G., Perry, S., Bangsberg, D., Clark, R., and Moss, A.R. (2002). Emergency department use among the homeless and marginally housed: Results from a community-based study. *American Journal of Public Health*, 92, 778-784.

Litrownik, A.J., Taussig, H.N., Landsverk, J.A., and Garland, A.F. (1999). Youth entering an emergency shelter care facility: Prior involvement in juvenile justice and mental health systems. *Journal of Social Service Research*, 25, 5-19.

McCarthy, B., and Hagan J. (1992). Surviving on the street: The experiences of homeless youth. *Journal of Adolescent Research*, 7, 412-430.

National Secretariat on Homelessness (2003). *Research and services related to mental illness and homelessness*. Federal Government of Canada.

Noell, J.W., and Ochs, L.M. (2001). Relationship of sexual orientation to substance use, suicidal ideation, suicide attempts and other factors in a population of homeless adolescents. *Journal of Adolescent Health*, 29, 31-36.

Nyamathi, A.M., Christiani, A., Windokun, F., Jones, T., Strehlow, A., and Shoptaw, S. (2005). Hepatitis C virus infection, substance use and mental illness among homeless youth: A review. *AIDS*, 19, S34-40.

Padgett, D.K., Stuening, E.L., Andrews, H.L., and Pittman, J. (1995). Predictors of emergency room use by homeless adults in New York City: The influence of predisposing, enabling and need factors. *Social Science Medicine*, 41, 547-556.

Perkins, J.M., Tryssenaar, J., and Moland, M.R. (1998). Health and rehabilitation needs of a shelter population. *Canadian Journal of Rehabilitation*, 11, 117-122.

Peterson, A.C., Compas, B.E., Brooks-Gunn, J., Stemmler, M., Ey, S., and Grant, K. (1993). Depression in adolescents. *American Psychologist*, 48, 155-168.

Radford, J.L., King, A.J.C., and Warren, W.K. (1989). Street youth and AIDS. Ottawa, Ontario: Health and Welfare Canada.

Rhode, P., Lewinsohn, P.M., and Seeley, J.R. (1991). Comorbidity of unipolar depression: Comorbidity with other mental disorders in adolescents and adults. *Journal of Abnormal Psychology*, 54, 653-660.

Robertson, J.J., Koegel, P., and Ferguson, L. (1989). Alcohol use and abuse among homeless adolescents in Hollywood. *Contemporary Drug Problems*, 16, 415-453.

Rotheram-Borus, M.J. (1993). Suicidal behaviour and risk factors among runaway youths. *American Journal of Psychiatry*, 150, 103-107.

Rotheram-Borus, M.J., Koopman, C., and Ehrhardt, A.A. (1991). Homeless youths and HIV infection. *American Psychologist*, 46, 1188-1197.

Rotheram-Borus, M.J., Parra, M., Cantwell, C., Gwadz, M., and Murphy, D.A. (1996). Runaway and homeless youth. In R.J. DiClemente, W.B. Hansen, and L. Ponton (Eds.), *Handbook of adolescent health risk behaviour* (pp. 369-391). New York: Plenum Press.

Rotheram-Borus, M.J., Rosario, M., and Koopman, C. (1991). Minority youths at high risk: Gay males and runaways. In M.C. Colten and S. Gore (Eds.), *Adolescent stress: Causes and consequences* (pp. 181-200). New York: Aldine de Gruyter, Inc.

Roy, E., Haley, N., Leclerc, P., Sochanski, B., Boudreau, J-F., and Boivin, J-F. (2004). Mortality in a cohort of street youth in Montreal. *Journal of the American Medical Association*, 292, 569-574.

Shaffer, D., and Caton, C. (1984). *Runaway and homeless youth in New York City. A report to the Ittleson Foundation.* New York: Division of Psychiatry, New York State Psychiatric Institute and Columbia University College of Physicians and Surgeons.

Shane, P.G. (1989). *What about America's homeless children?* London: Sage Publications.

Smart, R.G., and Adlaf, E.M. (1991). Substance use and problems among Toronto street youth. *British Journal of Addiction*, 86, 999-1010.

Smart, R.G., Adlaf, E.M., Walsh, G.W., and Zdanowicz, Y. (1994). Similarities in drug use and depression among runaway students and street youth. *Canadian Journal of Public Health*, 85, 17-18.

Smart R.G., and Ogborne, A.C. (1994). Street youth in substance abuse treatment: Characteristics and treatment compliance. *Adolescence*, 29, 733-745.

Smart, R.G., and Walsh, G.W. (1993). Predictors of depression in street youth. *Adolescence*, 28, 41-53.

SMARTRISK (1998). *The economic burden of unintentional injury in Canada.* Ontario Neurotrauma Foundation: Toronto, Ontario.

Smith, K., and Crawford, S. (1986). Suicidal behaviour among "normal" high school students. *Suicide and Life-Threatening Behaviours*, 16, 313-325.

Stiffman, A.R. (1989). Suicide attempts in runaway youths. *Suicide and Life-Threatening Behaviour*, 19, 147-159.

Sweeney, P., Lindegren, M.L., Buehler, J.W., Onorato, I.M., and Janssen, R.S. (1995). Teenagers at risk for Human Immunodeficiency Virus type 1 infection. *Archives of Pediatrics and Adolescents Medicine*, 149, 521-528.

Totten, M., and Quigley, W. (2003). *Canadian anti-bullying best practices.* Ottawa, ON. Canadian Public Health Association Conference.

Tyler, K.A., Whitbeck, L.B., Hoyt, D.R., and Johnson, K.D. (2003). Self-mutilation and homeless youth: The role of family abuse, street experiences and mental disorders. *Journal of Research on Adolescence*, 13, 457-474.

Tyler, K.A., and Cauce, A.M. (2002). Perpetrators of early physical and sexual abuse among homeless and runaway adolescents. *Child Abuse and Neglect*, 26, 1261-1274.

Unger, J.B., Kipke, M.D., Simon, T.R., Montgomery, S.B., and Johnson, C.J. (1997). Homeless youths and young adults in Los Angeles: Prevalence of mental health problems and the relationship between mental health and substance abuse disorders. *American Journal of Community Psychology*, 25, 371-394.

Unger, J.B., Kipke, M.D., Simon, T.R., Johnson, C.J., Montgomery, S.B., and Iversen, E. (1998). Stress and social support among homeless youth. *Journal of Adolescent Research*, 13, 134-157.

van der Ploeg, J.D., and Scholte, E. (1997). *Homeless youth.* London: Sage Publications.

Velez, C.N., and Cohen, P. (1988). Suicidal behaviour and ideation in a community sample of children: Maternal and youth reports. *Journal of American Academy of Child and Adolescent Psychiatry*, 27, 349-356.

Virley O'Connor, B., and MacDonald, B.J. (1999). A youth-friendly intervention for homeless and street-involved youth. *Reclaiming Children and Youth*, 8, 102 - 106.

Votta, E., and Farrell, S. (2005). *Physical and mental health outcomes in female youth: A follow-up study with homeless and non-homeless females.* Ottawa, ON: Final report prepared for the CHEO Research Institute.

Votta, E., and Manion, I. (2003). Factors in the psychological adjustment of homeless adolescent males: The role of coping style. *Journal of the American Academy of Child and Adolescent Psychiatry*, 7, 778-785.

Votta, E., and Manion, I. (2004). Suicide, high-risk behaviours and coping style in homeless adolescent males' adjustment. *Journal of the Adolescent Health, 34,* 237-243.

Whitbeck, L.B., Chen, X., Hoyt, D.R., Tyler, K.A., and Johnson, K.D. (2004). Mental disorder, subsistence strategies and victimization among gay, lesbian and bisexual homeless and runaway adolescents. *Journal of Sex Research, 41,* 329-42.

Whitbeck, L.B., Hoyt, D.R., Yoder, K.A., Cauce, A.M., and Paradise, M. (2001). Deviant behavior and victimization among homeless and runaway adolescents. *Journal of Interpersonal Violence, 16,* 1175-1204.

Whitbeck, L.B., Hoyt, D.R., and Bao, W-N. (2001). Depressive symptoms and co-occurring depressive symptoms, substance abuse, and conduct problems among runaway and homeless adolescents. *Child Development, 71,* 721-732.

Whitbeck, L.B., Hoyt, D.R., and Yoder, K.A. (1999). A risk-amplification model of victimization and depressive symptoms among runaway and homeless adolescents. *American Journal of Community Psychology, 27,* 273-296.

Yoder, K.A. (1999). Comparing suicide attempters, suicide ideators, and non-suicidal homeless and runaway adolescents. *Suicide and Life-Threatening Behaviour, 29,* 25-36.

Zide, M.R., and Cherry, A.L. (1992). A typology of runaway youths: An empirically based definition. *Child and Adolescent Social Work Journal, 9,* 155-168.

Plate 4 "Chrysallis" (J. LeClair)

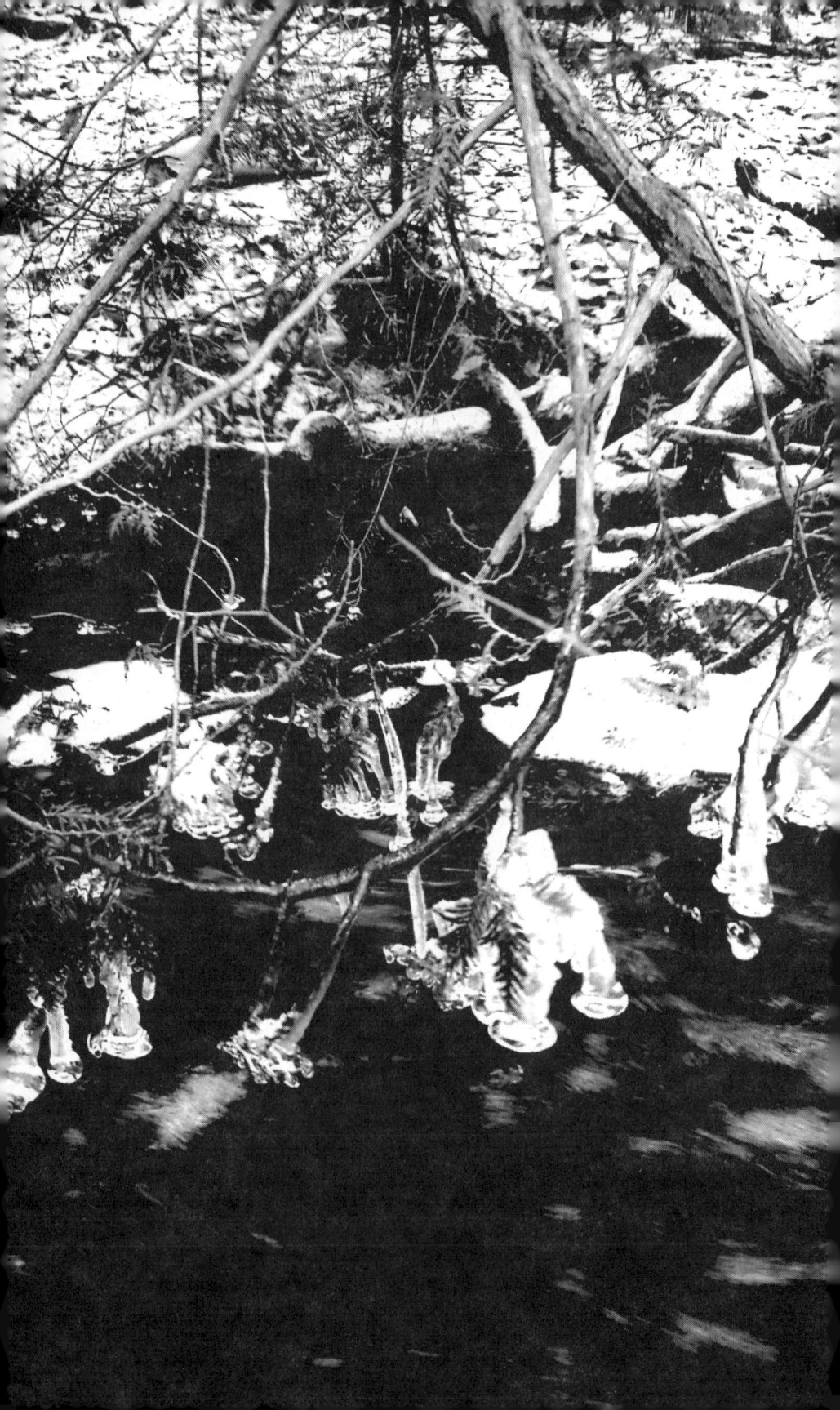

Cross-Disciplinary Perspectives on Children's Mental Health

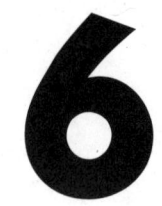

James A. LeClair
Department of Geography, Nipissing University

Introduction

While studies undertaken internationally report a relatively broad range of estimates for the prevalence of childhood mental health problems (Jensen, 1991), research completed in Canada suggests that 15-20% of children and adolescents suffer from *at least* one psychological disorder that may significantly impair day-to-day functioning (Offord, Boyle, Fleming, Munroe Blum, and Rae Grant, 1989; Offord and Lipman, 1996; Waddell and Shepherd, 2002; see also chapters by Waddell et al., and Tonkin, this volume). The potential long term importance of this problem is highlighted by a growing body of research that suggests that behavioural differences in early childhood can predict a variety of psychiatric disorders in adults (Zeitlin, 2000). Results from a longitudinal study undertaken by Caspi and co-authors (1996), for example, suggest that children who are impulsive, restless, and distractible at age 3 are more likely to be suicidal, show characteristics of antisocial personality disorder, and engage in criminal activity by age 21. Those who are observed to be shy, fearful, or easily upset as children are more prone to depression and suicide attempts as young adults. Pakiz and co-workers (1997) report the results of an 18 year follow-up study of 375 young adults: aggression and hostility, and disruptive behaviour at a young age are shown to be predictors of antisocial behaviour at age 21.

Thus, it is suggested that dysfunctional behaviour exists as a continuum throughout childhood and into young adulthood. Unresolved problem behaviours in childhood are likely to persist into later life, exacting high social and individual costs, such as antisocial and criminal behaviour, low educational attainment, substance abuse, and economic dependence. Young women with conduct disorder face additional obstacles to a positive life outcome, including high rates of pregnancy before the age of 17 (Zocolillo and Rogers, 1991).

Although the aetiology of childhood behavioural problems is not completely understood (Jensen, 1991), considerable research evidence, identifying a wide variety of potential causal pathways and mechanisms, has been compiled. In spite of the widespread acceptance of relatively holistic conceptualizations of the health-disease process [such as the 'determinants of health' (CIAR, 1991)], even a cursory examination of the literature would reveal that the potential causal factors chosen for consideration in any particular study are largely reflective of the discipline-specific belief systems of particular researchers.

From a biomedical perspective, for example, mental health problems in children might be conceptualized as a manifestation of some underlying, individually possessed neurological defect, perhaps caused by sub-optimal conditions of foetal development, trauma-related damage to the brain, or the presence of other physiological characteristics that impair normative neuropsychological function.

Low birth weight, for example, typically indicative of prematurity or impaired foetal development, has been identified as a potential risk factor for attention deficit-hyperactivity disorder (Szatmari, Saigal, Rosenbaum, Campbell, and King, 1990; Klebanov, Brooks-Gunn, and McCormick, 1994; Breslau et al., 1996), internalizing behaviours such as anxiousness and social insecurity, and overall behavioural difficulties (Weisglas-Kuperus, 1993; Sommerfelt, Troland, Ellertsen, and Markestad, 1996). Likewise, a history of brain trauma has been linked to an increased risk for psychiatric disorders in general (Max et al., 1997a; Max et al., 1997b), and attention deficit-hyperactivity disorder (Max et al., 1998) and schizophrenia (Templer, 1992) specifically. Those with an allergy to particular foods or food additives, typically identified through the use of elimination diets, may be at greater risk for a wide range of behavioural difficulties, including irritability, aggression (Werbach, 1992), depression (Werbach, 1991), and hyperactivity (Feingold, 1975; Crook, 1980).

Less reductionist explanations, such as those typically espoused by psychologists, may attribute such problems to excessive levels of stress, or the outcome of emotional, social, and material deprivation.

Children living in low income families, for instance, are at greater risk for psychiatric disorders in general, as well as specific problems including social impairment, poor school performance (Lipman, Offord, and Boyle, 1994), attentional problems, and hyperactivity (Offord, Boyle, and Racine, 1989a; Szatmari, Offord, and Boyle, 1989). As well, children living in a family where the main source of income is social assistance have a higher prevalence of conduct disorder, somatization, emotional disorder, and hyperactivity (Offord, Boyle, and Racine, 1989b) than do their peers.

Other examples of characteristics more commonly found among children with behavioural difficulties include living in a single parent family (Offord, Boyle, and Racine, 1989b; Szatmari et al., 1989; Lipman, Offord, and Dooley, 1996), a parental history of mental illness (Jensen, 1991; Cytryn, 1982; Weissman, Leckman, Merikangas, Gammon, and Prussof, 1984; Weissman, Prusoff, Gammon, Merikangas, Leckman, and Kidd, 1984; Offord, Boyle, and Racine,

1989a; Garralda, 2000), and residential instability (Mundy, Robertson, Greenblat, and Robertson, 1989; Simpson and Fowler, 1994; DeWit, Offord, and Braun, 1998).

Studies undertaken by geographers and sociologists suggest that mental health problems have a geographical dimension, the pattern of psychosocial morbidity perhaps resulting from spatial variations in a variety of potential risk or protective factors. To illustrate, Faris and Dunham (1939) found that overall rates of hospital admission for mental illness in Chicago were concentrated in the city centre, with incidence rates declining with increasing distance from the core. This pattern, and its association with areas of social and economic deprivation, was also observed for specific disorders, most notably for schizophrenia. Similar results were revealed in an examination of data for Providence, Rhode Island (Faris and Dunham, 1939), and in later work completed in Chicago (Levy and Rowitz, 1973), Nottingham (Giggs, 1973; Giggs, 1983; Giggs and Mather, 1983; Giggs, 1986; Giggs and Cooper, 1986), and Plymouth (Dean and James, 1981). Although most of the existing arealbased research has focused upon adult mental illness, similar spatial patterns and ecological correlates have been seen in studies of behavioural problems and psychiatric service utilization patterns in children (LeClair and Innes, 1997; LeClair, 2001).

While ecological research has consistently linked the geography of mental health problems to characteristics of the urban environment, explanations of the aetiological significance of this relationship are relatively underdeveloped. Increasingly, however, it is suggested that aggregate (neighbourhood-level) social conditions may play an independent role in the generation (or prevention) of mental health problems, most notably in children (see Chase-Lansdale and Gordon, 1996; Aneshensel and Sucoff, 1996; Boyle and Lipman, 1998; LeClair, 2001; Boyle and Lipman, 2002).

Considered in isolation, the discipline-specific explanations for childhood mental health status may seem mutually exclusive. However, the research evidence associated with each perspective reveals its potential explanatory value, and suggests that these seemingly competing paradigms are more properly conceptualized as components of a broadly defined system of human-environment interactions wherein risk and protective factors operate at a number of levels (individual, family, community, etc.) and (individually and synergistically) promote or diminish personal and aggregate states of mental (ill-) health.

In an attempt to consider each disciplinary perspective as a sub-component of such a system, the research presented in this chapter examines the relationships between the behavioural status of urban children and potential explanatory factors which reflect facets of each of the paradigms outlined above. More specifically, the roles of risk factors measured at three scales—that of the individual, the family, and the census tract—are considered in order to evaluate each of the explanatory paradigms proffered.

DATA COLLECTION AND BEHAVIOURAL ASSESSMENT

The research discussed in this chapter utilizes data collected during the period October to December, 1997, as part of a larger study of children's mental health. Employing a cross-sectional design, the study targeted children attending grades Kindergarten through 4 in the most highly urbanized portion of Greater Victoria, British Columbia. A total of 18 English-language public elementary schools were invited to take part in the study. Of these, Principals and/or Parent Action Committees at 15 of the schools agreed to participate (Figure 6.1). The study area considered in this chapter consists of 26 census tracts which correspond, in whole or in part, to the catchment areas of the participating schools (Figure 6.2).

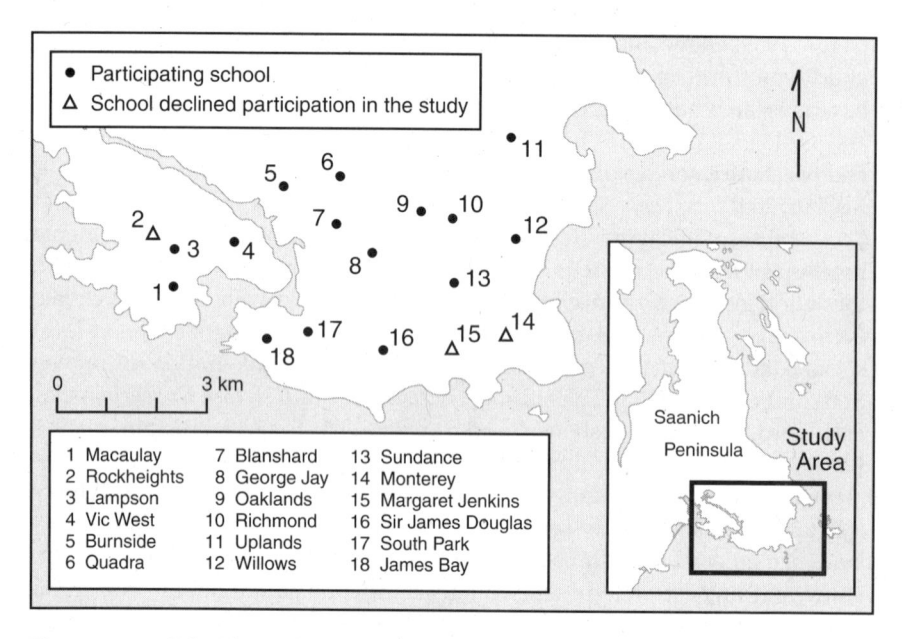

Figure 6.1 Schools in the study area

Implementation of the study, accomplished with the cooperation of the Greater Victoria School District and the Principals and Teachers of the participating schools, involved the distribution of a two-part self-administered questionnaire to the parents/guardians of the children in the study population. Parents were asked to complete the survey package and to return it in the addressed, postage-paid envelope provided.

The first part of the survey package, a socio-demographic and medical history questionnaire, was used to obtain each child's postal code (in order to determine the census tract of residence), as well as information about a

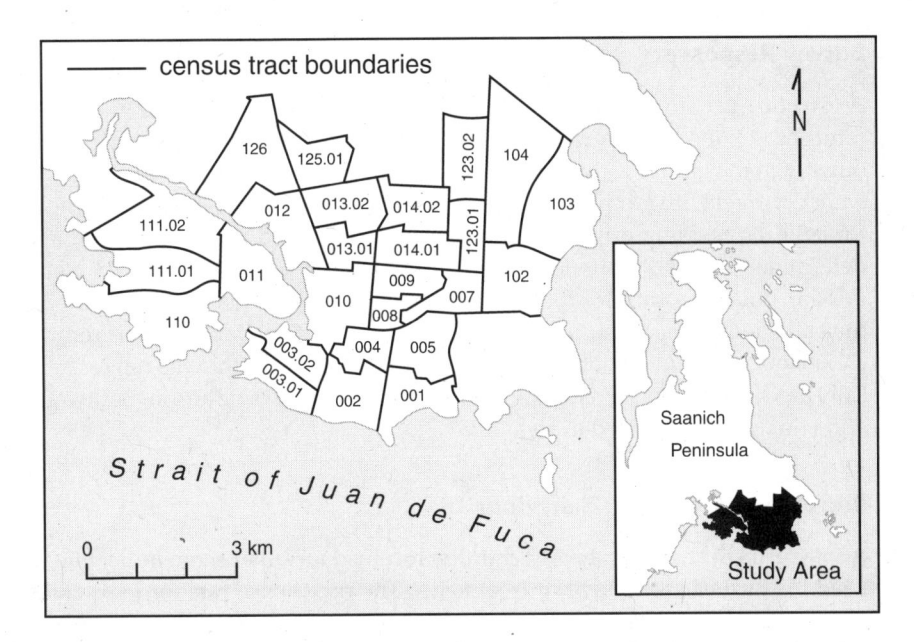

Figure 6.2 The study area

variety of factors that may be associated with the behavioural status of children, including those pertaining to birth and medical history, socio-economic status, dwelling characteristics, and family composition.

The second part of the survey package consisted of the Walker Problem Behavior Identification Checklist [revised] (Walker, 1983), a behavioural assessment tool that has been shown to be a reliable and effective means of differentiating between disturbed and non-disturbed behavioural patterns in children (Walker and Buckley, 1973; Greenwood, Walker, Todd, and Hops, 1976; Mash and Mercer, 1979) when completed by a teacher or a parent (Strain, Steele, Ellis, and Timm, 1982). The checklist is comprised of 50 items describing negative behaviours, each with an associated weight (ranging from 1 to 4) that reflects its relative importance in handicapping a child's normal behavioural functioning. Respondents selected the items that were characteristic of their child's behaviour in the preceding 2 month period.

For the purposes of this research, the checklist's Total scale, which provides a measure of overall behavioural functioning, is obtained by summing the weighted scores for each item selected. The checklist's sex and grade-range adjusted t-score distributions [a t-score of 60 or greater suggesting the need for further evaluation or treatment (Walker, 1983)] are used to dichotomize participating children into 'problem' and 'non-problem' behaviour groups.

Survey Response

A total of 3,121 survey packages were distributed, of which 622 (19.9%) were returned. Of these, 11 were returned completed for children attending grades other than the grades K through 4 study group established for the research, 11 were returned with no spatial data (no postal code reported), 40 were returned for children residing outside the study area established for this research (as determined by school attendance or census tract of residence), and 43 were missing data necessary for the completion of the present analyses (27 without the behavioural checklist; 16 missing responses to key variables). This return (517) yields a useful response rate of about 16.6%, a rate within the range typically associated with such mental health-oriented surveys (Johnson, Boutwell, and Hinkle, 1975, as cited in Kyle, 1981).

Prevalence of Problem Behaviour

A total of 141 (27.3%) of the 517 children received a Walker score indicating a need for further assessment or treatment. The prevalence rate for male children in the sample (26.0%) is slightly lower than that observed for the female children (28.7%). This difference is, however, statistically insignificant ($\chi^2=0.467$; $p>0.05$).

ECOLOGICAL ANALYSIS

Spatial data in the form of the children's postal codes of residence, obtained in the questionnaire, were used to identify the census tract of residence for each participating child using a Postal Code Conversion File available from Statistics Canada. This information was used to aggregate the data, and census tract rates of problem behaviour within the sample, expressed in percent, were calculated.

In order to allow for a simple visual assessment of the distribution of problem behaviour within the study area, census tract prevalence rates are mapped herein using location quotients. A descriptive spatial statistic, the location quotient (LQ) measures the relative concentration of a particular phenomenon in an areal unit with respect to the mean for the region as a whole. In this instance, because the data are expressed in percentages, the location quotient is calculated using the equation:

$$LQ_i = X_i / j$$

where: X_i = the prevalence rate in census tract i
j = the mean (study area-wide) prevalence rate

Thus, where LQ = 1, the census tract rate is equal to the mean rate for the study area as a whole. An LQ of less than 1 indicates that the census tract rate is lower than the mean rate (e.g., where LQ = 0.5, the census tract rate was one half that of the mean rate), while an LQ greater than 1 denotes a relative concentration of problem behaviour in that census tract (e.g., LQ = 2.0 indicates a rate twice that of the mean) (Shaw and Wheeler, 1985; Griffith, Amrhein, and Desloges, 1991).

The final step in the ecological analysis uses simple bivariate correlation analyses in order to identify which descriptors of the urban ecology of the study area have a significant statistical relationship with the distribution of problem behaviour. To this end, census tract prevalence rates of problem behaviour serve as the dependent variable in the bivariate analyses. The following census variables are employed as independent variables in the ecological correlation analyses:

Income and Employment
- average family income
- percent families with household income of less than $20,000
- percent census tract income from government transfer payments
- percent unemployed

Educational Attainment
- percent aged 15-24 not in school
- percent with less than a grade 9 education

Housing Characteristics
- average dwelling value
- percent dwellings requiring major repairs
- percent rented dwelling units

Population Mobility
- percent movers (1 year mobility status)

Family Status
- percent single parent families

Results

Distribution of Problem Behaviour

Rates of problem behaviour at the census tract level (Table 6.1) vary considerably. As shown in Figure 6.3, there is a marked concentration of high rates, with location quotients indicating that census tracts in the central and north-western-most portions of the study area have prevalence rates 1.6 times (or greater) than the mean rate. Lower rates are observed toward the fringes of the study area, with the lowest location quotients, indicating prevalence rates which are one half of the mean rate or less, found exclusively in the north-eastern-most tracts.

Table 6.1 Census tract prevalence of problem behaviour

Census tract	Number of children	Number in problem behaviour group	Prevalence of problem behaviour (%)	Location quotient
1.00	22	8	36.4	1.33
2.00	29	7	24.1	0.88
3.01	18	5	27.8	1.02
3.02	11	3	27.3	1.00
4.00	12	3	25.0	0.92
5.00	13	4	30.8	1.13
7.00	9	2	22.2	0.81
8.00	21	7	33.3	1.22
9.00	26	6	23.1	0.85
10.00	7	5	71.4	2.62
11.00	21	8	38.1	1.40
12.00	11	5	45.5	1.67
13.01	22	13	59.1	2.16
13.02	16	7	43.8	1.60
14.01	31	7	22.6	0.83
14.02	20	5	25.0	0.92
102.00	45	5	11.1	0.41
103.00	12	1	8.3	0.30
104.00	22	3	13.6	0.50
110.00	76	13	17.1	0.63
111.01	13	3	23.1	0.85
111.02	16	8	50.0	1.83
123.01	17	5	29.4	1.08
123.02	8	1	12.5	0.46
125.01	9	2	22.2	0.81
126.00	10	5	50.0	1.83
Total	517	141	27.3	1.00

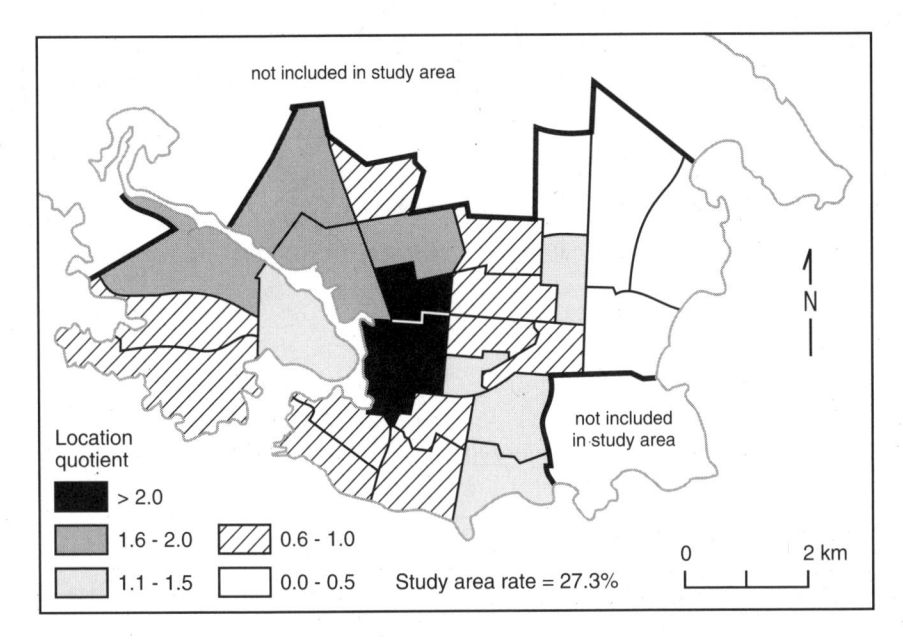

Figure 6.3   Distribution of problem behaviour

Ecological Correlations

Results of the bivariate ecological correlation analyses, shown in Table 6.2, suggest that the observed pattern of problem behaviour is related to the overall ecological structure of the study area. Two of the income-related variables considered (i.e., average income and percent with an income less than $20,000 per year) are significantly correlated with the distribution of problem behaviour; the direction of each relationship suggests that lower aggregate income levels are associated with a higher prevalence of problem behaviour. Likewise, both of the education-related variables (i.e., percent aged 15-24 not in school and percent with less than a grade 9 education) are significantly related to the pattern of problem behaviour, with lower levels of educational participation and attainment related to higher rates of behavioural difficulties in the children. The remaining significant ecological correlations suggest that higher rates of problem behaviour are associated with a greater census tract prevalence of lone parenthood, lower quality housing (in terms of both average value and state of repair), and higher rates of residential mobility.

INDIVIDUAL- AND FAMILY-LEVEL ANALYSES

Although they differ conceptually, individual- and family-level variables can be analysed in an identical fashion, with factors measured at both levels treated as individual attributes of the participating children. For the purposes of

Table 6.2 Ecological correlations

Variable	r
Average family income	-0.457*
Percent families with household income <$20,000	0.507**
Percent census tract income from government transfer payments	0.362
Percent unemployed	0.281
Percent aged 15-24 not in school	0.504**
Percent with less than a grade 9 education	0.543**
Average dwelling value	-0.487*
Percent dwellings requiring major repairs	0.424*
Percent rented dwelling units	0.402*
Percent movers (1 year mobility status)	0.587**
Percent single parent families	0.434*

*p<0.05   **p<0.01

this research, survey data were used to classify the children on the basis of 'exposure' to each of the potential risk and protective factors considered. This dichotomous classification, coupled with that obtained in the behavioural assessment portion of the research, allows for the identification of significant differences in exposure between the problem and non-problem behaviour groups through chi-square analyses of 2X2 contingency tables. Yates' Continuity Corrected Chi-Square statistic is reported when the expected frequency in one or more cells of the contingency table in question is less than five (Walsh, 1990; Munro and Page, 1993).

The following factors serve as predictors in the family- and individual-level analyses:

Housing Status
- living in rented housing
- living in subsidized housing

Income and Employment Status
- someone in the family is unemployed
- income less than $20,000 per year
- main income is from social assistance

Family Factors
- death in the family in the past 6 months
- someone left home in the past 6 months

- someone in the family with a chronic illness or physical disability
- lone parent family
- parental history of mental illness
- mother was under the age of 20 at the time of the child's birth

Biomedical Factors
- history of concussion
- low birth weight
- diagnosed food allergy
- diagnosed learning disability
- physical disability
- diagnosed neurological disorder

Results

Rates of exposure to the potential family- and individual-level risk factors, for both the problem and non-problem behaviour groups, as well as the results of the chi-square analyses of the 2X2 contingency tables, are shown in Table 6.3. The strength and direction of the observed associations are reported as odds ratios.

Housing Status

Although living in rented housing is a common characteristic within the sample as a whole, those in the problem behaviour group are almost three times as likely to do so than children in the comparison group. Tenure in subsidized housing has a slightly stronger association with behavioural status: those living in rent-assisted dwellings are at over three times greater risk for behavioural problems than those living in other forms of housing.

Income and Employment Status

Results obtained in the ecological analysis suggested a link between low income levels and higher rates of problem behaviour, a finding which is supported by the significant associations observed between behavioural status and the family-level income- and employment-related variables considered here. In each case, those children with a Walker score indicating a need for further evaluation or treatment are significantly more likely to be in the disadvantaged group. Children living in a family setting wherein someone is unemployed and seeking work, for instance, are over two times more likely to receive a Walker score which exceeds the problem behaviour threshold. Those living in a home with an annual income of less than $20,000 are at a similar risk. The strongest association is between behavioural status and receipt of welfare: children whose parent/guardian reports that the main

Table 6.3 Chi-Square analysis results

Variable	Percent exposed (of problem behaviour group)	Percent exposed (of non-problem behaviour group)	Chi-square	Odds ratio
Housing Status				
Renter	66.0	39.9	27.965**	2.919
Subsidised housing	22.0	7.7	20.364**	3.372
Income and Employment Status				
Someone unemployed	25.5	13.0	11.663**	2.288
Income <$20,000 per year	34.8	17.3	18.197**	2.548
On social assistance	25.5	5.6	41.592**	5.796
Family Factors				
Death in family	30.5	25.0	1.591	1.316
Someone left home	19.1	9.6	8.785**	2.237
Family disability	22.0	10.6	11.146**	2.367
Single parent family	39.0	24.2	11.091**	2.003
Parental mental illness	36.2	21.8	11.069**	2.032
Teen mother (at child's birth)	9.2	4.3	4.774*	2.285
Biomedical Factors				
History of concussion	3.5	2.9	0.717	1.220
Low birth weight	5.0	4.0	0.239	1.257
Food allergy	10.6	5.3	4.597*	2.119
Learning disability	14.2	1.3	36.822**	12.264
Physical disability	3.5	1.9	0.648	1.938
Neurological disorder	5.7	0.8	9.463**[a]	7.479

* $p<0.05$ ** $p<0.01$ [a] Yates' Continuity Corrected Chi-Square

source of family income is social assistance are almost six times as likely as other children to be identified as in need of further assessment or treatment for a behavioural problem.

Family Factors

Each of the family status-related factors selected for analysis is more prevalent among children in the problem behaviour group. For all but one of the variables—that identifying children who experienced the death of someone close to them in the past 6 months—the observed prevalence differs significantly between the behaviour status groups. Children who had a family member move out in the preceding 6 month period, those living with someone with a physical disability, those in lone parent families, and those born to a mother under the age of 20 are more than two times as likely as other children to receive a Walker score in the problem behaviour range. Likewise, children with one or both parents ever treated for a mental health problem are more than twice as likely as other children to exhibit signs of mental health problems themselves.

Biomedical Factors

Each of the biomedical risk factors considered is reported more frequently for children in the problem behaviour group. For three of these factors, the observed differences are statistically significant. Although diagnosed neurological disorders are relatively uncommon in the sample, those children so affected are over seven times as likely as other children to receive a Walker score above the problem behaviour threshold. Likewise, there is a pronounced difference between the groups with respect to the prevalence of diagnosed learning disabilities. Children in the problem behaviour group are reported to have such difficulties at a rate over 12 times that of the comparison group. One additional factor, the presence of a diagnosed food allergy, was reported more than twice as often for children with problem behaviour than for other children in the sample.

CONTEXTUAL ANALYSES

Results of the analyses undertaken at both the urban ecological and family level imply a relationship between socio-economic disadvantage and problem behaviour. Conceptually, the link between behavioural problems and family-level processes is relatively straightforward, and backed up by considerable research evidence. While the results of the ecological analyses are clearly consistent with those obtained at the family level, it is unclear whether the significant correlations observed are indicative of some *meaningful* underlying process, wherein characteristics of the urban environment influence mental health outcomes. In this portion of the research, contextual analyses are undertaken in order to identify census tract-level variables that may have an *independent* influence on behavioural status, beyond the effects of an equivalent variable measured at the family level. The methodological approach used to meet this objective is modelled after that employed by Brooks-Gunn, Duncan, Klebanov, and Sealand (1993) in their evaluation of neighbourhood effects on teenage births.

Three of the ecological variables which are significantly correlated with census tract rates of problem behaviour (i.e., percent single parent families, percent families with household income of less than $20,000, and percent rented dwelling units) have an equivalent family-level variable as collected in the survey questionnaire. Census tract (mean) values for each of the ecological variables in question were assigned to each child, based upon their census tract of residence. Contextual effects were assessed using two-stage hierarchical logistic regression models. For the first analytical stage, the strength of the association between behavioural status and the ecological variable in question was determined. In the second stage, the equivalent family characteristic was forced into the regression model along with the ecological variable. A contextual effect is suggested when the association between behavioural status and the ecological variable under consideration remains statistically significant after allowing for the effects of the family-level characteristic.

Results

Results of the contextual analyses are shown in Table 6.4. For two of the three significant ecological variables (i.e., percent single parent families, and percent families with household income of less than $20,000) a contextual effect is suggested by the results of the hierarchical logistic regression analyses. In both cases, the logistic regression coefficient remains statistically significant, with only a slight decrease in the value of the odds ratio, after allowing for the effect of the equivalent family-level variable. However, the coefficient observed for the remaining ecological variable (i.e., percent rented dwelling units) is no longer statistically significant following the inclusion of the family-level characteristic (living in a rented dwelling). This finding suggests that, while the result obtained at the urban ecological level reflects the family-level association between behavioural status and housing tenure, the census tract prevalence of rented dwellings does not independently influence behavioural outcomes through a contextual effect.

Table 6.4   Hierarchical logistic regression analysis results

Variable	Stage One (odds ratio)	Stage Two (odds ratio)
Percent families with household income <$20,000	1.054**	1.040**
Family income <$20,000 per year	—	2.070**
Percent single parent families	1.075**	1.066**
Single parent family	—	1.752**
Percent rented dwelling units	1.017**	1.007
Renter	—	2.711**

*$p<0.05$ **$p<0.01$

MULTIVARIATE ANALYSIS

In each of the preceding stages of analysis, a number of potential risk factors, measured at the level of the individual, the family, and the census tract, have been identified. With the exception of the few variables used in the contextual analyses, however, no consideration has been given to the potential for significant correlations/associations among the proposed explanatory variables themselves. In this, the final analytical stage of the research, an attempt is made to identify a parsimonious list of variables that collectively account, in part, for the effects of other, closely related variables.

Backward step-wise logistic regression analyses are used in order to determine which of the individual-, family-, and ecological-level characteristics have a significant independent relationship with behavioural status, beyond the effects of similar, inter-correlated variables. Criteria for removal from the logistic regression model was based upon the significance of the Wald statistic (p.[in]=0.05; p[out]=0.10).

Results

Results of the step-wise logistic regression analysis are shown in Table 6.5. The final model consists of seven variables, including those related to urban ecology (percent dwellings requiring major repairs), housing tenure (living in a rented dwelling), socio-economic and family status (main income from social assistance; someone in the family with a chronic illness or physical disability), and medical history (diagnosed learning disability; diagnosed neurological disorder).

Table 6.5   Multivariate analysis: Final model

Variable	Odds Ratio
Percent dwellings requiring major repairs	1.136[a]
Diagnosed learning disability	8.535**
Diagnosed food allergy	2.620*
Diagnosed neurological disorder	4.072[a]
On social assistance	3.643**
Living with someone with a physical illness or disability	1.863*
Living in a rented dwelling	1.855*

[a]$p<0.10$ *$p<0.05$ **$p<0.01$

DISCUSSION

The analyses undertaken in this study identified significant relationships between behavioural problems and potential risk factors measured at each of the levels considered.

The results of the ecological analyses, for example, suggest that the distribution of problem behaviour in the urban environment considered is not even. Rather, there is a pronounced spatial concentration of behavioural difficulties among children living in the central and western-most portions of the study area. While it is impossible to dismiss the possibility that this distribution is artifactual, the results of the ecological correlation analyses suggest that the observed spatial pattern is indicative of some underlying process, wherein children living in certain portions of the urban environment are at greater risk for developing behavioural problems than are other children. Specifically, the pattern of problem behaviour appears to be associated with variations in access to social and material resources, wherein socio-economically disadvantaged census tracts experience higher rates of dysfunctional behaviour. This finding is entirely consistent with the results reported in the existing body of ecological research, as reviewed earlier.

Although the interpretation of ecological analyses is usually hampered by a lack of associated data collected at the level of the individual or the family, the contextual analyses undertaken are to a degree helpful in elucidating the potential aetiological significance of the spatial pattern observed. Specifically, the contextual analyses identify two ecological variables (i.e., percent single parent families, and percent families with household income of less than $20,000) that are significantly associated with behavioural status both before and after controlling for the effects of equivalent variables measured at the level of the family.

While neither of the two proposed contextual factors were selected for inclusion in the final multivariate logistic regression model, a single ecological variable (i.e., percent dwellings requiring major repairs) remained marginally significant after allowing for the effects of variables measured at other levels. While the analytical approach utilized does little to elucidate the potential aetiological significance of any single factor, the inclusion of an ecological variable in the multivariate model further implies the potential for risk-enhancing processes occurring at the census tract level.

The ecological relationship observed between socio-economic disadvantage and behavioural problems is clearly mirrored in the results obtained from the family-level analyses. Each of the variables concerned with income and employment status are identified as strong predictors of problem behaviour in the bivariate analyses. This relationship is further emphasized by the findings reported for the housing status variables; an approximate three-fold increase in risk is associated with factors indicative of relative disadvantage in terms of housing tenure. Living in rented housing, a characteristic that remained in the final logistic regression model, appears to be a particularly important predictor of behavioural status. This notion is reinforced by the results of the contextual analysis involving this variable, wherein this family characteristic rendered the effect of the equivalent ecological variable statistically insignificant.

While it is impossible to determine what (if any) specific impact(s) living in rental housing may have on child health, speculative influences may include its association with lower socio-economic status, potential risk(s) connected to living in crowded conditions, or the operation of a 'peer effect'—a contextual influence—due to the clustering of 'at-risk' children in such housing. As well, an important question is raised when considering the results obtained for this factor alongside those of the ecological analyses: given the significant ecological relationship between problem behaviour and housing requiring major repairs, what is the relationship between living in rental housing and the quality of that housing? Unfortunately, the lack of an equivalent housing quality variable measured at the family level precludes further consideration of this question within the present data set.

A number of other factors measured at the family level are associated with an apparent increase in risk for behavioural problems among the participating children. In general terms, factors indicative of family disruption and diminished parenting resources, each of which may also be associated with social and material disadvantage, are strong predictors of problem behaviour among participating children. Of these characteristics, one factor (i.e., living with a parent who has a chronic illness or physical disability) remained in the final multivariate model.

Although not among those factors in the final logistic regression model, the observed association between behavioural status of the child and parental history of mental illness is of particular interest. This finding, consistent with results reported elsewhere (see Duncan and Reder, 2000; Fellow-Smith, 2000; Garralda, 2000), likely reflects a number of potential risk processes, among them the possibility of a transmitted genetic risk, or the impact of social and economic marginalization and/or diminished parental abilities. The latter influence is perhaps affecting only those children whose parent suffers from a chronic mental health problem. While this factor transcends the levels of analysis employed—it is simultaneously a biomedical as well as a family-level risk factor—it is also among the most difficult to interpret due to the cross-sectional nature of the data set, and the consequent inability to determine the temporal precedence of events. While the association itself is quite strong, and theoretically plausible from all of the perspectives considered, it may also reflect the risk that children with behavioural difficulties present to the well-being of their parent(s).

With respect to the medical history-related factors, three of the co-morbid conditions considered occurred significantly more frequently among those children with a Walker score in the problem behaviour range. For two of these factors the strength of the observed relationship with behavioural status is quite strong: an almost 7.5-fold increase in risk is observed for those with a neurological disorder, while those diagnosed with a learning disorder are at over 12 times the risk of other children in the sample. The potential importance of these variables is further suggested by their presence in the final, multivariate logistic regression model.

One additional biomedical factor (i.e., having a diagnosed food allergy) occurs more than twice as often in those receiving a score in the problem behaviour range than it does in other children. Although this finding should be viewed with caution since no attention was given to the nature or severity of the allergies in question, it does offer confirmation of the associations between behavioural status and food intolerance noted previously.

Taken together, the results obtained implicate a wide variety of potential risks to the psychosocial well-being of children, extending from the community, through to the family and biological levels. Although the methodological approach used to 'sort out' the significant correlates of problem behaviour identifies only those factors of the greatest statistical, rather than aetiological significance, the results obtained are useful in understanding the apparent importance of variables measured at each level of analysis. In this regard, the results obtained are suggestive of the validity of each disciplinary perspective considered.

Perhaps unsurprisingly, the impact of any particular risk factor appears to be a function of its 'distance' from the child. For instance, although certain ecological characteristics seem to have an independent influence on behavioural status, the effect is arguably weak. This interpretation is further borne out by the results of the multivariate analysis, wherein the single ecological variable that remained in the final model was of marginal statistical significance. The strongest relationships, on the other hand, were observed for two of the biomedical risk factors, as indicated by their strong bivariate associations with behavioural status, and by their inclusion in the final logistic regression model.

It should be noted, however, that the biomedical risk factors in question were relatively rare in the study sample, while behavioural problems were not. As a result, the importance of family and urban ecological characteristics should not be underestimated since, if the links observed are causal in nature, they likely account for the bulk of the psychosocial morbidity found in the participating children.

LIMITATIONS OF THE DATA

While the findings presented in this chapter provide interesting insight into the multi-level correlates of problem behaviour in urban children, the results obtained should be considered within the context of the limitations of the study methods employed and, consequently, of the data obtained.

An important limitation of the data utilized in this study stems from the sampling method employed. In undertaking this project, it was necessary to accommodate the needs of the school district and the participating schools, and to implement a study design compatible with the limited information about the student body which the schools could provide. As a result, a random sampling design was not possible. As well, constraints placed upon the involvement of school personnel necessitated the implementation of the study materials in one stage. Consequently, methods typically used to increase response rates, such as reminder cards, follow-up phone calls, and personalized cover letters (Sheskin, 1985), could not be used.

As a result of these limitations on the sampling design, a volunteer sample was obtained. Such samples may suffer from an interest bias, wherein potential respondents who feel that they have a particular reason to participate in the study are more likely to do so (Sheskin, 1985). Further, the lack of information about the families to whom the survey was distributed prevents an assessment of the characteristics of the non-respondent population. Thus, the results obtained using such a sample cannot be simply generalized to the population as a whole.

While, as noted earlier, the response rate obtained for this study was fairly typical of a voluntary mail-back survey, higher rates of return would have increased confidence in the validity of the sample. Factors that may have influenced the response rate in this instance include the sensitive nature of the study and the information requested, the need to rely upon the children to bring the survey package home to their parents, and an interruption in postal service that occurred as a result of a labour dispute during the data collection period.

With respect to the data collected in the survey, an assumption is made that the information provided by respondents is both complete and accurate. Although it seems unlikely that participants would knowingly provide incorrect information, a social desirability bias, or a desire to avoid 'labelling' their child may have influenced responses to the behaviour checklist. Alternately, those who experience difficult behaviour from their children may be given to overstate behavioural problems when selecting items on the Walker checklist.

The content of the survey was intended to provide information about a variety of factors theoretically linked to the behavioural well-being of children. While a relatively broad range of factors were considered, they were in no way comprehensive. Other factors that may have a significant impact upon children's mental health (e.g., those related to temperament, parenting style, drug use in the home, exposure to violence, etc.) were not considered, either as a result of difficulties in measurement, or the unlikelihood of receiving accurate information concerning illegal activities.

Further, survey items regarding the presence of specific medical problems were intended to identify those children with a *clinical diagnosis* consistent with the conditions in question. Some respondents may have identified conditions that they perceive as present in their child, regardless of the lack of a clinical diagnosis. As well, even in the absence of a clinical diagnosis, some children may have suffered from one or more of the conditions at the time of the study.

Regarding the ecological analysis, the division of the study sample by census tract of residence yielded, in some cases, relatively small numbers of children per areal unit. As a result, census tract rates of problem behaviour may vary considerably due to sampling fluctuations. This, coupled with the lack of information about the families that made up the pool of potential respondents, makes it impossible to establish response rates at the census tract level, or to assess the resulting spatial distributions probabilistically.

While the results obtained in the contextual analyses imply that the characteristics of the urban environment may have an independent impact on the psychosocial well-being of children in the study sample, the findings should be considered within the context of two important limitations of the analytical method employed. First, contextual models effectively use the same variable twice, measured once at the level of the individual, and again at the group (contextual) level. As a result, the observations made at each level of measurement may not be statistically independent when the contextual data describes the characteristics of a relatively homogeneous group. As well, such models may *imply* the existence of contextual effects on behaviour, but cannot reveal *how much* of the risk is attributable to these effects (Kreft and de Leeuw, 1998).

Finally, as noted in the discussion regarding the parent-child mental health link, this study was undertaken using a cross-sectional design. This approach offers a 'snap shot' view of problem behaviour in the study sample at the time that the data were collected. Because they compile information about ill-health conditions and theoretical risk and protective factors simultaneously, cross-sectional surveys "do not establish the temporal sequence of events necessary for the establishment of causal inferences" (Mausner and Kramer, 1985, p. 177). Consequently, the significant relationships identified in this study offer insight into a variety of factors that are *associated* with problem behaviour in the participating children; the advancement of causal hypotheses based upon such associations would require the use of longitudinal data.

CONCLUSION

Much of the research concerned with the aetiology of childhood mental health problems has focused primarily on the influence of a relatively narrow set of potential risk and protective factors. When considered collectively, however, it seems clear that there is a wide range of factors associated with behavioural problems in children, a notion that is, as noted earlier, wholly consistent with contemporary conceptualizations of the health-disease process. The seemingly divergent explanations for poor behavioural outcomes traditionally offered from each disciplinary perspective may, in fact, be complementary, with each filling a conceptual 'gap' found elsewhere. While a simple chain of cause and effect has arguably been the 'holy grail' of biomedicine, such uncomplicated explanatory paradigms seem unimaginable for mental health problems. Rather, child-specific outcomes are likely the result of a complex interplay of (external) social and environmental factors, mediated by temperament and other predisposing (and mitigating) internal characteristics.

From a clinical perspective, the implication of this suggestion—if it is, in fact, an accurate one—is significant. As indicated earlier in this chapter, it seems that the 'closer' the potential risk factor is to the individual child, the stronger its association with behavioural status. This is, perhaps, encouraging, as many neurological disorders are likely preventable, and the identification and amelioration of learning disorders may provide psychological relief to some children. On the other hand, while it is clearly desirable to aim at prevention, it is far from obvious how such interventions could occur with respect to those potential risk factors that occur at greater 'distance' from the child (e.g., low socio-economic status, contextual effects) without significant structural readjustments in society. This seems a heady goal indeed, when one considers the rather profound inertia in social policy development, and the oft-dwindling resources allocated to social welfare.

It could be argued, then, that the most pragmatic approach would involve focusing on treatment. In this regard, the results communicated herein are suggestive of the need to cast the clinical 'net' widely: when considering the underlying stimulus to pathology, those involved with treatment should consider far-reaching psychological stressors, including those related to the characteristics of not just the family, but also the community (unless, that is, their concern is merely the masking of symptomatology, in which case they can happily continue to prescribe psycho-active drugs).

Further research should be motivated by two key factors. First, greater attention needs to be given to the conceptual links between the proposed risk factors and negative health outcomes. For instance, it is very well documented that those of low socio-economic status are at increased risk for a wide variety of health problems, both physical and psychosocial. However, the actual link between the two—how socio-economic disadvantage *creates* ill health—is poorly developed. Only when such mechanisms are more clearly understood will the potential for prevention and treatment be apparent. Second, given the clear role for treatment regimes in mitigating the more serious outcomes of mental health problems, researchers should endeavour to inform the delivery of mental health services. Specifically, attention might be paid to the factors that are at play in determining who among the population in need of treatment actually receives it, and what social, economic, and cultural characteristics may be mediating need and uptake of such services. In each case, a more holistic approach to the study of children's mental health, encompassing investigators and perspectives from a variety of disciplines, seems justified.

Acknowledgements

The author would like to thank the Greater Victoria School District, the principals and teachers of the participating schools, and, most of all, the parents/guardians and children who agreed to take part in this study. Special thanks are also due to Dr. Harold D. Foster, Dr. Leslie T. Foster, Dr. Roy V. Ferguson, Ms. Johanna Mutch, Ms. Vanessa Houston, and the volunteers, too numerous to name, whose assistance, support, and encouragement helped make this study possible. Financial support for this research, provided by the *British Columbia Health Research Foundation* and the *Sara Spencer Foundation*, is most gratefully acknowledged.

References

Aneshensel, C.S., and Sucoff, C.A. (1996). The neighborhood context of adolescent mental health. *Journal of Health and Social Behavior*, 37, 293-310.

Boyle, M.H., and Lipman, E.L. (1998). *Do places matter? A multilevel analysis of geographic variations in child behaviour in Canada. Working paper W-98-16E.* Hull, PQ: Human Resources Development Canada.

Boyle, M.H., and Lipman, E.L. (2002). Do places matter? Socioeconomic disadvantage and behavioural problems of children in Canada. *Journal of Consulting and Clinical Psychiatry*, 70, 378-389.

Breslau, N., Brown, G.G., DelDotto, J.E., Kumar, S., Ezhuthachan, S., Andreski, P., and Hufnagle, K.G. (1996). Psychiatric sequelae of low birth weight at 6 years of age. *Journal of Abnormal Child Psychology*, 24, 385-399.

Brooks-Gunn, J., Duncan, G.J., Klebanov, P.K., and Sealand, N. (1993). Do neighborhoods influence child and adolescent development? *American Journal of Sociology*, 99, 353-395.

Caspi, A., Moffit, T.E., Newman, D.L., and Silva, P.A. (1996). Behavioral observations at age 3 years predict adult psychiatric disorders. *Archives of General Psychiatry*, 53, 1033-1039.

Chase-Lansdale, P.L., and Gordon, R.A. (1996). Economic hardship and the development of five- and six-year-olds: Neighborhood and regional perspectives. *Child Development*, 67, 3338-3367.

CIAR (1991). *The determinants of health.* Toronto: Canadian Institute for Advanced Research.

Cytryn, L., McKnew, D.H., Bartko, J.J., Lamour, M., and Hamovitt, J. (1982). Offspring of patients with affective disorders: II. *Journal of the American Academy of Child Psychiatry*, 21, 389-391.

Crook, W.G. (1980). Can what a child eats make him dull, stupid, or hyperactive? *Journal of Learning Disabilities*, 13, 281-286.

Dean, K.G., and James, H.D. (1981). Social factors and admission to psychiatric hospital: Schizophrenia in Plymouth. *Transactions of the Institute of British Geographers*, 6, 39-52.

DeWit, D.J., Offord, D.R., and Braun, K. (1998). *The relationship between geographic relocation and childhood problem behaviour.* Hull, PQ: Human Resources Development Canada.

Duncan, S., and Reder, P. (2000). Children's experience of major psychiatric disorder in their parent: An overview. In P. Reder, M. McClure, and A. Jolley (Eds.), *Family matters: Interfaces between child and adult mental health* (pp. 83-96). London: Routledge.

Faris, R.E.L., and Dunham, H.W. (1939). *Mental disorders in urban areas*. Chicago, IL: University of Chicago Press.

Feingold, B.F. (1975). Hyperkenesis and learning difficulties linked to artificial food flavors and colors. *American Journal of Nursing*, 75, 797-803.

Fellow-Smith, L. (2000). Impact of parental anxiety disorder on children. In P. Reder, M. McClure, and A. Jolley (Eds.), *Family matters: Interfaces between child and adult mental health* (pp. 96-106). London: Routledge.

Garralda, M.E. (2000). The links between somatization in children and adults. In P. Reder, M. McClure, and A. Jolley (Eds.), *Family matters: Interfaces between child and adult mental health* (pp. 122-134). London: Routledge.

Giggs, J.A. (1973). The distribution of schizophrenics in Nottingham. *Transactions of the Institute of British Geographers*, 59, 55-76.

Giggs, J.A. (1983). Schizophrenia and ecological structure in Nottingham. In J. Blunden and N. McGlashan (Eds.), *Geographical aspects of health* (pp. 197-222). London: Academic Press.

Giggs, J.A., and Mather, P.M. (1983). *Nottingham monographs in applied geography no. 3: Perspectives on mental health in urban areas*. Nottingham, England: Department of Geography, University of Nottingham.

Giggs, J.A. (1986). Mental disorders and ecological structure in Nottingham. *Social Science and Medicine*, 23, 945-961.

Giggs, J.A., and Cooper, J.E. (1986). Mental disorders and human ecological structure: A case study of schizophrenia and affective psychosis in Nottingham. *Cambria*, 13, 151-180.

Greenwood, C.R., Walker, H.M., Todd, N., and Hops, H. (1976). *SAMPLE: Social assessment manual for preschool Llevel*. Eugene, OR: CORBEH Center on Human Development, University of Oregon.

Griffith, D.A., Amrhein, C.G., and Desloges, J.R. (1991). *Statistical analysis for geographers*. Englewood Cliffs, NJ: Prentice Hall.

Jensen, P.S. (1991). Mental health and disorder in children and adolescents: Current status and research needs. *Family and Community Health*, 14, 1-11.

Johnson, T.I., Boutwell, C.R., and Hinkle, A.L. (1975). Community mental health center evaluation: A survey of mental health problems and professional services, *Evaluation*, 2, 18-19.

Klebanov, P.K., Brooks-Gunn, J., and McCormick, M.C. (1994). Classroom behavior of very low birth weight elementary school children. *Pediatrics*, 94, 700-708.

Kreft, I., and de Leeuw, J. (1998). *Introducing multilevel modelling*. London: Sage Publications.

Kyle, J.L. (1981). *The effect of incentives on mail survey response rate and content*. PhD Dissertation. Victoria, BC: Department of Psychology, University of Victoria.

LeClair, J.A., and Innes, F.C. (1997). Urban ecological structure and perceived child and adolescent psychological disorder. *Social Science and Medicine*, 44, 1649-1659.

LeClair, J.A. (2001). Children's behaviour and the urban environment: An ecological analysis. *Social Science and Medicine*, 53, 277-292.

Levy, L., and Rowitz, L. (1973). *The ecology of mental disorder*. New York, NY: Behavioral Publications.

Lipman, E.L., Offord, D.R., and Boyle, M.H. (1994). Relation between economic disadvantage and psychosocial morbidity in children. *Canadian Medical Association Journal*, 151, 431-437.

Lipman, E.L., Offord, D.R., and Dooley, M.D. (1996). What do we know about children from single-mother families? *Growing Up in Canada*. Ottawa: Human Resources Development Canada; Statistics Canada.

Mash, E., and Mercer, B.J. (1979). A comparison of the behavior of deviant and non-deviant boys while playing alone and interacting with a sibling. *Journal of Child Psychology and Psychiatry,* 20, 197-204.

Mausner, J.S., and Kramer, S. (1985). *Epidemiology: An introductory text.* Toronto: W.B. Saunders Company.

Max, J.E., Smith, W.L., Sato, Y., Mattheis, P.J., Castillo, C.S., Lindgren, S.D., Robin, D.A., and Stierwalt, J.A.G. (1997a). Traumatic brain injury in children and adolescents: Psychiatric disorders in the first three months. *Journal of the American Academy of Child and Adolescent Psychiatry,* 36, 94-102.

Max, J.E., Robin, D.A., Lindgren, S.D., Smith, W.L., Sato, Y., Mattheis, P.J., Stierwalt, J.A.G., and Castillo, C.S. (1997b). Traumatic brain injury in children and adolescents: Psychiatric disorders at two years. *Journal of the American Academy of Child and Adolescent Psychiatry,* 36, 1278-1285.

Max, J.E., Arndt, S., Castillo, C.S., Bokura, H., Robin, D.A., Lindgren, S.D., Smith, W.L., Sato, Y., and Mattheis, P.J. (1998). Attention deficit hyperactivity symptomology after traumatic brain injury: A prospective study. *Journal of the American Academy of Child and Adolescent Psychiatry,* 37, 841-847.

Mundy, P., Robertson, J., Greenblat, M., and Robertson, M. (1989). Residential instability in adolescent inpatients. *Journal of the American Academy of Child and Adolescent Psychiatry,* 28, 176-181.

Munro, B.H., and Page, E.B. (1993). *Statistical methods for health care research: Second edition.* Philadelphia: J.B. Lippincott Company.

Offord, D.R., Boyle, M.H., Fleming, J.E., Munroe Blum, H., and Rae Grant, N.I. (1989). Ontario Child Health Study: Summary of selected results. *Canadian Journal of Psychiatry,* 34, 483-491.

Offord, D.R., Boyle, M.H., and Racine, Y. (1989a). Ontario Child Health Study: Correlates of Disorder. *Journal of the American Academy of Child and Adolescent Psychiatry,* 28, 856-860.

Offord, D.R., Boyle, M.H., and Racine, Y. (1989b). *Ontario Child Health Study: Children at risk.* Toronto: Queen's Printer for Ontario.

Offord, D.R., and Lipman, E.L. (1996). Emotional and behavioural problems. *Growing Up in Canada: National Longitudinal Survey of Children and Youth.* Ottawa: Human Resources Development Canada; Statistics Canada.

Pakiz, B., Reinherz, H.Z., and Giacona, R.M. (1997). Early risk factors for serious antisocial behavior at age 21: A longitudinal community study. *American Journal of Orthopsychiatry,* 67, 92-101.

Shaw, G., and Wheeler, D. (1985). *Statistical techniques in geographical analysis.* New York: John Wiley and Sons.

Sheskin, I.M. (1985). *Survey research for geographers.* Washington, DC: Association of American Geographers.

Simpson, G.A., and Fowler, M.G. (1994). Geographic mobility and children's emotional/behavioral adjustment and school functioning. *Pediatrics,* 93, 303-309.

Sommerfelt, K., Troland, K., Ellertsen, B., and Markestad, T. (1996). Behavioral problems in low-birthweight preschoolers. *Developmental Medicine and Child Neurology,* 38, 927-940.

Strain, P., Steele, P., Ellis, T., and Timm, M. (1982). Long term effects of oppositional child treatment with mothers as therapists and therapist trainers. *Journal of Applied Behavior Analysis,* 15, 163-170.

Szatmari, P., Offord, D.R., and Boyle, M.H. (1989). Correlates, associated impairments, and patterns of service utilization of children with attention deficit disorder: Findings from the Ontario Child Health Study. *Journal of Child Psychology and Psychiatry,* 30, 205-217.

Szatmari, P., Saigal, S., Rosenbaum, P., Campbell, D., and King, S. (1990). Psychiatric disorders at five years among children with birthweights <1000g: A regional perspective. *Developmental Medicine and Child Neurology*, 32, 954-962.

Templer, D.I. (1992). Schizophrenia and the environment. In M.V. Hayes, L.T. Foster, and H.D. Foster (Eds.), *Community, environment and health: Geographic perspectives* (pp. 115-134). Victoria, BC: Western Geographical Press.

Waddell, C., and Shepherd, C. (2002). *Prevalence of mental disorders in children and youth*. Vancouver, BC: Mental Health Evaluation & Community Consultation Unit, University of British Columbia.

Walker, H.M., and Buckley, N. (1973). Free operant teacher attention to deviant child behavior after treatment in a special class. *Psychology in the Schools*, 8, 275-284.

Walker, H.M. (1983). *Walker problem behavior identification checklist*. Los Angeles: Western Psychological Services.

Weisglas-Kuperus, N., Koot, H.M., Baerts, W., Fetter, W.P.F., and Sauer, P.J.J. (1993). Behaviour problems of very low-birthweight children. *Developmental Medicine and Child Neurology*, 35, 406-416.

Weissman, M.M., Leckman, J.F., Merikangas, K.R., Gammon, G.D., and Prussof, B.A. (1984). Depression and anxiety disorders in parents and children. *Archives of General Psychiatry*, 41, 845-852.

Weissman, M.M., Prusoff, B.A., Gammon, G.D., Merikangas, K.R., Leckman, J.F., and Kidd, K.K. (1984). Psychopathology in children (ages 6-18) of depressed and normal parents. *Journal of the American Academy of Child Psychiatry*, 23, 78-84.

Werbach, M.R. (1991). *Nutritional influences on mental illness*. Tarzana, CA: Third Line Press.

Werbach, M.R. (1992). Nutritional influences on aggressive behaviour. *Journal of Orthomolecular Medicine*, 7, 45-51.

Zeitlin, H. (2000). Continuities of childhood disorders into adulthood. In P. Reder, M. McClure, and A. Jolley (Eds.), *Family matters: Interfaces between child and adult mental health* (pp. 21-37). London: Routledge.

Zocolillo, M., and Rogers, K. (1991). Characteristics and outcome of hospitalized adolescent girls with conduct disorder. *Journal of the American Academy of Child and Adolescent Psychiatry*, 30, 973-981.

Plate 5 "Involvement" (Ferruccio Sardella) ▶

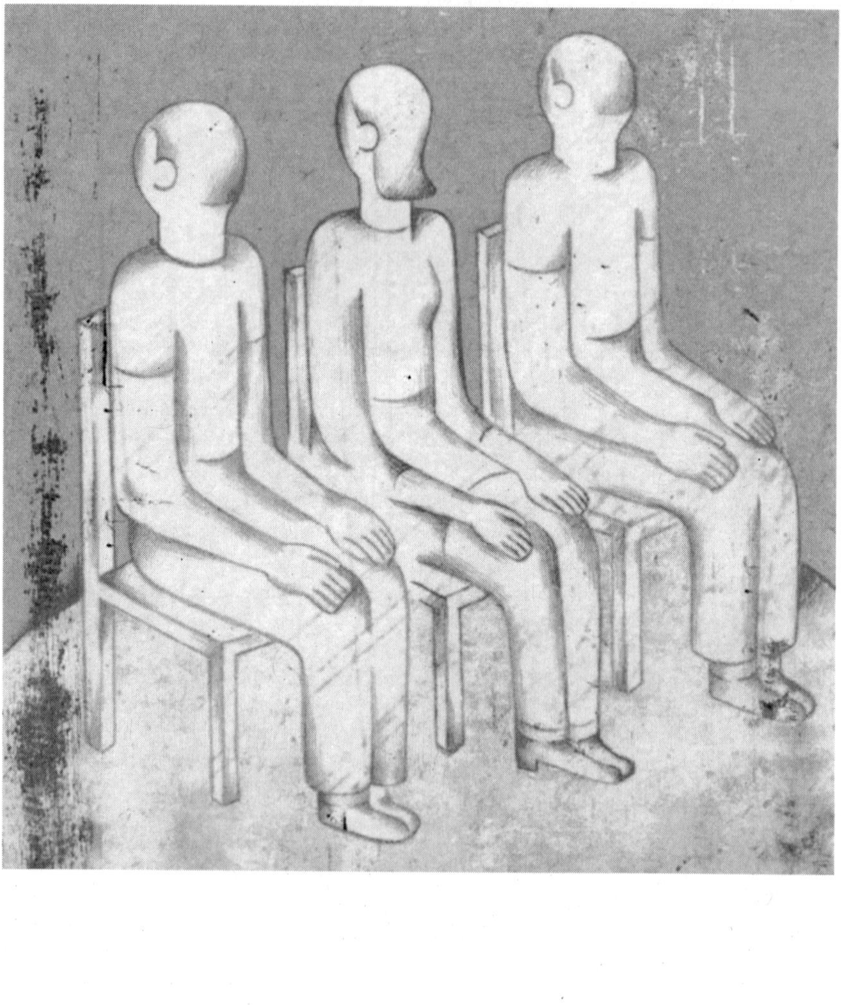

Psychosocial Influences of School Culture

Gord Miller
Centre for Community Health Promotion Research, University of Victoria

INTRODUCTION

School culture has emerged as an area worthy of research and can be attributed to changes in societal trends over the past 50 years in which schools fulfill roles previously deemed the responsibility of families and the community. Dual income and single parent families have become commonplace, distances between extended family members has increased resulting in decreased family support, and the spiritual guidance provided by churches has become less utilized. The shift away from family and community support has resulted in a focus on schools as a means of providing children and youth with "life lessons." Ministries of Education, school boards, and parents view schools as the optimal arena to develop our children and youth into informed and capable future citizens, adopting a lengthy and complex list of learning outcomes and directives that include many psychosocial aspects. Schools are now caring for children and youth by offering after school activities and programs, and providing training in career and personal planning at school on topics such as sexual health, dangers of drinking and driving, tolerance of cultural, gender, and sexuality differences, as well as other factors relating to mental well-being.

School culture affects students, staff, parents, administrators, and the community and can dramatically shape the school experience of children and youth. The following review of literature has been prepared to examine psychosocial factors that affect school culture, namely: the impact of effective leadership which embraces shared decision making, open and honest communication, and encourages community and family involvement; reducing teacher stress and providing teachers with opportunities to develop teacher collegiality and participate in professional development; having high expectations for academic achievement; ensuring equitable rules and high expectations for positive behaviour; addressing issues of violence and issues of difference; ensuring trust, sense of belonging, and emotional safety; and assessing school climate and culture.

This chapter also provides exemplars of best practices, such as the Western Australian School Health (WASH) project, involving over 70 elementary and secondary schools, trained school staff, and parents in a comprehensive approach to school health promotion. An effective survey and evaluation schemata is presented which assists practitioners and researchers in rating school culture. Recommendations include further research nationally to inform practice with evidence from schools across Canada that are currently successful and improving, and the development of a streamlined survey instrument which has the flexibility to be adapted to the local Canadian school context and maintain a balance between brevity for ease of respondents and comprehensiveness for gaining a clear understanding of a complex range of specific issues.

The relationship between the school environment and culture and the emotional well-being of young people is well documented (Bond, Glover, Godfrey, Butler, and Patton, 2001; McBride, Midford, and Cameron, 1995, 1999; Rutter, Maughan, Mortimer, Ouston, and Smith, 1979; Hargreaves, Earl, and Ryan, 1996). A positive school culture enhances young people's sense of security and trust, sense of social connectedness with teachers and peers, provides opportunities for meaningful engagement and valued participation in school life, and is related to a wide range of behavioural and mental health outcomes (Fullan, 1992; St. Leger, 1998; Salmon, James, and Smith, 1998; Lynch, 1996; House, Umgerson, and Landis, 1988). School culture is an ever-changing factor that can be a positive influence on the mental health and well-being of the learning environment or a significant barrier (Sprott, 2004). Furthermore, the impact of the school environment goes beyond that of academic achievement, with research also showing associations with adolescent health and health risk behaviours (Dykeman, Daehlin, Doyle, and Flamer, 1996; Lynch, 1996; Rutter, 1983; Vuille and Schenkel, 2001). Researchers have discovered common characteristics in schools where students report a positive school culture, including an emphasis on academic achievement, positive relationships among students and teachers, respect for all members of the school community, fair and consistent discipline policies, attention to safety issues, and family and community involvement (Dykeman et al., 1996; Griffith, 2000; Furlong and Morrison, 2000; Roach and Kratochwill, 2004). Furthermore, school culture has been identified as a key element in improving school effectiveness by a host of educational researchers (Deal and Petersen, 1994; Firestone and Wilson, 1993; Fraser and Walberg, 1991; Goodlad, 1994; Keefe and Howard, 1997; NASSP, 1996; Sashkin and Sashkin, 1993; Schmoker and Wilson, 1993; Sergiovanni, 1992, 1993; Stevens, 1990; Stolp and Smith, 1995; and Tarter et al., 1995).

This chapter firstly examines the psychosocial influences which affect school culture. Secondly, a number of approaches, programs, and strategies are considered in terms of their impact on school culture. Thirdly, examples of program innovations which support positive school culture are provided, and lastly, recommendations for future research are suggested.

DEFINITIONS OF KEY TERMS AND CONCEPTS

The purpose of providing a glossary of terms is to avoid confusion regarding terms that may be unfamiliar to readers or to clarify the usage of terms that may have multiple meanings throughout the various literatures.

School Climate

School climate refers to the perception school community members hold about the school learning environment which results from the underlying values, beliefs, and norms (Joyce and Slocum, 1990). School climate includes several key external indicators such as cohesiveness, collegiality, communication patterns, participation in decision-making, level of perceived safety, and trust. School climate is a quality of the entire school that is experienced by members, describes their collective perceptions of routine behaviour, and affects their attitudes and behavior in the school" (Hoy, Hannum, and Tschannen-Moran, 1998, p. 337).

The notion of school climate grew out of research on effective schools and is based upon the identification of a set of commonly observed internal characteristics of highly-effective schools. Descriptions of school climate, sometimes referred to as ethos, frequently include comments about the attitude or disposition of the administration, faculty, or students. Typically, school climate is measured through participant self-perceptual and/or attitudinal survey data. These data are aggregated at the school level and used to describe school values, beliefs, and processes; in fact the presence of a positive climate has itself become a widely accepted characteristic of effective schools.

School Culture

School culture is defined as the shared values, beliefs, and norms (Kilman, Saxton, and Serpa, 1985) of a school community which govern both its attitude and behaviour and which find expression through the overt and symbolic phenomena of that school community (Deal, 1993; Smircich, 1992). School culture finds expression through stated rules and policies and through artifacts such as news articles and parent newsletters. These common meanings provide an organizational identity and a framework that both motivates members of the school and helps them interpret their world (Denison, 1990).

"School culture is the underground stream of norms, values, beliefs, traditions, and rituals that has built up over time as people work together, solve problems, and confront challenges" (Peterson and Deal, 1998, p. 28).

School culture refers to what people believe, the assumptions they make about how schools work and what they consider to be true and real (Sergiovanni, 1996), and the way people do things (Barth, 2002; Bower, 1996; Deal and Peterson, 1999). School culture describes the holistic activities and ways of being and doing of those who work in or participate on a regular basis within a school. This is an organizational approach, which sees each individual school as having a unique and distinctive ethos or personality, comprised of the collective expressions of members of the school organization (Owens, 2001).

School Community

School community is a "collection of individuals who are bonded together by natural will and who are together bound to a set of shared ideas and ideals" (Sergiovanni, 1996, p. 48). School community of an individual school is composed of the various stakeholders that are involved with the function of that school, including the parents, teachers, students, administrators, and public and private sector community groups of the specific locale.

For the purpose of this chapter we have elected, for the most part, to utilize the term school culture to avoid confusion over the terms school culture and school climate. The rationale is that both concepts share a similar research problem and overlapping boundaries of the two concepts make a clear separation difficult. In addition, researchers who avoid expending energy differentiating between 'culture' and 'climate' will avert the intellectual fatigue that many scholars experience in this area and will focus more beneficially on the core problem of improving school effectiveness (Deal, 1995; Denison, 1990; Stolp and Smith, 1995).

PSYCHOSOCIAL FACTORS INFLUENCING SCHOOL CULTURE

There are signs that health and education agendas are converging (Patton et al., 2003) in an effort to counteract the negative impact on the mental health and well-being of youth, many of whom experience alienation and disengagement as they transition to middle and secondary schools (Hargreaves et al., 1996; Withers and Russell, 1998). In their 15,000-hour study, Rutter and co-workers (1979) concluded that differences in schools largely relate to a school's characteristics and culture, not the intake of students.

In a Canadian study, Wendel (2000) summarizes ineffective schools as having the following: lack of vision; unfocused leadership; dysfunctional staff relations; and, ineffective classroom practice. The literature identifies the importance of school culture, stating that researchers believe the culture of a school is often underestimated, overlooked, or ignored (Angelides and Ainscow, 2000; Barth, 2002). As a consequence, school improvement initiatives usually fail to reach maximum potential. Therefore, leaders must first devote extensive time and effort to assessing, shaping, and sustaining a healthy school culture before they can truly expect initiatives to reach maximum potential (Angelides and Ainscow, 2000; Deal and Peterson, 1999; Zmuda, Kukulis, and Kline, 2004).

This chapter reviews the current literature pertaining to psychosocial factors influencing school culture. These factors can serve to assist school learning communities in identifying aspects of school culture which may be in need of improvement.

Impact of Leadership

The impact of effective leadership in guiding and influencing psychosocial factors to positively influence school culture is well documented in the literature (Wendel, 2000; Stoll and Fink, 1996, 2001; Ginder, 2005; Fullan, 2002; Kotter, 2002; Uchiyama and Wolf, 2002).

In his comprehensive review, Ginder (2005) found that researchers have recently concluded that school leadership is a major influence on the school culture, stating that principals need to set an effective, as well as an affective course for the school. Principals who address the many factors affecting school culture improve the overall mental health outlook of all its members (Vuille and Schenkel, 2001). Kotter (2002) stated that a leader is so important that the winning process is 80% leadership and 20% other factors. The principal's greatest challenge and responsibility is to develop a caring community in the school, a place where strong character emerges from shared purpose that allows and encourages students to be successful learners (Sergiovanni, 1999; Furlong and Morrison, 2000). Bolman and Deal (2002) also believe in a shared purpose, saying that this starts with leaders who articulate their own beliefs and orchestrate a dialogue about mission and values. As noted by Flemming (2003), in a Canadian study, Hajnal, Walker, and Sackney (1998) surveyed 377 teachers in 93 Saskatchewan schools and found that those in which principals visited teachers in classrooms were more effective and successful in implementing the province's school improvement program.

Educational reformers affirm the importance of a principal's role in school improvement and change efforts (Deal and Peterson, 1999; Lambert, 2002; Leithwood and Jantzi, 2000; Senge et al., 2000; Sergiovanni, 1992; Southwest Educational Development Laboratory, 1997). Researchers continue to assert that the success of school improvement initiatives is dependent on the existence of a healthy school culture. Thus, principals must acknowledge culture as the most crucial aspect behind change and school improvement initiatives. Such initiatives need to support the behavioural and mental health outcomes of students by building a school culture which enhances a sense of belonging, including more supportive relationships with teachers, opportunities and skills to make a valued contribution to school life, a sense of security, and the availability of close and positive relationships (Hargreaves et al., 1996).

Principals effectively consult with others by involving the faculty and other groups in the school decision process. This process allows teachers to feel they are genuinely encouraged to exchange ideas and share a commitment to the academic mission of the school, as well as support the operation of the school (Sashkin and Sashkin, 1993; Stolp and Smith, 1995; Dalin, 1993; Covey, 1990).

Leadership which leads to improvement in the quality of the social environment has the capacity to influence mental health in a variety of ways. For example, students with strong social ties build a stronger self concept and sense of belonging and they tend to handle social stressors better (Heaney, 1997).

Ginder (2005) states that administrators effectively and efficiently mobilize resources such as materials, time, and support to enable the school and its personnel to most effectively meet academic goals. In addition, administrators need to recognize time as a scarce resource and create order and discipline by minimizing factors that may disrupt the learning process.

Teacher Stress

Teaching today is very stressful. One of the main causes of stress is the inability to direct stress toward a solution, which leads to energy loss (Ginder, 2005; Graves 2001). Three factors that drain energy according to Graves were (a) lack of control over time and space, (b) lack of support from administrators, and (c) difficult children.

Bluestone (2004) implied that a high level of teacher dissatisfaction with accountability processes is reflected in widespread reports of teacher stress, anxiety, and resentment. Additionally, Tye and O'Brien (2002) stated that the "main reason teachers leave the profession is the increased pressures from accountability" (p.24). Accountability is too often seen as synonymous with student performance on a single set of standardized tests and rarely measures realistic criteria. Reeves (2004) explains that teachers know that their jobs are far more complex than what can be measured on a single test. They resent the notion that the curriculum, energy, and attention to student needs can be summed up with a single number. There is growing evidence documenting that it is possible to raise standardized test scores quickly under high stakes accountability systems.

According to Farber (1991), what is most troubling to teachers is their feeling that society expects them to educate, socialize, and graduate virtually every student who comes to school, regardless of the social, economic, familial, or psychological difficulties some students bring with them. For many teachers, the public cry for accountability is no more than a more sophisticated way of expecting schools and teachers to cure all the ills of society. Nagel and Brown (2003) stated that one-third of all teachers would not enter the field of teaching if they had an opportunity to choose again, and 30% of novice teachers exit the profession prior to their fifth year.

Swick (1989) believed teacher stress might be related to poor psychological climate, ineffective leadership, and inadequate support staff resources. Other stressors mentioned were scheduling conflicts, constant interruptions of classroom teaching, excessive paperwork, lack of support from administrators, and excessive work demands. Also highlighted were new training requirements, increased job responsibilities, and the fact that the profession is under rapid change. Cox and Brockley (1984) concluded that "work appears as a major source of stress for working people, with teachers appearing to experience more stress through work than non-teachers" (p.84).

High Expectations for Academic Achievement

Saphier and King (1985) identify high expectations as an essential element of school culture which encourages excellence in teaching and learning (Barnett and McCormick, 2003). High expectations are representative of the following behaviours: a commitment to professionalism, a belief that all students could and should be given the opportunity to reach their potential, and a commitment to improvement in teaching and learning. Researchers have identified higher levels of student achievement when expectations are high (Barnett and McCormick, 2003; Saphier and King, 1985) and the focus is on academics (Hoy, Tarter, and Kottkamp, 1991, Licata and Harper, 1999; Hammun and Hoy, 1997).

Almeida (2005) states that teachers' perceptions of the health of their school strongly correlate with the measured, observed degree of organizational health within the school (Hoy et al., 1991, as cited in Licata and Harper, 1999; Hoy and Tarter, 1997, as cited in Licata and Harper, 1999). Their findings also suggest that healthy and robust schools are likely to be characterized by a dominant organizational theme emphasizing students' academic achievement.

Licata and Harper (1999) state: "When such a theme is in place, teachers feel that they are working in an unusual, challenging, important, meaningful, action-packed and powerful school environment. This emphasis on academics probably provides collective organizational meaning about purposes and a vehicle for integrating the behavior and sentiments of school administrators, teachers and students" (p. 473).

Equitable Rules and High Expectations for Positive Behaviour

School culture is strongly affected by the behaviour of all members of the school environment, who in turn are influenced by the related factors of attitude, feeling, and behaviour of individuals within the school system (Sherman, 1997). Welsh (2000) states that school culture is affected by "the unwritten beliefs, values, and attitudes that become the style of interaction between students, teachers, and administrators." He goes on to say that school culture sets the parameters of acceptable behaviour among all school actors, and it assigns individual and institutional responsibility for school safety.

Dorsey (2000) views school culture as involving four key relationships: a student to him or herself; a student to his or her peers; a student to his or her parents and community; and a student to his or her school workers, including teachers, administrators, and all staff.

Behaviour of students is influenced by the behaviour of adults in the school community, which ultimately reflects on school culture. Monitoring and modelling of positive behaviour by adults not only includes classroom situations, but also activities occurring at other times of day, such as recess, lunch hours, extra-curricular activities, sports and intramurals, and in places such as the cafeteria, school grounds, and the hallways. Welsh (2000) campaigns for a system where all members of the school understand which behaviours are acceptable and which are not. In addition, parameters of positive behaviour should be defined within the code of conduct and rules. Rules need to address areas like the fair treatment of others, standards of dress, physical touch, what teasing and joking is acceptable, and the consequences for transgressions of these behaviours. Rules need to be clear and fair and should be enforced consistently (Adams, 2000; Furlong and Morrison, 2000; Gottfredson, 1989; Sherman et al., 1997; Remboldt, 1994; Welsh, 2000). Further, codes of student conduct should set unambiguous and high expectations for student behaviour and should also specify the consequences for violations of the code clearly, in writing, providing specific procedures to be followed in the case of a violation (Cloud, 1997).

Issues of Violence

Welsh (2000) looked at the effects of school culture on school disorder and found major factors related to high levels of victimization including school size, inadequate resources for teaching, poor teacher-administration cooperation, inactive administrations, and punitive attitudes on the part of teachers.

Hernandez (2004) states that a major factor in the development of a safe school culture is the development of a clear definition of school violence. Remboldt (1994) asserts that such a definition must be clear, all-encompassing, and universally acceptable so that all students and educators can understand, accept, and use it to identify or recognize violent incidents. Remboldt (1994) goes on to explain that the absence of such a definition of violence in schools severely impairs the ability to create a safe school culture. A consensus agreement regarding the definition of violence determines the presence or lack and degree of acceptability or unacceptability of violence (Howell and Hawkins, 1998). Hernandez (2004) asserts that defining the parameters of acceptable behaviour is the responsibility of the entire school community. He suggests that students, faculty, staff, administration, parents, community members, and the school board should all be involved in this process. Even support personnel such as bus drivers, lunchroom attendants, crossing guards, and maintenance staff have a stake in the process of defining what is violence and what is acceptable behaviour.

Positive peer relationships can reduce disruptive or violent behaviours (Dykeman, Daehlin, Doyle, and Flamer, 1996; Nims, 2000); thus, it is important for students to develop strong interpersonal relationships with peers (Griffith,

2000) and adults (Furlong and Morrison, 2000). Locus of control refers to "an individual's expectations of ability to control his or her experiences" (Dykeman et al., 1996, p. 38). Dykeman and co-workers found an external locus of control, lack of empathy, and impulsivity to be antecedents to violent behaviour in schools. They argue that schools need to stimulate an internal locus of control in their students. Thus, student responsibility and an internal locus of control need to be encouraged (Baker, 1998) as a support of a safe school culture.

Levels of Communication and Cooperation

The way schools are run influences the school culture. The administration sets the tone for the kind of communication and cooperation that occurs in schools. Fostering "an atmosphere of inclusiveness, open communication, and shared decision-making on safety and other important issues with students, staff, and parents" (p. 159) is crucial to school culture (Anderson, 1998). For example, in a review of studies that examined school culture, Sherman and co-workers (1997) concluded that "schools in which the administration and faculty communicate and work together to plan for change and solve problems have higher teacher morale and less disorder" (p. 5). High morale among staff and students also contributes to effective schooling (Furlong and Morrison, 2000). While the administration sets the tone, all school members have an impact on the level of communication and cooperation within the school.

Issues of Difference

Difference refers to individual characteristics that impact how one experiences the world and how one is perceived and treated by others and society at large. This includes, but is not limited to, race, ethnicity, gender, sexual orientation, religion/spirituality, ability, weight and physical size, and national origin. All members of a school have the right to feel safe regardless of difference.

Kuperminc and co-workers (1997) examined the nature of the social culture of schools and how it is linked to student adjustment in an ethnically and socio-economically diverse middle school (ages 10-16). They found that a number of variables are linked to student risk for maladjustment. Those variables might include ethnic minority status, family poverty, and household composition. The authors stated that ethnic minorities may be at a greater risk of externalizing and internalizing school problems and failure. Interventions may be needed to increase a mutual understanding of the culturally linked expectations that teachers and students have about appropriate behaviour in the school setting (Zimmerman, Khoury, Vega, Gil, and Warheit, 1995). Similarly, psychological variables such as exposure to stressful events, academic self concept, self worth, and academic performance are linked to student risk for maladjustment and these can contribute to differing student perceptions of school culture (Kuperminc, Leadbeater, Emmons, and Blatt, 1997).

Rituals, Traditions, and Celebrations

Peterson and Deal (1998) suggest that traditions and rituals are an important part of a school's culture. In a study of 12 schools in Ontario, Leithwood and Jantzi (1990) concluded that using symbols and rituals to celebrate and recognize the work of the staff and students fostered a healthy culture. Dinham and co-workers (1995) found that recognition of work and achievement is essential to both effective leadership and a healthy school culture. Blase and Blase (2000) conducted a study on instructional leadership, specifically on teachers' perspectives on how principals promote teaching and learning in schools. They found that giving praise affected teacher motivation, self-esteem, and efficacy. It also fostered teacher reflective behaviour, including reinforcement of effective teaching strategies, risk taking, and innovation/creativity.

APPROACHES, PROGRAMS, AND STRATEGIES THAT IMPACT SCHOOL CULTURE

Building Capacity for Leadership and Building a Learning Community

Creating a Horizontal Stratification for Leadership

In a Canadian study, Mitchell and Sackney (2001) argued that school leadership is "better served by horizontal stratification than by vertical" (p. 7).

> In other words, hierarchical levels are reduced and power is dispersed throughout the school in that kind of arrangement, administrators serve facilitative functions rather than control functions, and performance appraisal ensues from a developmental perspective rather than an evaluative one. Leadership is also dispersed throughout the school, with different individuals taking on leadership roles in different situations. This kind of ubiquitous power and leadership serves to facilitate work rather than control people (Mitchell and Sackney, 2001, p. 7).

They went on to argue that

> This approach to power and leadership implies the development of a community of leaders. By this, we mean a condition whereby individuals feel a deep sense of empowerment and autonomy and a deep personal commitment to the work of the school (Mitchell and Sackney, 2001, p. 7).

Beck and Foster (1999) suggested that educational leaders have the opportunity to put in place conditions that "have the potential to harness forces within schools so that teachers, parents, students, and others from the outside world can begin to experience and enjoy community" (p. 350).

Professional Development

There is overwhelming agreement in the literature that professional learning, although not a magic bullet, is directly and persistently linked to educational improvement and school development (Bredeson and Scribner, 2000; Campos, 1993; Fullan, 1982, 1991; Louis, Toole, and Hargreaves; Putnam and Borko, 1997; Tschannen-Moran, 2001).

Within a positive school culture, the learning of the teachers is as important as that of the children. Stamps (1998), for example, indicates that one of the greatest surprises of recent years for human resource officers has been the notion of "informal workplace learning as a social phenomenon: the idea that humans learn within work-based groups called communities of practice" (p. 36). Sergiovanni (2001) positions that the development of a learning community comes about through the interplay among personal abilities, interpersonal relationships, and organizational structures. Growth occurs as personal, interpersonal, and organizational capacities increase; it is limited as they decrease.

Building personal capacity consequently entails searching one's professional networks to identify new and different ideas. Strong ties are likely to be forged when individuals spend considerable time together, when they participate in emotional or deeply engaging activities, when they share common knowledge, and when they receive mutual rewards (Mitchell and Sackney, 2001; Lick, 2000).

The processes of collective reflection and professional conversation engage educators in critical dialogue about the actions, behaviours, craft, and art of professional practice (Louis, Marks, and Kruse, 1999; Bryk, Lee, and Holland, 1993; Youngs and King, 2002). They also argue that releasing teachers from their isolation can be regarded as beneficial to supporting teacher collegiality.

According to Isaacs (1999), dialogue includes the skills of listening, respecting, suspending, and voicing. These skills provide the necessary safety for the deep disclosure and critical talk that characterize a learning community.

Mitchell and Sackney (2001) believe that too often educators and parents have said that classroom time cannot be sacrificed for professional development. The authors suggest enabling structures for professional development for teachers include (but are not limited to) collective reflection meetings, problem-solving think tanks, formal opportunities for collaboration, connections to educational research and development, and networking.

One way to keep the collaborative focus on teaching and learning is to institute a database approach to professional discourse (Hannay and Ross, 1997). In this approach, teams collect extensive and intensive data on a multitude of indicators, not the least of which are student retention, student achievement, student interest, and student perception measures. Data also can be collected from colleagues, parents, community members, other educators, or anyone else who might have a stake in a particular educational experience; data can be collected in relation to educational, social, financial, and political conditions.

Hargreaves (1993) warns that individualism and solitude also need to be embraced, even in the midst of community and collaboration. Organizational capacity is about building a system that invests heavily in professional learning and relationship building (Haskins, Liedtka, and Rosenblum, 1998). At the school level, it means placing "professional development at the core of teacher work to ingrain the value of continuous professional learning throughout teachers' careers" (Scribner, 1999, p. 261).

Teacher Collegiality

Teacher collegiality, as indicated by frequent communication and mutual support, is a strong indicator of implementation success; this has been validated by nearly every research study on this topic (Schmoker, 1996). In a school culture that "values collegiality and collaboration, there is a better climate for the social and professional exchange of ideas, the enhancement and spread of effective practices, and widespread professional problem solving" (Deal and Peterson, 1999; Hoffman, Sabo, Bliss, and Hoy, 1994).

Teachers stimulate, inspire, and motivate each other to contribute and implement best ideas, and best ideas mean greater overall coherence (Sergiovanni, 2001; Wolf, Borko, Elliot, and McIver, 2000; Uchiyama and Wolf, 2002). Supportive collegial interaction for sharing instructional strategy and developing learning goals was identified as a major construct associated with the operation of an effective school (Dalin, 1993; Keefe and Howard, 1997; NASSP, 1996; Schmoker and Wilson, 1993; Stolp and Smith, 1995; Sweeney, 1992). Gains in student achievement, higher quality solutions to problems, and increased confidence among school members have been attributed to positive levels of collegiality (Schmoker and Wilson, 1993). Collegiality also aids in strengthening cultural cohesion because collegial relationships make it likely that commonalities will be emphasized (Hannum and Hoy, 1997; Firestone and Wilson, 1985).

Kruse, Louis, and Bryk (1995) listed five structural conditions that must be present in schools to give rise to teacher community: 1) time to meet and talk; 2) physical proximity; 3) interdependent teacher roles; 4) communication structures; and 5) teacher empowerment and school autonomy (p.2). In addition, they noted five social and human resources that enhance professional community. They are: 1) openness to improvement; 2) trust and respect; 3) cognitive and skill base; 4) supportive leadership; and 5) socialization (Kruse, Louis, and Bryk, 1995, pp. 2-3). They argued that the social and human resources are more important than the structural conditions when building teacher collegiality toward a positive school climate (Kruse, Louis, and Bryk, 1995, p. 3).

Shared Decision-Making and Supportive Leadership

A recent Canadian study (Foster and St. Hilaire, 2003) suggests that "leadership that fosters successful schooling is a shared professional responsibility that involves skill and co-ordination of administrative goals, and teaching and learning goals" (p. 13). Foster and St. Hilaire (2003) drew upon the extensive review of literature conducted by Crowther and co-workers (2002) to suggest that both teacher and administrative leadership are critical to school success.

This is further supported in a 3-year longitudinal study by Johnson and Pajares (1996), who note that shared decision making results in "new voices speaking up and being heard, the breaking down of barriers of authority and of isolation, and changes in teacher beliefs and attitudes" (p. 623).

Campo (1993) found that sharing in the decision-making process gives teachers a greater feeling of ownership, which is essential for school improvement. When involved, teachers are also motivated and committed to their shared school vision. Attention must be given to roles in decision making and increased opportunities for meaningful, collective participation in the critical areas that likely determine the organizational goals (Campo, 1993).

According to Covey (1990), all of the stakeholders in the learning environment have their own contribution to make and a responsibility to be part of the decision-making process. Participation in decision making by the members of the school community has been consistently found to have a positive correlation to effectiveness in school settings (Bolman and Deal, 1991; Howard, Howell, and Brainard, 1987; NASSP, 1996; Stevens, 1990; Stolp and Smith, 1995; Sweeney, 1992).

Dinham and co-workers (1995) state that principals need to recognize the efforts and achievements of others, embrace the process of shared decision making, facilitate problem solving, and develop informal and formal avenues of communication. Clearly, such attributes exemplify shared/supportive leadership behaviour.

"It is not only the formal leadership of the principal that sustains and continuously reshapes culture but the leadership of everyone. Deep, shared leadership builds strong cohesive cultures" (Deal and Peterson, 1999, p. 87). Such leadership is also known as transformational leadership in which the purpose and vision serve the common good, meet the needs of the followers, and elevate them to a higher moral level (Burns, 1978, as cited in Sergiovanni, 1996). Fullan (2001) notes, "good leaders foster good leadership at other levels. Leadership at other levels produces a steady stream of future leaders for the system as a whole" (p. 10).

Trust, Sense of Belonging, and Emotional Safety

Trust

Trust and respect from colleagues, parents, and the school community as a whole is essential to the establishment of an effective school community (Barth, 2002; Deal and Peterson, 1999; Kruse and Louis, 1998; Senge, 2000; Sergiovanni, 1996). Trust is also a crucial ingredient of collegiality because it enhances a sense of loyalty, commitment, and effectiveness necessary to maintain a shared focus on students (Hoy, et al., 1996, as cited in Hoy and Hannum, 1997; Kruse and Louis, 1998).

"Increasingly, trust is seen as a vital element in well functioning organizations," creating greater levels of communication (Tschannen-Moran, 1998, p. 334). Evans (1997) found that offering teachers opportunities to collaborate with superiors and colleagues about teaching and learning builds a level of comfort and trust and relationships are fostered. Members learn to trust one another by discussing, debating, encouraging, sharing, helping, and, most importantly, adding to their knowledge base through nurturing each other's ideas (Evans, 1997; Wignalf, 1992, as cited in Hord, 1997). Such behaviour in a school community is exemplified by colleagues reviewing one another's teaching practices (Kruse and Louis, 1995; Hord, 1997).

Sweeney (1992) surveyed 600 schools and found that trust, the belief that people are fair and honest, is a prerequisite for positive action and change. Group effectiveness develops from openness and trust, which is a prerequisite for successful change (Dalin, 1993). Trust is also necessary to develop a climate for successful shared decision-making and it is the key to effective working relationships among school staff (Stolp and Smith, 1995). Consequently, school relationships that are built on trust help to develop cohesion (Stockard and Mayberry, 1992).

Data from a study of 2,777 middle school teachers indicated that principal behaviour of support toward staff developed and promoted the level of trust in the school (Tartar, Sabo, and Hoy, 1995). Lack of trust inhibits collaboration, risk taking, and school improvement, and reduces the efficient operation of a school (Schmoker and Wilson, 1993).

Building a Sense of Belonging and Emotional Safety

Hargreaves, Earl, and Ryan (1996) suggested that "one of the most fundamental reforms needed in secondary or high school education is to make schools into better communities of caring and support for young people" (p. 77). Osterman (2002) argued that school culture is not present until members experience feelings of belonging, trust in others, and safety (p. 167). According to Osterman (2002), the "need for relatedness involves the need to feel securely connected with others in the environment and to experience oneself as worthy of love and respect" (p. 167). Belonging evokes emotions of happiness, elation, contentment, and calm (Osterman, 2002, p. 168).

When contemplating the notions of school culture and school community, there is a discussion about listening to a common voice or the "collective we" of commonly held beliefs (Sergiovanni, 1994), and considering a community of difference (Fine, Weis, and Powell, 1997; Furman, 1998; Shields and Seltzer, 1997; Shields, 2002). Shields stated that school communities of difference will move away from basing what they do on traditions, stereotypes, or unchallenged assumptions about their members; rather, they will emerge through carefully seeking out, and listening to, the various voices of those who, together, make up each school community. This is particularly important in a country like Canada, where we embrace multiculturalism and seek

Psycho-Social Influences of School Culture

to support a diverse student body whose members may represent the various sociocultural and economic factions from the wider community (Shields, 2002, p.197).

Numerous researchers have expressed the importance of emotional safety in creating a positive school culture (Wood, 1998; Bluestein, 2001; Goleman, Boyatzis, and McKee, 2002; Ginnis, 2002). Bluestein (2001, p. 10) suggested that students in emotionally safe schools experience all of the following:

1. A sense of belonging, of being welcomed and valued; being treated with respect and dignity; acceptance.
2. The freedom to not be good at a particular skill, make mistakes, forget, or need additional practice and still be treated respectfully and with acceptance.
3. Encouragement and success; recognition; instruction, guidance and resources according to need and regardless of need.
4. Having one's own unique talents, skills, and qualities valued, recognized, and acknowledged.
5. Understanding and clarity (about requirements and expectations); predictability (consistency of follow-through); freedom from arbitrary, indiscriminate, and unexpected punishment and reactivity.
6. The freedom from harassment, intimidation (including labelling, name-calling, ridicule, teasing, criticism, or contempt), and threat of physical harm from adults or peers.
7. The freedom to make choices and influence one's own learning, pursue personal interests, and control various factors in the process of learning (such as content, presentations, media, and location; social context; direction; specific assignments or approaches) based upon personal needs and preferences.
8. The freedom from prejudice, judgment, and discrimination based on: physical characteristics and general appearance; religion, race, or cultural background; sexual orientation.
9. The freedom from prejudice, judgment, and discrimination based on academic, athletic, creative, or social capabilities; modality or learning-style preferences and temperament.
10. The freedom to have (and express) one's own feelings and opinions without fear of recrimination.

Managing Change

Chenoweth and Everhart (2002) assert that healthy organizations encourage and support a diversity of information to be gathered and shared throughout the organization where all organizational members have access to critical information and have the opportunity to use the information to make decisions.

Dinham and co-workers (1995) conducted in-depth case studies on three secondary schools and identified that principals need to be a source, facilitator and conduit for both formal and informal communication within and without the school. Short and co-workers (1994) noted similar findings in their study of school climate, that communication must flow across all boundaries and in all directions, including dialogue both within the school and outside the school. Both studies found that a variety of communication means must be employed to support the necessary flow of information (Dinham, Cairney, Craigie, and Wilson, 1995; Short, Greer, and Melvin, 1994).

School leaders must structure the communication process if it is to reach the level of effectiveness needed to achieve consensus. Several important features are: a) communication that is free of domination by any single group; b) provides equal access to all members; and c) is genuinely open and expressive (Heckman, 1993).

Principals spend 70-80% of their day in oral communication (Deal and Petersen, 1993), thus they are the central communicators of the school climate and culture and have hundreds of interactions every day (Firestone and Wilson, 1993). Each of these interactions is an opportunity to develop, promote, or reinforce key school values. When competing points of view or values are in conflict, principals are in an advantageous position to resolve the situation in a positive way because they control the communication resources of the school and can provide sanctions and rewards for behaviour (Sergiovanni, 1996).

Open and Honest Communication

Understanding change cultivates change, innovation, and improvement in schools (Tobergte and Curtis, 2002). The process begins with relationships built upon trust, time spent together, and respect and passion for each child. This process moves forward based on knowledge, research, and experience, and is driven by data (Tobergte and Curtis, 2002). Fundamental change often involves altering the school's culture. This essential transformation is an inherently slow process (Patterson, Purkey, and Parker, 1986; Boyd, 1992). Due to the fact that the change process takes time, it creates temporary chaos and is uncomfortable (Tobergte and Curtis, 2002). It is important to remember that the major impediment to successful change is that people may understand and accept change but lack the skills and ability to carry out the new plan (Boyd, 1992). In order to change the culture, educational leaders must understand the core values and beliefs that provide both direction and stability (Piperato and Roy, 2002).

Family and Community Involvement

For more than 30 years, studies have shown that when parents are involved at home and at school, their children are more successful and stay in school longer and often the school improves (Jordan and Rodriguez, 2004). Henderson and Mapp (2002) looked in depth at 51 recent research studies published between 1995 and 2002 to identify evidence that could support efforts to design and implement family and community connections leading to increased student success and positive school culture. They found that when schools, families, and community groups work together to support learning, children tend to be more successful in school, stay in school longer, and adapt to school more readily. The studies reviewed suggest that parent and community involvement was linked to higher student grade point averages, enrolment in more challenging academic programs, better attendance, improved behaviour at home and at school, and better social skills (Henderson and Mapp, 2002). What is important for parents, teachers, and administrators to know is that according to the studies, this relationship holds across families of all economic, racial/ethnic, and educational backgrounds and for students of all ages, including secondary students. Although there is less research available on the effects of community involvement, study results suggest benefits from community involvement for schools, families, and students including improved achievement and behaviour (Henderson and Mapp, 2002).

Assessing School Climate and Culture

Measuring and studying school culture is a difficult task. It is nonetheless crucial in informing students, parents, and school professionals as to their efforts in creating an optimal learning environment for students. Numerous empirical assessment instruments have been developed and administered, each with a specific purpose, in school systems to include the following: Organizational Climate Description Questionnaire (Halpin and Croft, 1962, as cited in Webb and Norton, 2003); The High School Characteristics Index (Stern, 1964, as cited in Webb and Norton, 2003); The Purdue Teacher Opinionaire (Bentiey and Rempel, 1980, as cited in Webb and Norton, 2003); The CFK Ltd. "School Climate" Profile (Phi Delta Kappan, 1973, as cited in Webb and Norton, 2003); The Harrison Instrument for Diagnosing Organizational Ideology (Harrison, 1985, as cited in Webb and Norton, 2003); Organizational Health Inventory (Hoy, Tarter, and Kottkamp, 1991); Organizational Climate Description Questionnaire - Revised (Hoy, Tarter, and Kottkamp, 2000); School Climate and Context Inventory (Bobbett and French, 1991); Group Openness and Trust Scale (Bulach, 1993); Tennessee School Climate Inventory (Butler and Albery, 1991); and Comprehensive Assessment of School Environments (National Association of Secondary School Principals, 1987).

In many cases, both corporate organizations and schools (Richardson, 2001; Webb and Norton, 2003) have taken an informal approach, developing their own assessment tools to analyse their culture. Due to the uniqueness of each school's culture, the lack of resources, and the issues of ensuring an assessment tool is reliable and valid, many researchers advocate for such an approach

(Center for School Improvement, 2002; Miller, 2003; Peterson, 2004; Richardson, 2001; Masden and Wagner, 2000).

In order to conduct a thorough and credible assessment of an organization's culture, a multifaceted, qualitative and quantitative approach must be taken (Center for Improving School Culture, 2002; Miller, 2003). In addition, the data collected should be triangulated. To ensure the data collected can be triangulated through both qualitative and quantitative measures, assessors must consider gathering data through each of the following: survey(s), interviews, observations, and reviewing school documents (Center for Improving School Culture, 2002; Miller, 2003; Richardson, 1998). Furthermore, it is important that essential elements of a healthy school culture be identified prior to selecting the strategy and tools to conduct an assessment. In doing so, the essential elements will determine appropriate strategies and assessment tools (Miller, 2003; Peterson, 2004; Richardson, 2001).

EXAMPLES OF PROGRAM INNOVATIONS AND A DATA MEASURING TOOL

Successful School Improvement in United Kingdom and Canada

Harris (2000) discusses the Improving the Quality of All Project (IQEA) in the United Kingdom and the Manitoba School Improvement Program (MSIP) in Canada, which have both demonstrated considerable success in their work with schools (Earl and Lee, 1998; Hopkins and Harris, 1997). These projects are well known within the international research community and provide a basis for comparing what works in different countries and in contrasting educational contexts. The IQEA model of school improvement is based upon a fundamental belief in the relationship between teachers' professional growth and school development.

The MSIP differs from the IQEA in that it pre-dated government reform aimed at schools, it originated from an independent charitable foundation, it draws more upon the professional knowledge of teachers than on the expertise of academics, and its focus is exclusively on high school reform in the province in contrast to the IQEA's national and international activity. Projects are defined locally by the school improvement team. Some schools have focused on curriculum reforms (e.g., improving participation rates and marks for girls and young women in mathematics and science), others on personal and social development (e.g., personalizing the high school through models of schools within schools', and teacher advisory groups), while others have focused on school improvement processes. Whatever the focus, attention is given to the potential of the project to engage the whole school community in a dialogue on improvement and to pay particular attention to supporting "students at risk."

Harris (2000) explains that multi-year funding is provided ($10,000 - $30,000 per year for 3 to 5 years) to support teachers in taking coordinating roles and allowing teachers time during the school day to work together in teams, to visit other schools, and engage in other related professional development activities. Each school had access to the Manitoba-based MSIP staff, who provided a readily available source of expertise on school-based change and the measurement of improvement, as well as an external source of accountability. In addition, all schools participated in a provincial MSIP network of educators that provided a support structure for professional growth and risk-taking.

Harris (2000) states that the process of school improvement remains a 'black box' for many school improvement projects. Clearly, this is a difficult area to traverse, as there are no universals, no recipes for success. However, both the IQEA and the MSIP are able to articulate the process of change and to provide concrete examples of what the improvement process looks like in action. Some common features of effective school improvement emerge from this analysis. In both programs, the emphasis is upon teaching and learning developmental goals. In the MSIP, teachers spend a great deal of time refining their goals and developing a related evaluation strategy. Each of the projects has a set of related goals directly related to improving student learning outcomes, and systems in place for recording change and progress in these areas.

The twin processes of formative and summative evaluation are evident and transparent within all IQEA and MSIP schools. The feedback loop provided by formative evaluation mechanisms enables teachers to take stock of innovation and development. This allows changes to be made using data to inform development. Similarly, external evaluation procedures allow for a check on the program and provide data that allows judgements to be made about the impact of the program as a whole. The emphasis placed on internal and external evaluation in both projects establishes enquiry and reflection as central to school development.

The CATCH Program

Parcel and co-workers (2003) studied the effectiveness of school culture on the institutionalization of the Child and Adolescent Trial for Cardiovascular Health program (CATCH). CATCH was the largest field trial of school-based health promotion in the US. It was conducted in 96 schools in four geographic areas. Data were collected from classroom teachers, physical education specialists, food services workers, and administrators through two different school climate questionnaires that measured principal and teacher behaviour (42 item questionnaire), organizational health (37 item questionnaire), principal/teacher openness, and school health composite scores. The study included 56 intervention schools and 40 control schools. This study demonstrated that interventions that help schools maintain and institutionalize a health promotion program may be more effective if they take into consideration the school culture and address those aspects that may not support continued implementation of an innovative program. Findings demonstrate that practitioners can use instruments to assess the organizational climate to evaluate the readiness of the school to implement and sustain an innovative program. Following this evaluation, they can then initiate interventions to help the schools develop more supportive cultures before investing time and resources to implement a program that might not be sustained. Once an innovative program has been implemented, assisting the school in addressing and maintaining a supportive culture could also improve the sustainability of a program.

The Gatehouse Project

Bond and co-workers (2001) presented program evaluation findings of the Gatehouse Project, a comprehensive approach to mental health promotion in secondary schools. This intervention is based on an understanding of individual and social risk processes for adolescent depression and emotional well-being. The focus ranges from aspects of the school's social environment and school culture (e.g., conflict, bullying, isolation, and alienation) to aspects of an individual's cognitive and social skills. Young people who experience difficulties in their social interactions and are exposed to adverse environments are at higher risk of experiencing emotional difficulties. Furthermore, those students who are socially isolated are more likely to engage in health risk behaviours. The conceptual framework of the project emphasizes the importance of applying an ecological approach and of healthy attachments (sense of positive connection with teachers and peers). The project has identified three priority areas for action: building a sense of security and trust, enhancing skills and opportunities for good communication, and building a sense of positive regard through valued participation in aspects of school life. The intervention is a multilevel strategy designed to promote change in the school climate, in the social and learning environments of the school, and at an individual level. The strategy seeks to make changes in the schools' social and learning environments and school culture, to introduce relevant and important skills through the curriculum, and to strengthen the structures within the school that promote links between the school and its community. The project evaluation used a cluster-randomized controlled trial design involving 26 schools. Analysis of data from field notes, key informant interviews, and school background audits revealed that the major elements that contributed to system changes within the schools and positive school culture were feedback of the school social climate profile, establishment of the adolescent health teams, input of the critical friend, and identification of appropriate intervention strategies for each school.

The WASH Project

McBride, Midford, and Cameron (1999) studied the effects of the Western Australian School Health (WASH) project. This project involved over 70 elementary and secondary schools, trained school staff and parents in school health promotion, provided access to central health/educational professionals, and provided time for school-based representatives to plan and implement school health promotion activity. The model used in the WASH project is loosely based on Kolbe's (1986) model 'School Health Promotion Components and Outcomes' and also draws on systems theory related to school organizational change and enhancing school climate. The key components of the WASH model include:

1. *School Health Education* — curriculum, health teaching, teacher training, resources

2. *School Physical Education* — curriculum, sport, daily physical activity

3. *School Health Environment* — physical environment, policies, and procedures

4. *School Nutrition and Food Service* — healthy canteen or food service, healthy fundraising, healthy food eating incentives/competitions

5. *School Health Services* — access to nurse, dental hygienist, vaccinations, screenings

6. *School Counselling Services* — pastoral care, counselling support

7. *School Staff Health Promotion Activities* — healthy food options, personal health information, regular physical activity opportunities at work

8. *Integrated School and Community Health Promotion Activities* — school links with school agencies and professionals, involvement with the local and extended community

9. *Parental Involvement* — extending the time and effort dedicated to health promotion by alleviating some tasks of school staff and by providing alternative areas of health related expertise (i.e., parents as helpers/organizers, training in health promotion, parents as school health promotion planners, parent group funding health promotion activity)

10. *School Health Management* — organizational support plays a vital role in extending the time and scope of school health promotion activity (i.e., providing an adequate budget, personnel, and resources for school health promotion, training staff, and the school's planning, review, and evaluation processes of health promotion activities).

SUMMARY

Societal trends are resulting in communities and families being less able to support children and youth because of work commitments, distances separating family members, less involvement of churches, and the influence of mass media. To bridge this gap, schools are adding emotional, physical, and vocational training to their academic curriculae. This has put a great deal of pressure on teachers and requires an administrative style that builds trust, open communication, and shared leadership at all levels, and invests in teachers' professional development and collegiality, as well as celebrates success. These complex psychosocial factors of school culture have been presented along with evidence to improve school effectiveness in a way that positively affects the mental well-being of students, staff, administrators, parents, and the community. Given the constant change and innovation that occurs within the educational system, the practical exemplars provided within the chapter and recommendations for further research and evaluation are timely.

RECOMMENDATIONS FOR FUTURE RESEARCH

The research clearly demonstrates that building an effective school culture is beneficial to all members of the local school community. In 2003, the Learning Commission in Alberta released its report that included reference to the importance of school environment and culture in improving effectiveness and creating a learning community. This shows the importance and timeliness of this literature review and also the need for further Canadian research in this area.

The following recommendations are based on gaps in the literature and the critical need for further research pertaining to both a Canadian and local school context:

1. Conduct a national study following up on the 1995 investigation of what makes a school successful, commissioned by the Canadian Federal Government. The new study would inform practice with evidence from schools across Canada that are currently successful and improving. The scope would be broadened to a whole school "settings approach" by measuring the perception of culture and the importance of culture in the school environment of students, teachers, administrators, and parents, along with local community groups. In addition, a comparative study between the school administrator and teacher perceptions dealing with the major factors of school culture would be measured. Key factors could be determined that lead to a positive school climate where students experience academic and social success, where teachers find challenging, rewarding work, and parents and the community are meaningfully involved.

2. Development of a streamlined survey instrument which has the flexibility to be adapted to the local Canadian school context and maintains a balance

between brevity for ease of respondents and comprehensiveness for gaining a clear understanding of a complex range of specific issues. In addition, this survey tool needs to be user friendly and include perspectives from staff, students, parents, and community groups.

3. Conduct a longitudinal study of school culture to document intended and unintended cultural changes occurring in schools over time. This research would inform practice of the links between school culture and school effectiveness and improvement.

4. Study the applicability of Schoen's Schematic Framework as a guide to support Canadian schools in defining and conceptualizing school culture's impact on school improvement efforts and its use as an evaluation tool (Table 7.1).

In conclusion, research needs to be supported that illuminates how different elements or factors (i.e., cultural cohesion, collegiality, positive communication, participatory decision-making, safety, trust, etc.) facilitate a positive school culture within a Canadian and local school context. In addition, research efforts need to investigate a whole school or systems approach and the relative effects of various levels of the system (staff relations; school, parent, and community links; administrative leadership; school district and Ministry of Education policy, etc.) in order to yield valuable results in shaping policy and practice and thus improving the quality of school cultures within Canada. Finally, much can be gained by examining findings from best and promising practices, along with province-wide assessments of what is working and what is not.

Table 7.1 Schematic framework for examining factors which influence school culture (Schoen, 2005)

I. Professional Orientation	II. Organization Structure
• Formal goals/plan for improvement • Instructional support available for teachers • Staff attitude/teacher efficacy regarding professional growth, and change • The extent of professional inquiry and problem solving • Degree of collegiality and teamwork in instructional planning • Focused on-going professional development for teachers • Mentoring of new teachers • Individual teachers involved routinely in reflective practice, and personalized professional growth	• Principal leadership style • Informal leadership and communication structure • School policies, procedures, rules, routines, traditions • Internal accountability norms • Implementation of external policies • Shared sense of mission, faculty cohesion • Vehicles for involvement of multiple stakeholders • Formal support structures for change • Formal structure for problem solving and conflict resolution
III. Quality of the Learning Environment	IV. Student-Centred Focus
• All students routinely involved in higher order thinking • Student assessment practices reflect school goals, teacher objectives and student needs • Learning activities require active involvement of students and have value beyond school • Multiple modes of learning activities and assessments are used • Student involvement and learning is effectively monitored • Interdisciplinary approach to curriculum, with occasional teaming of teachers/classes • Curriculum meets state standards and provides for student exploration of personal interests • Students work in non-static groups on co-operative projects • Teachers maintain a report with parents and communicate frequently	• Mechanism exists for identifying student needs, and providing interventions on an individual has is • School sponsored support services are provided for students and families • Student motivation / academic futility addressed • School-wide approach to student discipline emphasizes personal responsibility and achievement • Active involvement of parents is sought • Formal recognition of student achievement • Emphasis on standards based instruction is balanced with a mutual focus on individualization and well-being of students • Scheduling reinforces the development of personal relationships between students, and among students and teachers

REFERENCES

Adams, T. (2000). The status of school discipline and violence. *Annals of the American Academy of Political and Social Sciences*, 567, 140-156.

Almeida, M. (2003). School culture survey. Unpublished manuscript.

Angelides, P., and Ainscow, M. (2000). Making sense of the role of culture in school improvement. *School Effectiveness and School Improvement*, 11(2), 145-163.

Anderson, D.C. (1998). Curriculum, culture and community: The challenge of school violence. In M. Tonry and M. Moore (Eds.), *Youth violence* (pp. 317-363). Chicago: University of Chicago Press.

Baker, J. (1998). Are we missing the forest for the trees? Considering the social context of school violence. *Journal of Social Psychology*, 36, 29-44.

Barnett, K., and McCormick, J. (2003). Vision, relationship, and teacher motivation: A case study. *Journal of Educational Administration*, 41(1), 55-73.

Barth, R. (2002). The culture builder. *Educational Leadership*, 59(8), 6.

Beck, L.G., and Foster, W. (1999). Administration and community: Considering challenges, exploring possibilities. In J. Murphy and K.S. Louis (Eds.), *Handbook of research on educational administration* (2nd ed.) (pp. 337-358). San Francisco: Jossey-Bass.

Binda, K. (2001). Decentralization and the development of an aboriginal education system: New genesis. In K. Binda and S. Calliou (Eds.), *Aboriginal education in Canada: A study in decolonization* (pp. 35-58). Mississauga, ON: Canadian Educators' Press.

Blasé, J., and Blasé, J. (2000). Effective instructional leadership: Teachers' perspectives on how principals promote teaching and learning in schools. *Journal of Educational Administration*, 38(2), 130-141.

Bluestein, J. (2001). *Creating emotionally safe schools: A guide for educators and parents.* Deerfield Beach, FL: Health Communications.

Bluestone, J. (2004). Acountability for teachers and schools. *http://www.handle.org/miscinfo/account.html*. Accessed February 2007.

Bobbett & French, 1992 School Climate and Context Inventory

Bobbett, G., and French, R. (1991) *Assessing school climate*. Paper presented at the Annual Meeting of the Mid-South Educational Research Association, November 12-15, 1991.

Bolman, L., and Deal, T. (1991). *Reframing organizations*. San Francisco: Jossey-Bass.

Bolman, L., and Deal, T. (1992). The organization as theatre. In H. Tsoukas (Ed.), *New thinking in organizational behaviour* (pp. 104-107). Oxford, UK: Butterworth-Heineman, Ltd.

Bolman, L., and Deal, T. (1994). *Becoming a teacher leader. From isolation to collaboration*. Thousand Oaks, CA: Corwin Press.

Bolman, L., and Deal, T. (2002). *Reframing the path to school leadership: A guide for teachers and principals*. Thousand Oaks, CA: Corwin Press.

Bond, L., Glover, S., Godfrey, C., Butler, H., and Patton, G.C. (2001). Building capacity for system-level change in schools: Lessons from the Gatehouse Project. *Health Education & Behavior*, 28(3), 368-383.

Bower, M. (1996). *Will to manage*. New York: McGraw-Hill

Boyd, V. (1992). School context: Bridge or barrier to change. Southwest Educational Development Laboratory. *http://www.sedl.org/change/school/*. Accessed February 2007.

Bredeson, P.V., and Scribner, J.P. (2000). A statewide professional development conference: Useful strategy for learning or inefficient use of resources? *Educational Evaluation and Policy Analysis*, 8(13). Online: *http://epaa.asu.edu/epaa/v8n13.html*. Accessed February 2007.

Bryk, A.S., Lee, V.E., and Holland, P.B. (1993). *Catholic schools and the common good.* Cambridge, MA: Harvard University Press.

Bryk, A.S., and Schneider, B. (2002). *Trust in schools: A core resource for improvement.* New York: Russell Sage Foundation.

Bulach, 1993 Group Openness and Trust Scale

Butler, E.D., and Alberg, M.J. (1991). *The Tennessee School Climate Inventory: Resource Manual.* Memphis, TN: Center for Research in Educational Policy, The University of Memphis.

Caldwell, B. (1998). Strategic leadership, resource management and effective school reform. *Educational Leadership,* 36(5), 445-461.

Campo, C. (1993). Collaborative school cultures: How principals make a difference [Electronic version]. *School Organization,* 13(2), 119.

Chavre, E.W., Cummins, C., and Wood, F. (1996). A middle approach to developing an effective school work culture. *National Association of Secondary School Principals Bulletin,* 80, 43-49.

Center for Improving School Culture (2002). Bowling Green, KY. Retrieved March 20, 2004 from *http://www.schoolculture.net/schoeye.html.*

Chenoweth, T.G., and Everhart, R.B. (2002). *Navigating comprehensive school change: A guide for the perplexed.* Larchmont, NY. *http://www.eyeoneducation.com.*

Cloud, R. (1997). *Solutions for youth violence for schools and communities: Resource guide.* Waco, TX: Health EDXO, a division of WRS Group.

Corson, D. (1999). Community-based education for indigenous cultures. In S. May (Ed.), *Indigenous community-based education* (pp. 8-19). North York, ON: Multilingual Matters Limited.

Corwin, R.G., and Borman, K.M. (1988). The school as a workplace: Structural constraints on administration. In N.J. Boyan (Ed.), *Handbook of research on educational administration* (pp. 209-237). New York: Longman.

Covey, S.R. (1990). *Principle-centered leadership.* New York: Summit Books.

Cox, T., and Brockley, T. (1984). The experience and effects of stress in teachers. *British Educational Research Journal,* 10(1), 83-87.

Crowther, F., Kaagan, S., Ferguson, M., and Hann, L. (2002). *Developing teacher leaders: How teacher leadership enhances school success.* Thousand Oaks, CA: Corwin Press.

Dalin, P. (1993). *Changing the school culture.* London: Cassell Publishing.

Deal, T. (1993). The culture of schools. In M. Sashkin and H.J. Wahlberg (Eds.) *Educational leadership and school culture* (pp. 85-95). Berkeley, CA: McCutchan Publishing.

Deal, T. (1995). Symbols and symbolic activity. In S.B. Bacharach and B. Mundell (Eds.), *Images of schools. Structures and roles in organizational behavior* (pp. 108-136.) Thousand Oaks, CA: Corwin Press

Deal, T.E., and Petersen, K.D. (1993). Strategies for building school cultures: Principals as symbolic leaders. In M. Sashkin and H. Wahlberg (Eds.), *Educational leadership and school culture* (pp.85-95). Berkeley, CA: McCutchan Publishing.

Deal, T.E., and Petersen, K.D. (1994). *The leadership papadox. Balancing logic and artistry in schools.* San Francisco: Jossey-Bass Publishers.

Deal, T.E., and Petersen, K.D. (1999). *Shaping school culture: The heart of leadership.* San Francisco: Jossey-Bass.

Denison, D.R. (1990). *Corporate culture and organizational effectiveness. The Wiley Series on Organizational Assessment and Change.* New York: John Wiley & Sons.

Dinham, S., Cairney, T., Craigie, D., and Wilson, S. (1995). School climate and leadership: Reseach into three secondary schools. *Journal of Educational Administration,* 33(4), 36-58.

Dorsey, J. (2000). Institute to End School Violence. Online: *http://www.endschoolviolence.com/strategy/*.

Dufour, R. (1999). Help wanted: Principals who can lead professional learning communities. *National Association of Secondary School Principals Bulletin*, 83(604), 12-17.

Dykeman, C., Daehlin, W., Doyle, S., and Flamer, H.S. (1996). Psychological predictors of school-based violence: Implications for school counselors. *The School Counselor*, 44, 35-47.

Earl, L., and Lee, L. (1998). *Evaluation of the Manitoba School Improvement Program*. Winnipeg: Manitoba School Improvement.

Evans, M. (1997). Shifting the leadership focus from control to empowerment: A case study. *School Leadership and Management*, 17(2), 273.

Farber, B. (1991). *Crisis in education*. San Francisco: Jossey-Bass Publishers.

Fine, M., Weis, L., and Powell, L.C. (1997). Communities of difference: A critical look at desegregated spaces created for and by youth. *Harvard Educational Review*, 67, 247-284.

Firestone, W.A., and Wilson, B.L. (1993). Bureaucratic and cultural linkages: Implications for the principal. In M. Sashkin and H. Wahlberg (Eds.), *Educational leadership and school culture* (pp. 85-95). Berkeley, CA: McCutchan Publishing.

Fleming, T. (1997). Provincial initiatives to restructure Canadian school governance in the 1990s. *Canadian Journal of Educational Administration and Policy*, 11, November 28.

Fleming, T., and Raptis, H. (2003). Reframing education: How to create effective schools. Commentary – C.D. Howe Institute, Issue 188.

Foster, R., and Goddard, T. (2003). Leadership and culture in schools in northern British Columbia: Bridge building and/or re-balancing act? *Canadian Journal of Educational Administration and Policy*, 27, July 25.

Foster, R., and St. Hilaire, B. (2003). Leadership for school improvement: Principals' and teachers' perspectives. *International Electronic Journal for Leadership and Learning*, 7(3). http://www.ucalgary.ca.

Friesen, J., and Friesen, V. (2002). *Aboriginal education in Canada: A plea for integration*. Calgary, AB: Detselig Enterprises Limited.

Fraser, B.J., and Walberg, H.J. (1991). *Educational environments. Evaluation, antecedents, and consequences*. Oxford, England: Pergamon Press

Fullan, M. (1982, 1991). *The meaning of educational change*. NY: Teachers College Columbia University.

Fullan, M. (1992). *The new meaning of educational change*. NY: Teachers College Columbia University.

Fullan, M. (2002). The change leader. *Educational Leadership*, 59(8), 16-20.

Furlong, M., and Morrison, G. (2000). The school in school violence: Definitions and facts. *Journal of Educational and Behavioral Disorders*, 8, 71-82.

Furman, G.C. (1998). Postmodernism and community in schools: Unraveling the paradox. *Educational Administration Quarterly*, 34(2), 298-328.

Ginder, D.L. (2005). *The impact of school climate on success*. A dissertation submitted to the faculty of Immaculata University.

Ginnis, P. (2002). *The teacher's toolkit: Raise classroom achievement with strategies for every learner*. Williston, VT: Crown House.

Goleman, D., Boyatzis, R., and McKee, A. (2002). *Primal leadership: Learning to lead with emotional intelligence*. Boston: Harvard Business School Press.

Goodlad, J. (1994). *Educational renewal. Better teachers, better schools.* San Francisco: Jossey-Bass Publishers.

Gottfredson, D. (1989). Developing effective organizations to reduce school disorder. In O. Moles (Ed.), *Strategies to reduce student misbehavior* (pp. 87-104). Washington, DC: Office of Educational Research and Improvement. (ERIC Document Reproduction Service No. ED 311 608).

Graves, D. (2001). *The energy to teach.* Portsmouth, NH: Heinemann.

Griffith, J. (2000). School climate as group evaluation and group consensus: Student and parent perceptions of the elementary school environment. *The Elementary School Journal*, 101(1), 35-61.

Hajnal, V., Walker, K., and Sackney, L. (1998). Leadership, organizational learning, and selected factors relating to the institutionalization of school improvement initiatives. *The Alberta Journal of Educational Research*, XLIV(1), 70-89.

Hammun, J., and Hoy, W. (1997). Middle school climate: An empirical assessment of organizational health and student achievement [Electronic Version]. *Educational Administration Quarterly*, (33)3, 290.

Hannay, L.M., and Ross, J.A. (1997). Initiating secondary school reform: The dynamic relationship between restructuring, reculturing, and retiming. *Educational Administration Quarterly*, 33 (Supplement), 576-603.

Hargreaves, A. (1993). Individualism and individuality: Reinterpreting the teacher culture. In J.W. Little and M.W. McLaughlin (Eds.), *Teachers' work: Individuals, colleagues, and contexts* (pp. 51-76). New York: Teachers College Press.

Hargreaves, A. (1994). *Changing teachers changing times: Teachers' work and culture in the post modern age.* London: Cassell.

Hargreaves, A., Earl, L.M., and Ryan, J. (1996). *Schooling for change: Reinventing education for early adolescents.* London: Falmer Press.

Harris, A. (2000). Successful school improvement in United Kingdom and Canada. *Canadian Journal of Educational Administration and Policy*, 15, April 13.

Haskins, M.E., Liedtka, J., and Rosenblum, J. (1998). Beyond teams: Toward an ethic of collaboration. *Organizational Dynamics*, 26(4), 34-50.

Heaney, C.A., and Israel, B.A. (1997). Social networks and social support. In K. Glanz, F.M. Lewis, and B.K. Rimer (Eds.), *Health behaviour and health education: Theory, research and practice* (pp. 179-205). San Fransisco: Jossey-Bass.

Heckman, P. (1993). School restructuring in practice: Reckoning with the culture of the school. *International Journal of Educational Reform*, 2(3), 263-272.

Henderson, A., and Mapp, K.L. (2002). *A new wave of evidence: The impact of school, family, and community connections on student achievement.* Austin, TX: National Center for Family and Community Connections with Schools.

Hernandez, T.J. (2004). A safe school climate: A systematic approach and the school counselor. *Professional School Counseling*, 7(4), 257.

Hoffman, J., Sabo, D., Bliss, J., and Hoy, W. (1994). Building a culture of trust. *Journal of School Leadership*, 4(5), 484-501.

Hopkins, D., and Harris, A. (1997). Improving the quality of education for all. *Support for Learning*, 12(4), 147-151.

Hord, S.M. (1992). *Facilitative leadership: The imperative for change.* Austin, TX: Southwest Educational Development Laboratory (SEDL).

Hord, S.M. (1997). *Professional learning communities: Communities of continuous inquiry and improvement.* Austin: Southwest Educational Development Laboratory.

House, J.S., Umgerson, D., and Landis, K.R. (1988). Structures and processes of social support. *Annual Review of Sociology*, 14, 293-318.

Howard, E., Howell,B., and Brainard, E. (1987). *Handbook for conducting school improvement projects*. Bloomington, IN: The Phi Kappa Delta Foundation.

Howell, J.C., and Hawkins, F.D. (1998). Prevention of youth violence. In M. Torry and M.H. Moore (Eds.), *Youth violence* (pp. 263-315). Chicago: The University of Chicago Press.

Hoy, W., Tarter, C.J., and Kottkamp, R.B. (1991). *Open schools/healthy schools: Measuring organizational climate*. Newbury Park, CA: Sage Publications.

Hoy, W.K., Sabo, D., and Barnes, K. (1996). Organizational health and faculty trust: A view from the middle level. *Research in Middle Level Education Quarterly*, 19, 21-39.

Hoy, W.K., and Hannum, J.W. (1997). Middle school climate: An empirical assessment of organizational health and student achievement. *Educational Administration Quarterly*, 33, 290-311.

Hoy, W., Hannum, J., and Tschannen-Moran, M. (1998). Organizational climate and student achievement: A parsimonious and longitudinal view. *Journal of School Leadership*, 8, 337.

Isaacs, W. (1999). *Dialogue and the art of thinking together*. New York: Doubleday.

Isbister, W. (2002). A piece of the pie: The inclusion of aboriginal pedagogy into the structures of public education. In L. Stiffarm (Ed.), *As we see...Aboriginal pedagogy* (pp. 77-85). Saskatoon, SK: University of Extension Press.

James, C. (1999). Culture, multiculturalism and the ideology of integration. In C. James (Ed.), *Seeing ourselves: Exploring race, ethnicity, and culture* (pp. 193-217). Toronto: Thompson Educational Publishing.

Johnson, M., and Pajares, F. (1996). When shared decision-making works: A 3-year longitudinal study. *American Educational Research Journal*, 33(3), 599-627.

Joyce, W.F., and Slocum, J.W. Jr. (1990). Strategic context and organizational climate. In B. Schneider (Ed.), *Organizational climate and culture* (pp. 130-150). San Francisco: Jossey-Bass.

Jull, S. (2000). Youth violence, schools, and the management question: A discussion of zero tolerance and equity in public schooling. *Canadian Journal of Educational Administration and Policy*, 17, November 30.

Kanu, Y. (2001). In their own voices: First Nations students identify some cultural mediators of their learning in the formal school system. *Alberta Journal of Educational Research*, 68(2), 98-121.

Keefe, J.W., and Howard, E. (1997). *Redesigning schools for the new century: A systems approach*. Reston, VA: National Association of Secondary School Principals.

Keefe, J.W., and Howard, E. (1997). The school as a learning organization. *National Association of Secondary School Principals Bulletin*, 80(589), 35-44.

Kilman, R., Saxton, M., and Serpa. R. (EDS.) (1985). *Gaining control of the corporate culture*. San Francisco: Jossey-Bass Publishers.

Kotter, J. (2002). *The heart of change*. Boston: Harvard Press.

Kruse, S., and Louis, K. (1998). Creating the conditions of empowerment: Resilient teachers and resilient students. *Research/Practice*, 6(1). http://education.umn.edu/CAREl/Reports/Rpractice/Fall98/empowerment.html.

Kruse, S., Louis, K., and Bryk, A. (1995). Building professional community in schools. http://www.learner.org/channel/workshops/principals/materials/pdf/kruse.pdf.

Kuperminc, G.P., Leadbeater, B.J., Emmons, C., and Blatt, S.J. (1997). Perceived school climate and difficulties in the social adjustment of middle school students. *Applied Developmental Science*, 1, 76-88.

Lambert, L. (2000). Framing reform for the new millenium: Leadership capacity in schools and districts. *Canadian Journal of Educational Administration and Policy*, 14, April 12.

Lambert, L. (2002). A framework for shared leadership. *Educational Leadership*, 59(8), 37-40.

Leithwood, K., and Jantzi, D. (1990). Transformational leadership: How principals can help reform school culture. Paper presented at the annual meeting of the *American Educational Research Association*.

Leithwood, K., and Jantzi, D. (2000). Principal and teacher leadership effects: A replication. *School Leadership and Management*, 20(4), 415-434.

Licata, J.W., and Harper, G.W. (1999). Healthy schools, robust schools and academic emphasis as an organizational theme. *Journal of Educational Administration*, 37(5), 463-475.

Lick, D. (2000). Whole-faculty study groups: Facilitating mentoring for school-wide change [Electronic Verions]. *Theory into Practice*, 39(1), 43.

Louis, K.S., Marks, H., and Kruse, S. (1996). Teachers' professional community in restructuring schools [Electronic Verions]. *American Education Research Journal*, 33(4), 757-798.

Louis, K.R., Toole, J., and Hargreaves, A. (1999). Rethinking school improvement. In K. Seashore-Louis and J. Murphy (Eds.), *Handbook of research on educational administration* (pp. 251-276). San Francisco: Jossey-Bass.

Lynch, Y. (1996). *Preventing violence in secondary schools and community action for full service schools: Making it work*. Sydney: Australian Centre for Equity through Education.

Marks, H., and Louis, K.S. (1999). Teacher empowerment and capacity for organisational learning. *Educational Administration Quarterly*, 35(5), 707-750.

Masden, P., and Wagner, C. (2004). School culture triage. Issaquah, WA: National School Improvement Project and Gary Phillips. http://www.Garyphillips.com

McBride, N., Midford, R., and Cameron, I. (1999). An empirical model for school health promotion: The Western Australian school health project model. *Health Promotion International*, 14(1), 17-25.

Miller, K. (2003). Assessing your institution's culture. The RMA Journal, 86(4), 32. http://www.rmahq.org/News_PR/Features/feat1_12_04.htm.

Mitchell, C., and Sackney, L. (2001). Building capacity for a learning community. *Canadian Journal of Educational Administration and Policy*, 19, February 24.

Nagel, L., and Brown, S. (2003). The abc's of managing teacher stress. *The Clearing House*, 76(5), 255.

Nash, J.K. (2002). Neighborhood effects on sense of school coherence and educational behavior in students at risk of school failure. *Journal of Children and Schools*, 24(2), 73-89.

National Association of Secondary School Principals (1987). *Assessment of School Environments*. Reston, VA: NASSP

National Association of Secondary School Principals (1996). *Breaking ranks: Changing an American Institution*. Reston, VA: NASSP.

Nims, D.R. (2000). Violence in our schools: A national crisis. In D.S. Sandhu and C.B Aspy (Eds.), *Violence in American schools: A practical guide for counselors* (pp. 3-20). Alexandria, VA: American Counselling Association.

Osterman, K. (2000). Students' need for belonging in the school community. *Review of Educational Research*, 70(3), 323-367.

Osterman, K. (2002). Schools as communities for students. In G. Furman (Ed.), *Schools as community: From promise to practice* (pp. 143-163). New York: State University of New York Press.

Owens, R. (2001). *Organizational behavior in education: Instructional leadership and school reform*. Needham Heights, MA: Allyn & Bacon.

Parcel, G.S., Perry, C.L., Kelder, S.H., Elder, J.P., Mitchell, P.D., Lytle, L.A., Johnson, C.C., and Stone, E.J. (2003). School climate and the institutionalization of the CATCH Program. *Health Education and Behavior*, 30(4), 489-502.

Patterson, J., Purkey, S., and Parker, J. (1986). *Productive school systems for a nonrational world.* Alexandria, VA: Association for Supervision and Curriculum Development.

Patton, G., Bond, L., Butler, H., and Glover, S. (2003). Changing schools, changing health? Design and implementation of the Gatehouse Project. *Journal of Adolescent Health*, 33(4), 231-239.

Peterson, K. (2004). *Personal interview*. Marborough, MA.

Peterson, K., and Deal, T. (1998). How leaders influence the culture of schools. *Educational Leadership*, 56(1), 28-30.

Piperato, D., and Roy, J. (2002). Transforming school culture. http://www.iirp.org/library/mn02/mn02_roypip.html.

Reeves, D. (2004). *Accountability for learning: How teachers and school leaders can take charge.* Alexandria, VA: Association for Supervision and Curriculum.

Remboldt, C. (1994). *Solving violence problems in your school: Why a systematic approach is necessary.* Minneapolis, MN: Johnson Institute.

Richardson, J. (1998). *Student learning grows in professional cultures. Tools for Schools.* Oxford, OH: National Staff Development Council. http://www.nsdc.org/library/publications/tools/8-98lead.cfm.

Richardson, J. (2001). *Educator, know thyself. Tools for Schools.* Oxford, OH: National Staff Development Council. http://www.nsdc.org/library/publications/tools/tools5-01rich.cfm.

Roach, A., and Kratochwill, T. (2004). Evaluating school climate and school culture. *Teaching Exceptional Children*, 37(1), 10.

Rutter, M. (1983). School effects on pupil progress: Research findings and policy implications. *Child Development*, 54, 1-29.

Rutter, M., Maughan, B., Mortimer, P., Ouston, J., and Smith, A. (1979). *Fifteen thousand hours: Secondary schools and their effects on children.* London: Falmer.

St. Leger, L. (1998). Australian teachers' understanding of the health promoting school concept and the implications for the development of school health. *Health Promotion International*, 13, 223-236.

Salmon, G., James, A., and Smith, D.M. (1998). Bullying in schools: Self reported anxiety, depression and self esteem in secondary school children. *British Medical Journal*, 317, 924-925.

Saphier, J., and King, M. (1985). Good seeds grow in strong cultures. *Educational Leadership*, 42(6), 67-74.

Sashkin, M., and Sashkin, M.G. (1993). Principals and their school cultures: Understanding from quantitative and qualitative research. In M. Sashkin and H. Walberg (Eds.), *Educational Leadership and school culture* (pp. 101-120). Berkeley, CA: McCutchan Publishing.

Schmoker, M.J. (1996). *Results: The key to continuous school improvement.* Alexandria, VA: Association for Supervision and Curriculum Development.

Schmoker, M.J., and Wilson, R.B. (1993). *Total quality education – Profiles of schools that demonstrate the power of Derning's management principles.* Bloomington, ID: Phi Delta Kappa Educational Foundation.

Schoen, L. (in press). *Conceptualizing, describing, and comparing school cultures: A comparative case study.* Lanham, MD: University Press of America.

Scribner, J.P. (1999). Professional development: Untangling the influence of work context on teacher learning. *Educational Administration Quarterly*, 35(2), 238-266.

Senge, P., Cambron-McCabe, N., Luca, T., Smith, B., Dutton, J., and Kleiner, A. (2000). *Schools that learn*. New York: Doubleday.

Sergiovanni, T. (1992). *Moral leadership. Getting to the heart of school improvement*. San Francisco: Jossey-Bass.

Sergiovanni, T. (1993). New sources of leadership authority. In M. Sashkin and H. Walberg (Eds.), *Educational leadership and school culture* (pp. 70-73). Berkeley, CA: McCutchan Publishing.

Sergiovanni, T. (1994). *Building community in schools*. San Francisco: Jossey-Bass.

Sergiovanni, T. (1996). *Leadership for the schoolhouse*. San Francisco: Jossey-Bass.

Sergiovanni, T.J. (2000). Leadership as stewardship. In The Jossey-Bass Reader on *Educational Leadership*. New York: John Wiley and Sons, Inc.

Sergiovanni, T.J. (2001). *Leadership: What's in it for schools?* London: Routledge.

Sergiovanni, T.J. (2005). *The principalship: A reflective practice perspective* (5th ed.). Needham Heights, MD: Allyn and Bacon.

Sherman, L.W., Gottfredson, D., MacKenzie, D., Eck, J., Reuter, P., and Bushway, S. (Eds.) (1997). *Preventing crime: What works, what doesn't, what's promising*. Washington, DC: US Department of Justice, Office of Justice Programs.

Shields, C.M. (2002). Learning from educators: Insights into building communities of difference. In G. Furman (Ed.), *School as community: From promise to practice* (pp. 143-163). New York: State University of New York Press.

Shields, C.M., and Seltzer, P.A. (1997). Complexities and paradoxes of community: Toward a more useful conceptualization of community. *Educational Administration Quarterly*, 33(4), 413-439.

Short, P., Greer, J., and Melvin, W. (1994). Creating empowered schools: Lessons in change. *Journal of Educational Administration*, 32(4), 38-52.

Smircich, L. (1983). Organization as shared meanings. In J. Shafritz and J.S. Ott (Eds.) (1992). *Classic of organization theory* (3rd ed.). Belmont, CA: Wadsworth Publishing Company.

Smith, M. (2001). Relevant curricula and school knowledge: New horizons. In K. Binda and S. Calliou (Eds.), *Aboriginal education in Canada: A study in decolonization* (pp. 77-88). Mississauga, ON: Canadian Educators' Press.

Southwest Educational Development Laboratory (1997). Assessing a school staff as a community of professional learners. Retreived October 5, 2002 from http://www.sedl.org/change/issues/issues71/welcome.html.

Sprott, J. (2004). The development of early delinquency: Can classroom and school climates make a difference? *Canadian Journal of Criminolgy & Criminal Justice*, 46(5), 553.

Stamps, D. (1998). Learning ecologies. *Training*, 35(1), 32-38.

Stevens, M.P. (1990). School climate and staff development: Keys to school reform. *National Association of Secondary School Principals Bulletin*, 74(529), 66-70.

Stockard, D.J., and Mayberry, M. (1992). *Effective educational environments*. Newbury Park, CA: Corwin Press, Inc.

Stoll, L., and Fink, D. (1996). *Changing our schools*. Philadelphia: Open University Press.

Stolp, S., and Smith, S.M. (1995). *Transforming school culture: Stories, symbols, values, and the leader's role*. Eugene, OR: Clearinghouse on Educational Management, U. of Oregon.

Sweeney, J. (1992). School climate: The key to excellence. *National Association of Secondary School Principals Bulletin*, 76(547), 69-73.

Swick, K.J. (1989). *Stress and the classroom teacher: What research says to the teacher*. Washington, DC: National Education Association.

Tarter, C.J., Sabo, D., and Hoy, W.K. (1995). Middle school climate, faculty trust and effectiveness: A path analysis. *Journal of Research and Development in Education*, 29(1), 41-49.

Tobergte, D., and Curtis, S. (2002). There is a crisis! And failure is not an option. *Education*, 122(4), 770-777.

Tschannen-Moran, M. (1998). Trust in schools: A conceptual and empirical analysis. *Journal of Educational Administration*, 36(4), 334-352.

Tschannen-Moran, M. (2001). Collaboration and the need for trust. *Journal of Educational Administration*, 39(4), 308-331.

Tye, B., and O'Brien, L. (2002). Why experienced teachers are leaving the profession. *Phi Delta Kappan*, 84(1), 24.

Uchiyama, K., and Wolf, S. (2002). The best way to lead them. *Educational Leadership*, 59(8), 80.

Vuille, J., and Schenkel, M. (2001). Social equalisation in the health of youth: The role of the school. *European Journal of Public Health*, 11, 287-293.

Webb, D., and Norton, S. (2003). *Human resources administration: Personal issues and needs in education*. Upper Saddle River, NJ: Pearson Education.

Weber-Pillwax, C. (1999). Indigenous research methodology: Exploratory discussion of an elusive subject. *Journal of Educational Thought*, 33(11), 31-46.

Welsh, W.N. (2000). Teen violence in the USA. In R. Summers and A. Hoffman (Eds.), *Teen violence: A global perspective* (pp. 183-200). Westport, CT: Greenwood Press.

Wendel, T. (2000). *Creating equity and quality: A literature review of school effectiveness and improvement*. Kelowna, BC: Society for the Advancement of Excellence in Education Research Series 6.

Withers, G., and Russell, J. (1998). *Educating for resilience: Prevention and intervention strategies for young people at risk*. Melbourne: Catholic Education Office.

Wolf, S., Borko, H., Elliot, R., and McIver, M. (2000). "That dog won't hunt!": Exemplary school change efforts within the Kentucky reform. *American Educational Research Journal*, 37(2), 349-393.

Wood, G.H. (1998). *A time to learn*. New York: Dutton.

Wyner, N.B. (1991). *Current perspectives on the culture of schools*. Stanfors, CA: Brookline Books.

Young, J., and Levin, B. (1999). The origins of Educational reform: A comparative perspective. *Canadian Journal of Educational Administration and Policy*, 12, January 19.

Youngs, P., and King, M. (2002). Principal leadership for professional development to build school capacity. *Educational Administration Quarterly*, 38(5), 643-670.

Zimmerman, R.S., Khoury, E.L., Vega, W.A., Gil, A.G., and Warheit, G.J. (1995). Teacher and parent perceptions of behaviour problems among a sample of African American, Hispanic and Non-Hispanic White students. *American Journal of Community Psychology*, 23, 181-198.

Zmuda, A., Kukulis, R., and Kline, E. (2004). *Transforming schools: Creating a culture of continuous improvement*. Alexandria, VA: Association for Supervision and Curriculum Development.

Plate 6 "Genome" (Ferruccio Sardella)

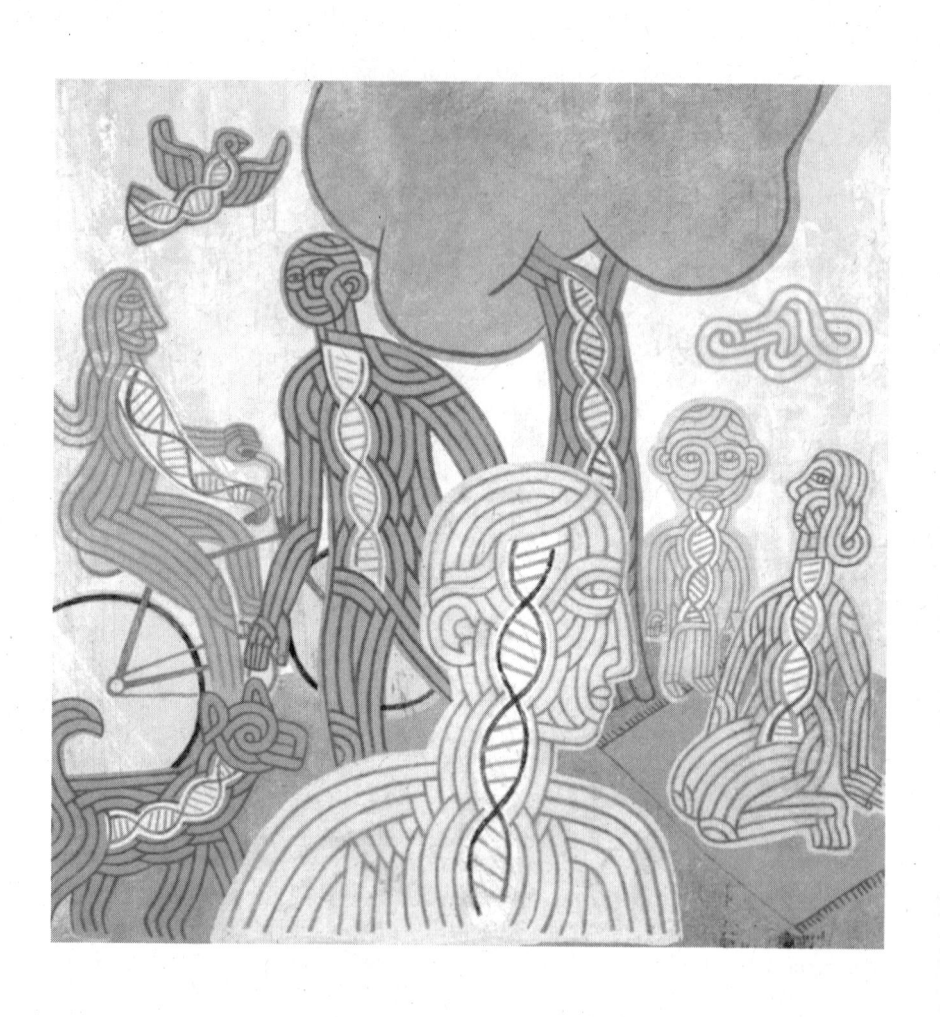

Elder Abuse: A Consequence of Risk and Anxiety in Everyday Life

Kari Brozowski
Department of Sociology, Criminal Justice and Social Welfare, Nipissing University

INTRODUCTION

The elusive nature of elder abuse and neglect in the late modern family is reflected in 25 years of research devoted to eliminating this serious social problem. Sadly, the embarrassment and shame surrounding this devastating experience comprise part of the reason researchers have had difficulty accessing information from elders being abused and the family caregivers who abuse them. Several theoretical frameworks have been applied to numerous data sets, yet none captures the enormous complexities that encompass the abuse of elders. This poses a challenge for researchers in motivating policy makers and health care professionals to construct appropriate safety provisions for elders and their families.

In an attempt to shed light on the challenges faced by the modern family's caring for aged relatives, I draw upon the ideas of risk in everyday life in order to elucidate the realities of living in an advanced modern society. At the core of these risks are the ever-pervasive societal fears of ageing, placing ageism at the forefront of our cultural value system. These values imbue risks to our intimate relationships with older kin. They are juxtaposed with the multitude of risks in everyday life, so that many elders are exposed to dangerous circumstances. Situated in a late modern context, families and religion are eclipsed by corporate capitalism, which encourages the development of an immature self-concept based on superficial personal choices and the overconsumption of material goods. This is compounded by the difficulties inherent in raising children, a volatile labour market, uncertainties about financial security in later life, divorce, separation, remarriage, reconstructed families, and novel family systems.

These dynamics can lead to feelings of depression, frustration, anxiety, and a diminished ability to care for ageing relatives. In addition, systemic inadequacies prevent elders from escaping these harmful situations and encourage their subjugation in abusive environments. Feelings of a lack of control, perhaps leading to depression, are reinforced. As one community health professional communicated to me, "Getting elders out of an abusive situation is often an impossible task and is, in my opinion, systemic abuse." Progressive federal health care policies and community action are imperative for eradicating elder abuse in families. Greater awareness of the effects of ageism in a late modern, ageing society can incite positive social changes for both the elders and their caregivers.

In this chapter, I delineate the historical and cultural context of a capitalist-driven, late modern society in order to trace the development of ageism and the heightened propensity for the social problem of elder abuse. This occurs in conjunction with our growing obsession with individuality and protection of self, due to the risks inherent in advanced modernity. The risks we encounter in everyday life are generally financial, health-related, and safety-oriented. They are subject to frequent manipulation by those in positions of power through the media and popular culture, promoting a state of constant fear. Consequently, the serious side effect of a pervasive fear of poverty, disability, illness, or victimization is the increasing feeling of mistrust of neighbours, community, and even our family members.

Mistrust of others persuades us to disconnect from community and social networks as we move deeper into isolation and fear. A range of mental health problems can surface when isolated individuals develop symptoms of anxiety and depression as well as borderline and narcissistic personality disorders. Distress in our relationships with family members could be the result, setting the foundation for increased abuse and neglect of elders. I conclude by offering ideas to reconstruct our communities and family dynamics, allowing us to connect with other humans through the re-establishment of trust. This should help alleviate such mental health issues as anxiety and depression and, thus, the potential for elder abuse in the late modern society.

OVERVIEW OF THE RESEARCH ON ELDER ABUSE

Elder abuse went unacknowledged by the medical community until the mid-1970s (Douglass, 1983). However, the first systematic research studies were not conducted until the beginning of the next decade (Reece, Walz, and Hageboeck, 1983; Douglass, 1983; Sengstock and Hwalek, 1987; Wolf and Pillemer, 1989). These studies demonstrate the difficulty of capturing this phenomenon accurately because of the hidden nature of elder abuse (Wolf and Pillemer, 1989). The obstacles inherent in accessing potential victims and their abusers produce research results that reveal inconsistent definitions of abuse, prevalence of types of abuse, and risk factors associated with abuse (Bonnie and Wallace, 2003; National Center for Elder Abuse, 2003).

In the early 1990s, more rigorous national surveys were completed, presenting some population characteristics concerning who is suffering from elder abuse (Podnieks, Pillemer, Nicholson, Shillington, and Frizzel, 1990; Pittaway et al., 1995). Unfortunately, the authors of much of the research generated in this decade continue to reinforce the premise that it is difficult to fully comprehend the phenomenon of elder abuse (Podnieks et al., 1990; Pittaway and Westhues, 1993; Anetzberger, 1997; Cyphers 1999). Along with the shame attached to being abused, much of the lack of understanding is due to the complexity that exists within the dynamics of the family, including the surrounding societal structural changes that lead to difficult interpersonal relations in families today (Reece et al., 1983; Power and Maluccio, 1999). Ultimately, it is a challenge for researchers to capture all of these intricacies in research designs. The result is a lack of appropriate action necessary for the reduction of elder abuse in the family (Kozak, Elmslie, and Verdon, 1995).

In the field of elder abuse research over the last decade, some patterns have developed among the victim, the abuser, and the type of abuse. Commonly, the spouse is more likely to commit physical abuse, while adult children tend to be more neglectful and emotionally abusive (Wolf, 1996a). Problems with emotional health and social isolation, and some dependence on others to carry out daily living activities are common characteristics for the abused elder, while the abusers tend to be financially dependent on the victim and are often substance abusers (Iecovich, Lankri, and Drori, 2004). In a study drawn from the General Social Survey of 1999, Brozowski and Hall (2004) report that isolation from external supports through health limitations, and isolated rural living conditions are key factors in emotional abuse. Risk factors connected to intimate relationships appear to be associated with these types of abuse (Wolf, 1996a; Brozowski and Hall, 2004). Whether such emotional challenges and social isolation are present before or after the abuse requires further investigation.

With regard to all forms of abuse, unmarried women who live alone are often victimized (Iecovich et al., 2004). Nevertheless, studies concur that among the elderly, gender is not a risk factor for physical or psychological abuse (Podnieks et al., 1990; Pittaway et al., 1995; Bond, Cuddy, Dixon, Duncan, and Smith, 1999). Not surprisingly, these conclusions have stimulated feminist theorists to examine the issue of gender as a construct of power relations between men and women. For example, Whittaker (1995) states that 'hairsplitting' arguments obscure evidence that a significantly greater number of older women are exposed to unacceptable forms of violence in comparison to adult men (p. 35). She elaborates further by claiming that research "reflects a growing anxiety about the nature of the 'family' and a concern to enshrine and safeguard 'normal family' relationships" (p. 39).

An analysis of the literature leads Whittaker (1995) to decry the tendency for researchers to absolve the abuser, reinforcing the social structural position of women in our society. Chrichton supports this argument, claiming that feminist and ageist perspectives explain the greater likelihood of women to be victims of male perpetrators (1999). Furthermore, through the secondary analysis of those who accessed health care services in London, Ontario in 1991, a feminist view was found to better explain physical abuse (Pittaway et al., 1995). Kosberg (1998) disagrees with the tendency to concentrate only on women when examining elder abuse and neglect, claiming that the abuse of elderly men has been given limited attention and, therefore, merits further research. Brozowski and Hall (2004) suggest that men are more likely to report being victims of emotional abuse. It is possible that men are more sensitive than women to real or perceived emotional abuse, as they negotiate the process of ageing (Brozowski and Hall, 2004).

There is no scarcity of theories in relation to elder abuse (Wolf, 1997), due to the multidimensional nature of elder mistreatment. This multi-theoretical framework has subsequently required different theories to explain particular forms of abuse (Pittaway et al., 1995; Wolf, 1997). Theories of social exchange, the situational model, symbolic interaction, and the feminist view are predominant in the field of elder abuse. However, Pittaway and co-workers (1995) report that none of the prevailing theories explain abuse or neglect well. Sciamberg and Gans (2000) call for a more encompassing theory to examine the intricate micro and macro aspects of family relationships as well as the surrounding structures. Accordingly, they explore an applied ecological framework and a life course perspective to ascertain the possibility of a more robust understanding of elder abuse by adult children. Wolf (1997) urges researchers to engage in more rigorous, scientific studies to test the myriad of theories that can be applied to the study of elder mistreatment.

In addition to the aforementioned obstacles, recent research examines the issue of cultural diversity in North American society. These studies produce a consensus about the discrepancy among cultures concerning the meaning of elder abuse (Wolf, 1996b; Anetzberger, Korbin, and Tomita, 1996; Anetzberger, 1997; Hudson and Beasley, 1999; Pittaway et al., 1995). For instance, using qualitative interviews, Hudson and Beasley (1999) conclude that African Americans are less tolerant of the abuse of elders and more likely to report the abuse than White or Native Americans. Employing a similar methodology, Anetzberger (1997) concludes that Appalachian elders are less likely to report abuse than Korean Americans, African Americans, Puerto Ricans, European Americans, Japanese Americans, or Navaho elders because family loyalty outweighs abuse. These distinct cultural issues need to be addressed by researchers and by policy and program makers (Pittaway et al., 1995).

The deficiencies in the research, due to problems of encapsulating the intricacies of elder abuse in late modern family life, reproduce the predominance of ageism in an advanced modern social world. This extends to the ambiguity of formulating effective public policy and community action (Podnieks and Pillemer, 1990; Sharon, 1991; Penhale, 1993). The uncertainty is linked to the belief that the older person is difficult and excessively stress-inducing (Sengtock and Hivaleck, 1987; Wolf and Pillemer, 1989; Penhale, 1993). Furthermore, elders who experience abuse have a tendency to hold themselves responsible for this treatment (Podnieks and Pillemer, 1990; Pittaway et al., 1995).

Effective health care policies to support families caring for older relatives are consistently avoided by politicians and policy makers in addressing an ageing society (Bolaria and Dickenson, 2002). This laissez-faire attitude results in a lack of publicly funded services and programs to support families caring for elders (Podnieks and Pillemer, 1990; Pittaway et al., 1995; Rosenthal, 2000). The potential for heightened anxiety and tension in the ageing family could lead to explosive neglectful behaviour at the expense of an older person (Brozowski and Hall, 2004). Clearly, more research is required to expose the multifaceted family dynamics surrounding elder abuse and neglect.

The Risk of Ageing in an Ageist Society

In late modern society, we generally consider risk as a signifier of danger. Because of this negative view, it is a contradiction to speak of something as a 'good risk' (Douglas, 1990). As reflected in the media, the prevalence of risk in everyday life is increasingly obvious. It is difficult to escape news reports on television or in the newspaper on the multitude of risks that confront us on a daily basis; such reports elicit fear and anxiety about the way we live our lives and conduct ourselves. From the risk of terrorism, avian flu, child abductions by strangers, and financial troubles, to the risk of ageing and death, we have become afraid of the future (Giddens, 1990). This state of hyper-reflexivity is manipulated by a neo-liberal agenda set by the global corporate forces inherent in an advanced modern society (Crook, 1999). Movies, television, magazines, and other forms of popular culture reinforce these fears, compelling us to buy such products as security systems, anti-flu agents, and ageing creams from companies capitalizing on 'future fear.'

One risk that plagues us today, according to science, health officials, and popular culture, is the progressive decay of the body manifested by the dreaded signs of ageing. Wrinkles, grey hair, cellulite, and shortening of stature expose the body's fragility to time, and signify our increasing connection to death. The fantasy of controlling our destiny through science leads us to a quixotic quest for youth and immortality through the practice of a healthy lifestyle and the use of advances in technology to defend against, or even reverse, the body's natural decline (Lupton, 1995; Featherstone and Wernick, 1995; Katz, 1996).

Historically, western society's focus on controlling health was intended to maintain order and support profit in industry (Lupton, 1995). Lupton argues that, over time, 'healthiness' has replaced 'Godliness' as a measure of an individual's self-discipline and goodness. According to Katz (1996), 'enlightenment' thinkers provided the impetus toward re-inscribing the body as an outward symbol of control over the future, as well as a marker of the self's capacity to project inner beauty through positive health practices. Francis Bacon viewed youth and old age as a continual life process related to moral, physical, and behavioural attributes and their ills. He proposed that this age continuum could be treated with life-prolonging medicines, such as poppy juice and tobacco, to strengthen the spirit. Moreover, the life-enhancing emotional states of joy, sorrow, and compassion would enhance the process while fear, anger, and envy would surely shorten life (Katz, 1996). Not surprisingly, these ideas were targeted at the white, educated male of the time, whose health and well-being were of interest to the state in its mission to create a prosperous and stable capitalist economy (Katz, 1996). Subsequently, as the modern public health movement established itself as an apparatus of government, the health of workers was viewed as a means to support a productive workforce (Tesh, 1988).

Mothers were promoted as servants of society expected, in caring for their children, to voice the popular health discourse of the day to ensure the future of the workforce. Children were to display and practice proper hygiene and manners in order to demonstrate their successful moral integration into society (Lupton, 1995). Those individuals and families whose appearance lacked the image of good health were viewed as undisciplined and sinful; this slovenly lifestyle was to be expected from the lower classes, deemed to be lacking in education and grace. The science of epidemiology helped identify the 'problem' populations of both the poor and working class immigrants, constructing them as 'other,' connoting dirtiness and the need for training to bestow the correct skills to achieve 'good health' (Lupton, 1995). Although health authorities regarded these deviant sub-populations as having ameliorative characteristics, another group, the elderly, was considered chronically unproductive. Furthermore, the failure of elderly people to show the self's true beauty through the control of the body over mortality rendered them morally lacking and even disgusting (Lupton, 1995). However, in creating the welfare state during early industrialism, society attempted to target needy sub-groups, such that financially destitute elders deserved basic life necessities. The Poor Law, established during the colonial period in America, was mandated to be inclusive of all persons suffering from misfortune, regardless of age. This permitted the poor elderly to be taken into one of the many established almshouses or poorhouses. These practices of classification provided justification for labelling the elderly as a social problem, with the concomitant legitimacy of health promotional discourses to exert control over the ageing body (Katz, 1996).

Health promotional risk discourses are embedded in everyday lifestyle practices in society, ranging from adequate nutrition and exercise to limiting the intake of alcohol and encouraging non-smoking. Those who choose to risk their health by ignoring such information are often confronted with the strong disapproval of friends, family, and strangers (Lupton, 1995). Lack of self-discipline and indulgence in risky activities connote a need for extensive re-training concerning the customs for achieving purity of the body and its possessor, the soul (Douglas, 1960; Lupton, 1995). Within this system of ideas is the belief that ageing is a curable disease (Featherstone and Hepworth, 1991). Social structural constraints for people who are not capable of buying themselves out of a risky lifestyle, leading to a more rapid ageing of the body, are of no consequence to the prevailing attitude of youthfulness over old age (Lupton, 1995; Featherstone and Wernick, 1995). For those who do reveal the signs of a decaying, ageing body, and who further demonstrate their dependency through some form of disability, there is often intolerance and disdain. Featherstone and Wernick (1995) label this stage 'deep old age.'

Health promotional discourses further cast a shadow of fear toward these individuals, reducing them to a status of uncleanliness and disease (Douglas, 1960; Lupton, 1995). Within this discourse is the fear of being around the older person in a state of 'deep old age,' since there is a risk of exposure to the toxic sight of mortality. This can generate feelings of disillusionment and despair among the elderly, since the self must reflexively confront the reality of not having control over nature. Further reinforcement of this belief is apparent in the older person's projection of shame and frustration as the dark side of the ageing process is exposed. The ageing body becomes a symbol of the imprisonment of the person, who is no longer capable of expressing their 'true self' (Featherstone and Wernick, 1995). Blaming the victim in this context is an illustration of systemic ageism, which serves the purpose of maintaining a cohesive society through bolstering loyalty and promoting internal social control of the members (Douglas, 1986).

Much of the communication of how to incorporate healthy practices into one's lifestyle is presented in the form of advertisements, with frightening messages to induce compliance. For example, a number of years ago a television ad portrayed a teenage girl smoking in front of a mirror, revealing the transformation of a once young, vital woman into a feeble, old woman, in an effective campaign to portray the dangers of smoking by adolescent girls. The risk of death and decay are frequently the theme for these health promotion advertisements, tapping into people's anxieties about not being healthy and provoking action on the part of individuals to adopt a proper lifestyle. In addition, the ads magnify the positive image of health officials by demonstrating their knowledge and concern for the health of the population (Lupton, 1995).

The likelihood of an individual receiving health discourses that produce conflicting messages is high. Accordingly, it is common for prescribed health customs to encounter resistance by many who may feel frustrated or alienated by practices that challenge their individuality. Diversity, in the form of class, gender, sexual orientation, race, ethnicity, and position in the life course, presents a daunting challenge to government health officials when they choose a health promotion discourse that speaks to this range of social locations (Lupton, 1995). As Lupton states:

> *The ways in which discourses are taken up and integrated into self-identity are at least partially contingent on the flux of individual positions in the workforce, lifestyle and interactions of institutions such as the economy, family and school"* (p. 149).

Irrationality is a consequence of the attempt by health promoters to control the population's health through the employment of rational health discourses (Lupton, 1995; Lupton, 1999; Katz, 1996). Competing discourses exist and are often found in everyday contexts, such as families caring for ageing relatives.

Family members must negotiate culturally accepted norms of compassionate care for the elderly who require some form of physical, emotional, or material assistance, but in doing so, they must address their own denial and face their own ageing process and the fear that this engenders. Consequently, these conflicting cultural values might induce anxiety and frustration in the family caregiver, resulting in a frustrated reaction in the form of physical, emotional, or financial abuse and in active or passive neglect.

Health promotional discourses, formulated around a capitalist, profit-making agenda, filter down into individual lives through the belief that death, and the process of ageing, can someday be healed. Within this context, the individual is accountable for overall 'good health' and the prerequisite 'youthful' image encouraged by society. A general fear of a decaying body creates a cultural climate that supports anxiety about ageing, resulting in an ageist society, and negative treatment of elders who require physical and/or social assistance.

INTERPERSONAL RISK AND ELDER ABUSE

Interpersonal risk has been identified by researchers as having the potential to contribute to the social problem of elder abuse (Brozowski and Hall, 2003; Brozowski and Hall, 2004). Interpersonal risk is fuelled by the process of individualization in late modernity, wherein people are enticed to become 'half-adult,' and subsequently removed from a sense of responsibility for others and their community (Cote, 2000). According to Cote (2000), late modern maturity has transformed from more traditional and obligatory behaviours to ones left open to individual preference, overwhelmingly dictated by market forces where self-concepts are often saturated by a superficial and ageist popular culture. The life course becomes a difficult trajectory in this context, wherein we can choose between the path of least resistance or 'default individualization,' involving circumstance and folly and little agentic assertion, or 'developmental individualization,' wherein continual and deliberate growth is pursued (Cote, 2000, p. 33).

Unfortunately, in an advanced modern time, most people choose the former type of individualization, producing serious consequences for intergenerational relations and caring. Many people are encouraged, through dominance of corporate capitalism, to develop character traits involving immediate gratification, self-absorption, and a poor sense of past and future. This results in a society in which mental problems such as borderline and narcissistic personality disorders thrive. An obsessive focus on the self and its protection can also cultivate anxiety and panic disorders (Cote, 2000). A neo-liberal, increasingly authoritarian political model encourages this hyper-individualism which leads many in their local spaces to feel socially disconnected and isolated from each other. An atmosphere of mistrust of others in our community and, in some cases family members, reinforces the reduction of personal connections (Bauman, 2003).

Feelings of extreme isolation, where powerful and wealthy others are controlling how we connect to the social world through the market and media, can result in increasing numbers of people afflicted with such mental states as depression and anxiety, often requiring the use of prescription drugs that might not be necessary if appropriate social interventions are implemented. In general, there is evidence that younger and older people tend to suffer more from depression, as opposed to those who are middle-aged, because of their lack of power in society. Furthermore, anger and anxiety can be more prevalent for younger adults, as they establish their lives and raise families. On the other hand, middle-aged adults' depression is less common in comparison to older and younger people, while older adults are the least angry and anxious. In addition, the barriers to power and personal resources for women and minorities can produce a sense of lacking control over life's circumstances, leading to mental conditions of depression and anxiety. For women and minorities, these maladies are due to life course experiences of discrimination. Ageing can compound these obstacles, as older women and minorities perceive a lowering of their status due to personal losses such as jobs, friends, partners, networks, and the limited powers once possessed in society (Mirowsky and Ross, 2003).

Relationships between elders and caregivers, conceivably made more difficult due to a growing dissatisfaction with life and personal connections, can produce neglectful or explosive scenarios. Moreover, an older person is more likely to maintain secrecy about the abuse, since they are often feeling powerless to change their living situations. Although this might lead one to be cynical about the future, Cote (2000) offers the possibility of the late modern forces permitting individuals to transform their self-identities collectively toward a universal caring model, wherein generational continuity is achievable. The bonds between generations can only benefit the younger citizens of today, as we have opportunities to draw on past knowledge of our elders to help us navigate the late modern world toward a fruitful future. This could be in the form of elders as teachers, justices of the peace, community activists, voluntary workers, and spiritual guides (Blaikie, 1999).

Giddens (1992) describes late modern society as involved in a movement toward the revolution of the self and its power to act reflexively, marking a break from a traditional society where religion and rules guided our behaviour and preserved kinship ties. Although this reflection of community connections is praised as an example of love and caring in families and among neighbours, the reality is it was out of necessity due to an awareness of mutual dependence (Beck and Beck-Gernsheim, 2002). The new, late modern self is engaged in an emancipatory project wherein intimate ties no longer obligate a person to follow traditional rules, but rather are chosen and negotiated in the pursuit of democratic relations. Giddens conceptualizes this as the *pure relationship*:

> Where a social relationship is entered into for its own sake, for what can be derived by each person from a sustained association with

> another; and which is contained only in so far as it is thought by both parties to deliver enough satisfactions for each individual to stay within it (1992, p. 58).

However, as our communal solidarity loosens, a probable side effect to the emancipated self has been disorganization, isolation, and a fragile self-identity (Bauman, 2003). Giddens goes on to argue that trust is the foundation for intimacy where, in the past, trust was taken for granted in kinship ties between adult children and ageing parents; yet now this trust is negotiated and bargained for:

> Take the case of the obligations adult children assume towards ageing parents. In some circumstances and cultural contexts it is more or less taken for granted that the parents can count on their children for material and social support. But the clear trend of development is for such support to depend on the quality of relationships forged (1992, p. 97).

In addition, the intricacies presented in advanced modern families, including the possibilities of separation, divorce, remarriage, blended families, stepfamilies, and a multitude of novel family forms wherein new intimate ties are reformulated and negotiated, can introduce strains in a relationship (Giddens, 1992). Beck and Beck-Gernsheim (1995) conceptualize the late modern family as a democratic site of individuals pursuing personal emancipation through discussion and cooperation. These strains within the family can be amplified through global economic changes, wherein uncertainties in employment and the wider socio-cultural environment are widespread (Crook, 1999, p. 181). As Giddens admits: "No one knows how far the advent of the pure relationship will prove more explosive than integrating in its consequences" (1992, p. 156).

The utopian ideal of the pure relationship may, in itself, set up many relationships to fail as individuals bargain for the emotional bonds that enhance their self-development. If this self-actualization is rooted in 'default-individualization,' wherein self-development is paramount, the care-giving relationship will be set up to fail.

Consequences to hyper-individualism can be a reaction of disconnection from family and community, fostering strenuous mental states of depression and anxiety for many, as well as the potential for some to develop maladaptive personality disorders. Furthermore, in a late modern society that devalues age and embraces ageism, many care-giving relationships with elder relatives are tenuous. Confounding these unstable relationships are the perceptions of a risky modern world, including a volatile labour market and uncertainties about financial security in later life. This serves to contribute to the need for hyper-individualism, presenting difficulties for caregivers of ageing relatives and leading to a heightened possibility of abuse. The ageing of the population promises to intensify this problem unless there is increasing support from the state and local communities.

These relationships may differ for elder women and men because, although ageism targets any aged body, the existence of economic and social inequality for women initiates unique relationship dilemmas (Woodward, 1995). Kathleen Woodward criticizes the theoretical shortcomings of psychoanalysis and feminism for including only two generations in their frameworks, and for neglecting to conceptualize the generational position of the older woman, implying that the older woman simply does not exist. She refers to the critique of Baba Copper as a movement toward rectifying this deficiency. For instance, Copper contends that ageism generates through the traditional pattern of the nuclear family, wherein the mother cares for others, but no one reciprocates and cares for the mother (Woodward, 1995). Woodward calls on feminism to incorporate age into its critique of patriarchy in order to improve the status of the older woman.

Giddens (1992) decries violence against others as anathema to the pure relationship, and maintains that its perpetrators are predominantly men in the patriarchal structure of advanced modern society. His framework suggests that the revolutionary movement toward more egalitarian relations will penetrate into late modern institutions to emancipate us from this social problem. However, the cultural support for a disdain of the ageing body and the prevalence of ageism in our institutions goes unconsidered in his construction of a personal democracy. This has negative implications for elders in their relations with members of their family. The inherently risky and unstable family tie, systematically sustained, provides the impetus for violence against elder family members. More specifically, the form of violence might be physical, emotional, financial, or neglectful, depending upon the individual circumstances and contexts within which they attempt to negotiate ties with their senior relatives. In general, systemic abuse of the aged provides the foundation for the surfacing of destructive behaviour. Concomitantly, if caregivers are pursuing a path of 'default individualization' and/or have characteristics of a personality disorder, the likelihood of elder abuse among family members magnifies.

Giddens (1992) embraces a dialectical phenomenon between people and institutions, where personal and collective resistance to coercive systemic power is an underlying principle of late modernity. In this vein, the possibility of transforming state structures to support democratic and egalitarian ideals for older people might be achievable.

THE ROLE OF PUBLIC POLICY AND INSTITUTIONAL SUPPORT IN AN AGEING SOCIETY

Given that productive citizens are important in health promotion discourse, an ageing society becomes a burden to the capitalist objective of making a profit (Lupton, 1995). Lupton maintains that the emergence of health promotion has its roots in the avoidance of revolution by capitalist reformers and not in humanitarian ethics. As a result, we encounter a state-supported hierarchy of action, wherein the top is self-care and individual responsibility for health, since this is the least expensive way of improving public health. The bottom is a 'safety net' of health care delivery, because of the financial costs associated with it (Lupton, 1995; Crook, 1999).

What follows is a climate of politically neo-liberal standards around the issue of health care support for an ageing population. In an attempt to 'download' the responsibilities of caring for older relatives onto families, neo-liberal politicians, often rhetorically, suggest that an ageing population will drain the current health care system (Crook, 1999). Individual family members, as discussed earlier, are often not equipped to take on this arrangement, requiring the state to take responsibility through policy improvements such as universal home care, progressive and affordable public transportation, and an array of housing alternatives for older people. Furthermore, nursing homes must be re-conceptualized and re-constructed to treat elders with greater respect through more and better-trained health care professionals, as well as by providing programs and an atmosphere of admiration for the aged. For instance, by dressing the elderly up in Donald Duck hats for tea parties in old people's homes, we contribute to the discourse that the elderly go into a second childhood; a notion that must be deconstructed (Hockey and James, 1995). A greater sensitivity to cultural differences of elders and their families within communities and nursing homes is also important (Featherstone and Wernick, 1995).

Finally, the re-design of cities and towns to become more inclusive of women, children, and seniors supports a more humanitarian and democratic environment for those groups often referred to as special populations (Eichler, 1995). For example, the augmentation of recreation and community centres to provide conflict resolution training would aid individual family members who are caring for elders. These centres could also provide education and counselling on advanced forms of maturity and growth, where the principles of universal caring are promoted (Cote, 2000). In addition, the move in some urban areas to strengthen community bonds through activist-based community ownership of parks can establish a safe haven for all ages. Initiatives such as the creation of a community garden and the provision of public benches in parks may encourage local seniors to have garden plots, and can attract neighbours to interact with each other, supporting positive community ties (Whitzman, 1995). Local schools can also participate in programs funded by non-profit environmental organizations such as Evergreen, by employing ecological education for their students, through the building and maintenance of gardens, bird and butterfly habitats, and promoting the involvement of elders in neighbourhoods to enhance relations between the generations. As people in communities forge new connections through these centres and initiatives, there is an opportunity to provide many with a global sense of community wherein our social roles find a greater purpose in the larger world order. Those with depression and anxiety, due to feelings of isolation and minimal control over their lives, might gain some relief, as relations with family and community are re-created. The prevalence of mental disorders might then be decreased through supportive, non-profit, social networks, rather than through such questionable interventions as the use of prescription drugs (Mirowsky and Ross, 2003). Fortunately, the late modern age of hyper-reflexivity is fertile ground for 'neo-traditional' community groups to emerge and transform our self-identities and social order (Crook, 1999).

Seniors associations and groups, as well as other activist groups involved with feminism and race and cultural relations, should have a voice in the political system and play an active part in the policies and community programs that serve to democratize an ageing society. It is also important that individual members in society become aware of these issues and demand social change to improve living conditions for everyone.

Conclusion

Elder abuse in the context of the family is a serious and growing social problem in an increasingly complex, hyper-reflexive, neo-liberal social order. The likelihood of violence against elders in the family is increased by a fragile and potentially volatile personal connection between family members and elders. This difficult relationship is fuelled by diminishing personal and emotional resources, wherein mental health problems including depression and anxiety can flourish, as the elder and caregiver attempt to negotiate the terms of their ties to each other. The caregiver may be grappling with a difficult financial and/or mental state, leaving the elder relative in the care of someone who is not capable of offering effective support. If the tension in this risky relationship becomes untenable, the elder will ultimately suffer in the descent toward a crisis, and a lack of community and social supports for the family will serve to reinforce this consequence. Transformation of our state and community structures through individual and collective action is imperative for the rights of our elders and the movement toward generational continuity. It is only when we can reach a social order of meaningful relations between generations that our world will shift toward a more sustainable and humanitarian existence.

In this millennium, the unprecedented ageing of our population presents challenges to our capacity for embracing and institutionalizing human rights for older people. Ageism is an ingrained belief system that must be recognized and eradicated if we are truly committed to the practice of democracy.

Risk in late modern society permeates our lives. Although, at first glance, this may instill a pessimistic view about improving personal relationships with older kin, our ability to react in a collective fashion toward democratizing our relations with elders is hopeful. A concerted effort is crucial on the part of seniors, feminists, race relations groups, and cultural groups. Greater involvement by communities to reconstruct their living spaces and create a more humanitarian and democratic order is paramount. Bolstering our personal connections to others in the neighbourhood and family reduces feelings of powerlessness and social isolation and appropriately addresses mental health issues for some individuals who may otherwise resort to behaviours such as abusing elder relatives. We can no longer ignore the violation of an elder's fundamental human rights, manifested in the persistence of elder abuse. It is the responsibility of us all to challenge and remove discrimination against older people.

ACKNOWLEDGEMENT

I am grateful to the anonymous reviewer who provided me with important suggestions for this manuscript.

REFERENCES

Anetzberger, G.J., and Korbin, J.E. (1994). Alcoholism and elder abuse. *Journal of Interpersonal Violence*, 9(2), 184-194.

Anetzberger, G.J., Korbin, J.E., and Tomita, S.K. (1996). Defining elder mistreatment in four ethnic groups across two generations. *Journal of Cross Cultural Gerontology*, 11(2), 187-212.

Anetzberger, G.J. (1997). Elderly adult survivors of family violence: Implications for clinical practice. *Violence Against Women*, 3(5), 499-605.

Bauman, Z. (2003). *Liquid love*. Cambridge: Polity Press.

Beck, U., and Beck-Gernsheim, E. (1995). *The normal chaos of love*. Cambridge: Polity Press.

Beck, U., and Beck-Gernsheim, E. (2002). *Individualization*. London: Sage Publications.

Blaikie, A. (1999). *Ageing and popular culture*. Cambridge: Cambridge Press.

Bond, J.B., Cuddy, R., Dixon, G.L., Duncan, K.A., and Smith, D. (1999). The financial abuse of mentally incompetent older adults: A Canadian study. *Journal of Elder Abuse and Neglect*, 11(4), 23-38.

Bolaria, S., and Dickinson, H.D. (2002). Sociology, health, illness, and the health care system: Current issues and future prospects. In S. Bolaria and H.D. Dickinson (Eds.), *Health, illness and health care in Canada*, Third Edition (pp. 506-514). Scarborough: Nelson.

Bonnie, R.J., and Wallace, R.B. (2003). *Elder mistreatment: Abuse, neglect and exploitation in America*. Washington: The National Academies Press.

Brozowski, K., and Hall, D. (2003). Elder abuse in a risk society. *Geriatrics Today: The Journal of the Canadian Geriatrics Society*, 6(3), 167-172.

Brozowski, K., and Hall, D. (2004). Growing old in a risk society: Elder abuse in Canada. *Journal of Elder Abuse and Neglect*, 16(3), 65-81.

Chrichton, S.J. (1999). Elder abuse: Feminist and ageist perspectives. *Journal of Elder Abuse and Neglect*, 10(3/4), 115-130.

Comijs, H.C., Jonker, C., van Tilburg, W., and Smit, J.H. (1999). Hostility and coping capacity as risk factors of elder mistreatment. *Social Psychiatric Epidemiology*, 34, 48-52.

Cote, J. (2000). *Arrested adulthood: The changing nature of maturity and identity*. New York: New York University Press.

Crook, S. (1999). Ordering risks. In D. Lupton (Ed.), *Risk and sociocultural theory: New directions and perspectives* (pp. 160-185). Cambridge: Cambridge University Press.

Cyphers, G.C. (1999). Elder abuse and neglect. *Policy and Practice of Public Human Services*, 57(3), 25-30.

Douglas, M. (1960). *Purity and danger*. London: Routledge and Kegan Paul

Douglas, M. (1986). *Risk acceptability according to the social sciences*. London: Routledge and Kegan Paul.

Douglas, M. (1990). Risk as a forensic resource. *Daedalus*, Fall, 1-16.

Douglass, R.L. (1983). Opportunities for prevention of domestic neglect and abuse of the elderly. *Aging and Prevention*, 135-150.

Eichler, M. (1995). Designing the eco-city in North America. In M. Eichler (Ed.), *Change of plans: Towards a non-sexist sustainable city* (pp. 1-24). Toronto: Garamond Press.

Featherstone, M., and Hepworth, M. (1991). The mask of ageing and the postmodern life course. In M. Featherstone, M. Hepworth, and B.S. Turner (Eds.), *The body: Social process and cultural theory* (pp. 371-389). London: Sage.

Featherstone, M., and Wernick, A. (1995). Introduction. In M. Featherstone and A. Wernick (Eds.), *Images of ageing: Cultural representations of later life* (pp. 1-??). London: Routledge.

Giddens, A. (1990). *The consequences of modernity*. Stanford: Stanford University Press.

Giddens, A. (1991). *Modernity and self-identity: Self and society in the late modern age*. Stanford: Stanford University Press.

Giddens, A. (1992). *The transformation of intimacy: Sexuality, love and eroticism in modern societies*. Stanford: Stanford University Press.

Hockey, J., and James, A. (1995). Back to our futures: Imaging second childhood. In M. Featherstone and A. Wernick (Eds.), *Images of ageing: Cultural representations of later life* (pp. 135-148). London: Routledge.

Hudson, M.F., and Beasley, C.M. (1999). Elder abuse: Some African American views. *Journal of Interpersonal Violence*, 14(9), 915-1119.

Iecovich, E., Lankri, M., and Drori, D. (2004). Elder abuse and neglect—A pilot incidence study in Israel. *Journal of Elder Abuse and Neglect*, 16(3), 45-63.

Katz, S. (1996). *Disciplining old age: The formation of gerontological knowledge*. Charlottetown: The University Press of Virginia.

Kosberg, J.I. (1998). The abuse of elderly men. *Journal of Elder Abuse and Neglect*, 9(3), 69-88.

Kozak, J. F., Elmslie, T., and Verdon, J. (1995). Epidemiological perspectives on the abuse and neglect of seniors: A review of the national and international literature. In M.J. Maclean (Ed.), *Abuse and neglect of older Canadians* (pp. 129-142). Ottawa: Canadian Association on Gerontology.

Lupton, D. (1995). *The imperative of health: Public health and the regulated body*. London: Sage.

Lupton, D. (1999). *Risk*. London: Routledge.

Mirowski, J., and Ross, C.E. (2003). *Social causes of psychological distress*, Second Edition. New York: Walter de Gruyter, Inc.

National Center for Elder Abuse (2003). Retrieved November 18, 2006 from http://www.elderabusecenter.org/default.cfm?p=faqs.cfm#seven.

Penhale, B. (1993). The abuse of elderly people: Considerations for practice. *British Journal of Social Work*, 23, 95-112.

Pillemer, K.A., and Finkelhor, D. (1988). The prevalence of elder abuse: A random sample survey. *The Gerontologist*, 28(1), 51-57.

Pittaway, E.D., and Westhues, A. (1993). The prevalence of elder abuse and neglect of older adults who access health and social services in London, Ontario, Canada. *Journal of Elder Abuse and Neglect*, 5(4), 77-93.

Pittaway, E.D., Gallagher, E., Stones, M.S., Kosberg, J., Nahmiash, D., Podnieks, E., Strain, L., and Bond, J. (1995). *Enhancing services for abused older Canadians*. Victoria: Ministry of Health.

Podnieks, E., Pillemer, K., Nicholson, J., Shillington, T., and Frizzel, A. (1990). *National survey on abuse of elderly in Canada*. Toronto: Ryerson Polytechnical Institute.

Power, M., and Maluccio, A.N. (1999). Intergenerational approaches to helping families at risk. *Generations*, 22(4), 37-42.

Reece, D., Walz, T., and Hageboeck, H. (1983). Intergenerational care providers of non-institutionalized frail elderly: Characteristics and consequences. *Journal of Gerontological Social Work*, 5(3), 21-34.

Rosenthal, C. (2000). Aging families: Have current changes and challenges been oversold? In E.M. Gee and G.M. Gutman (Eds.), *The overselling of population aging: Apocalyptic demography, intergenerational challenges, and social policy* (pp. 45-63). Don Mills: Oxford University Press.

Sengstock, M.C., and Hivalek, M. (1987). A review and analysis of measures for identification of elder abuse. *Journal of Gerontological Social Work*, 10(3/4), 21-36.

Sciamberg, L.B., and Gans, D. (2000). Elder abuse by adult children: An applied ecological framework. *International Journal of Aging and Human Development*, 50(4), 329-359.

Sharon, N. (1991). Elder abuse and neglect substantiations: What they tell us about the problem. *Journal of Elder Abuse and Neglect*, 3(3), 19-43.

Tesh, S.N. (1988). *Hidden arguments: Political ideology and disease prevention policy*. New Brunswick: Rutgers University Press.

Whittaker, T. (1995). Violence, gender and elder abuse: Towards a feminist analysis and practice. *Journal of Gender Studies*, 4(1), 35-45.

Whitzman, C. (1995). What do you want to do? Pave parks?: Urban planning and the prevention of violence. In M. Eichler (Ed.), *Change of plans: Towards a non-sexist sustainable city* (pp. 89-109). Toronto: Garamond Press.

Wolf, R.S., and Pillemer, K.A. (1989). *Helping elderly victims: The reality of elder abuse*. New York: Columbia University Press.

Wolf, R.S. (1996a). Understanding elder abuse and neglect. *Aging 367*, 4+, 4-9.

Wolf, R.S. (1996b). Elder abuse and family violence: Testimony presented before the US Senate Special Committee on Aging. *Journal of Elder Abuse and Neglect*, 8(1), 81-96.

Wolf, R.S. (1997). Elder abuse and neglect: Causes and consequences. *Journal of Geriatric Psychiatry*, 30(1), 153-174.

Woodward, K. (1995). Tribute to the older woman: Psychoanalysis, feminism, and ageism. In M. Featherstone and A. Wernick (Eds.), *Images of ageing: Cultural representations of later life* (pp. 79-96). London: Routledge.

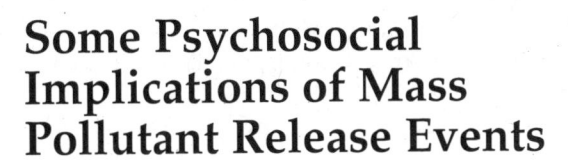

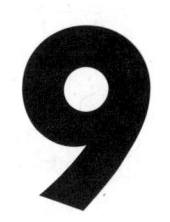

Some Psychosocial Implications of Mass Pollutant Release Events

Lisa Kadonaga

Department of Geography, University of Victoria

INTRODUCTION

Over the past half-century, concerns about hazardous pollutants have become widely recognized by scientists, the public, and policymakers. Publications such as Rachel Carson's 1962 landmark *Silent Spring* contributed to this rising awareness. Also, media coverage of the controversies surrounding toxic sites, such as Love Canal in New York state and Times Beach in Missouri, and the mercury contamination of the English-Wabigoon river system in northwestern Ontario, helped bring these issues to people's attention ("Love Canal probe 'botched,'" 1991; Schmidt, 1990; Reid, 1986). Through the 1970s and 1980s, industrial accidents caused the mass release of contaminants in various places around the world, such as Seveso in Italy and Bhopal in India (Charlton, 1988). There were also chemical train derailments, for example, Ontario's "Mississauga Miracle," and serious nuclear plant malfunctions at Three Mile Island in Pennsylvania, and Chernobyl in the then-USSR (Schachter, 1990; Shaw, 1999). The health risks posed by these types of events caused widespread concerns among professionals and the public.

Despite pressure on authorities for stricter laws to regulate the production, storage, transportation, and disposal of hazardous chemicals, incidents continued to occur. The increasing popularity of recycling, through the 1990s, created new dangers: pollutants could be released by massive fires in stockpiles of materials, such as plastics (Plastimet in Hamilton, Ontario) and discarded automobile tires (Hagarsville, Ontario, and Westley, California, among many others).

The problem assumed an ominous new form in 2001, with the possibility of deliberate destruction. The terrorist attacks of September 11th released large amounts of pollution from burning buildings. Whether or not this was the primary intent of the perpetrators, toxic emissions were being indirectly used as a weapon.

At the time of writing, another crisis looms: the disposal of millions of litres of New Orleans floodwater contaminated with sewage and industrial waste, such as heavy metals. Officials faced the dilemma of letting it remain in the city, posing a major health hazard (and possibly seeping into the local groundwater), or releasing it into Lake Pontchartrain, potentially threatening the area's lucrative seafood industry.

In this chapter, some of the possible connections between pollution events and mental health are examined. It has become apparent that toxic pollutants may have psychological as well as physiological implications. Recently, the mental health effects of exposure to environmental contaminants, in both the short- and long-term, have attracted research attention. The results have sometimes been controversial, since psychological and sociological causes and impacts may be viewed, if not with outright skepticism, as being less solid than measurable physical phenomena. The situation is complicated, with many different factors involved, on a continuum ranging from physical to mental. For psychological impacts, there is an additional difficulty—pollution events are frequently associated with other traumatic situations, such as mass evacuations, and reports of terrorism or military assaults, which can themselves generate symptoms.

Types of Pollutant Release Situations

Mass pollutant release events (MPREs) can be categorized in a number of different ways. They can be entirely anthropogenic (like factory spills), have a natural component (like forest fires which can blanket regions with vast amounts of haze), or be entirely natural, like volcanic activity. They can be relatively localized, or can have global effects, as was observed after the Mt. Pinatubo eruption. Releases of pollutants into the air or water are of particular concern, because of their ability to enter the atmosphere or hydrological system rapidly, often irreversibly, despite the mobilization of cleanup efforts. Air releases could potentially affect a wider area in a shorter time interval, depending on wind conditions. Browning and co-authors (1992) suggested that the smoke from oil well fires in Kuwait during the Gulf War reached thousands of kilometres, and caused detectable temperature changes due to reduction of incoming sunlight for 750 kilometres and more.

It is useful to identify rapid mass pollutant release events (RMPREs), occurring on a scale of hours or days, such as the Exxon Valdez oil spill, the Union Carbide disaster at Bhopal, and the World Trade Center collapse. By comparison, extended mass pollutant release events (EMPREs) may take place over years or even decades. These include emissions of sour gas (containing hydrogen sulphide), chronic urban smog, chemicals leaching from dumpsites, the releases from solid waste incinerators, and ongoing toxic dust storms (such as around the Aral Sea basin). A midrange group, lasting for weeks or months, would include the Gulf War oil fires, and the periodic Indonesian forest fires sometimes associated with slash-and-burn agriculture and logging operations. Due to space constraints, this discussion will mainly focus on anthropogenic

MPREs, with particular attention to the rapid type, which result in short-term acute exposure. Events such as these attract considerable media attention (a factor which will be examined later).

COMPLEXITY AND UNCERTAINTY

The frequency and intensity of exposure to pollutants, such as the formation of photochemical smog at certain times of year, can be affected not only by biophysical variables (e.g., topography, light intensity, wind flow, temperature, and vegetation cover), but also by socio-economic conditions within an area. The impacts of pollution are shaped by many different factors.

Elliott and co-authors (1993) report that the psychosocial effects of solid-waste facilities on nearby populations are governed by a complex, diverse set of variables. This observation is consistent with Mitchell's perspective on complexity: for environmental problems, it can be extremely difficult to sort out cause-and-effect patterns, due to the number of variables, and interactions among them (2002). For example, in their study of Gulf War veterans, Wolfe and colleagues (2002) list a wide range of risk factors for multisymptom illness, including gender, level of education, vaccination against anthrax, medication against nerve gas, and the use of a tent heater, in addition to possible exposure to the smoke from burning oil wells.

Mitchell (2002) describes the role of uncertainty in environmental decision-making, citing the example of arsenic contamination of groundwater in Bangladesh and India. Not enough was understood about the geological and hydrological aspects of arsenic toxicity, or the long-term health effects of ingesting that element in drinking water, or food grown using that water.

Another factor which can obscure the issue is that the negative effects on human health after exposure to particular contaminants might take decades to develop, so even now we might not be completely aware of the hazards posed. It took decades for authorities to recognize the connection between asbestos and cancer; regarding a recent high-profile case, Matas (2005) notes that an increasing number of claims are being submitted to the British Columbia government more than 20 years after exposure in the workplace.

PHYSIOLOGICAL IMPACTS OF POLLUTION

Various air pollutants are linked to respiratory problems and trouble breathing. The compounds given off by the Gulf War oil fires—"oxides of carbon, sulphur, and nitrogen, and unburnt hydrocarbons and particulates" (Browning et al., 1992)—are also released by industrial processes, and during the combustion of fossil fuels by stationary or mobile sources. Concentrations may be particularly high in urban settings, and areas with industrial activity. In their

Calcutta study, Chattopadhyay and colleagues (1995) find that, when compared to the inhabitants of residential areas, those living in industrial parts of the city report having more respiratory ailments and irritation of the mucous membranes.

Rising air pollution levels in urban areas around the world, for example, Iran (Masjedi et al., 2003) and the United States (Eggleston, Buckley, Breysse, Wills-Karp, Kleeberger, and Jaakkola, 1999), have been implicated in the increase of ailments such as asthma. Regarding specific Rapid Mass Pollution Release Events, numerous studies (Fagan, Galea, Ahern, Bonner, and Vlahov, 2002; McKinney, Benson, Lempert, Singal, Wallingford, and Snyder, 2002; Prezant et al., 2002; Levin et al., 2004; US Government Accountability Office, 2004; and others) reveal the respiratory effects of heavy, short-term exposure to dust, smoke, and other contaminants at the World Trade Center.

Respiratory health is crucial for maintaining the body's other systems. Brook and co-authors (2002) demonstrate that high concentrations of ground-level ozone and fine particulate matter can have a rapid effect on the heart, even for healthy people. This can affect oxygen supply to the brain, and under extreme conditions could have implications for mental functioning. Lack of oxygen, or hypoxia, is a stressor that can stimulate the adrenal glands (Foster, 2003).

Interestingly, a number of researchers have documented situations where the symptoms experienced by some of the affected population do not appear to match what might be expected from the quantitative pollution measurements. For example, the mental symptoms reported by community members during one pollution event could not be explained by the levels of pollutants found in blood samples (Bowie, Hill, and Murray, 1998). Likewise, Brody and colleagues (2004) report that perceptions of air quality do not necessarily match air quality as measured at monitoring stations, but instead seem to vary depending on access to information and socio-economic background. Dayal and co-workers (1994) document reports of physical symptoms that could not be explained by exposure to the known pollutants.

Luginaah and co-authors note that residents of an area near a petroleum refinery in Southern Ontario still reported health concerns after emissions had been reduced (2002a), and attribute the difference to odour perception (2000). The authors conclude that environmental stress in that case was due not only to actual emissions, but to perceived ones as well (2002a,b).

Rotko and colleagues (2002) suggest that the psychological impacts of air pollution are more important to health than the actual physical ones. However, the responses are not identical for everyone. In their European study, what determines annoyance levels seems to vary considerably depending on observer characteristics, such as gender. Ruback and Pandey (2002), in their consideration of mental distress and physical symptoms associated with air pollution in the poorer areas of New Delhi, India, also report some apparent gender effects.

PSYCHOLOGICAL AND PSYCHOSOCIAL SYMPTOMS

In their Calcutta study, Chattopadhyay and co-authors (1995) note that the residents of industrial areas report not only physical symptoms linked with pollution, but higher levels of tension and anxiety as well. Some research has been done on the relationship between particular ailments and psychosocial stresses, such as depression (Jacobs, Evans, Catalano, and Dooley, 1984; Bowler, Mergler, Huel, and Cone, 1994) and asthma (Eggleston et al., 1999; Pongracic and Evans, 2001; Kimes, Levine, Timmins, Weiss, Bollinger, and Blaisdell, 2004).

Schauer and Dornow (2001) note that it is important to attempt to distinguish between physical symptoms, for example those directly induced by exposure to contaminants, and psychological ones. However, Sellers points out that many investigations undertaken so far, such as the studies on 9/11 survivors, have preferentially looked at variables that have already been associated with particular physical or mental symptoms, and that could be quantified. "Other senses of hazard" tend to be overlooked (Sellers, 2003). Both Ooi and Goh (1997) and Rotko and colleagues (2002) conclude that the psychological aspects of air pollution could be of considerable importance.

As far as specific disasters, in the years after the Three Mile Island nuclear accident many researchers studied the psychological impacts (e.g., Dohrenwend, 1983; Cleary and Houts, 1984; Princeembury, 1988). Not as much time has elapsed since Chernobyl, but findings suggest that considerable stress and anxiety were generated by that event as well (e.g., Ginzburg, 1993; Huppe and Janke, 1994; Foster, 2002). The Bhopal accident also had serious psychological repercussions (Dhara and Dhara, 2002). This is not surprising, given that both accidents resulted in immediate loss of life (thousands of victims, in the case of Bhopal), and were associated with other traumatic experiences such as mass evacuations. There is a growing body of work chronicling the long-term physical and psychological impacts of the terrorist attacks on the World Trade Center (Melnik et al., 2002; Levin et al., 2004).

PERCEPTIONS OF POLLUTION

Apparently, the perception of contaminants may be as significant to health as empirically-measured variables, such as atmospheric concentrations. Given its significance in occupational health and safety and resource management decisions, pollution is a major element of environmental perception. There is considerable research in the related area of environmental hazards (e.g., Smith, 1996 and Bryant, 2004, among other comprehensive works), so public attitudes towards pollution, and which social and cultural factors affect them, have been a topic of interest for researchers (e.g., Wakefield, Elliott, Cole, and Eyles, 2001; Rotko, Oglesby, Kunzli, Carrer, Nieuwenhuijsen, and Jantunen, 2002; Bickerstaff 2004; Brody, Peck, and Highfield, 2004). Psychologists have also been contributing to this area, since fear of contamination is already recognized as a condition (Rachman, 2004).

It can be difficult to separate out so many overlapping physical and psychological factors (Chattopadhyay, Som, and Mukhopadhyay, 1995) when considering hazards and perceptions. Porteous (1996), in his work on environmental aesthetics, explores some profound spiritual and cultural linkages. There are many different facets to the ways in which landscapes are perceived —artistic, spiritual, historical, ethical—and it seems likely that a mass pollutant release event could have significant impacts on the relationship between people and the environment. Changes could occur over a number of years, and persist for even longer. The socio-economic aftereffects of major catastrophes like Bhopal and Chernobyl are still being felt, years and even decades later (e.g., Dhara and Dhara, 2002; Foster, 2002; Havenaar, de Wilde, van den Bout, Drozzt-Sjoberg, and van den Brink, 2003).

Pongracic and Evans (2001) identify low income groups as having a higher risk of morbidity and mortality for asthma; in addition, Schell and Denham (2003) argue that disadvantaged groups tend to receive more exposure to harmful pollutants. Gee and Payne-Sturges (2004) suggest that disadvantaged communities are particularly vulnerable to environmental hazards. Being affected can leave them even more suspectible, through displacement and poverty. Once started, this cycle would be difficult to break.

Some researchers have speculated that shifts in environmental perception, based on natural MPREs, may have occurred as far back as prehistoric times. Concepts such as personal safety and security, and sense of place, can be influenced by these types of events. Lake Nyos, in the Cameroon, experienced an eruption of carbon dioxide in 1986 which asphyxiated more than 1,700 local residents (Ladbury, 1996). Anthropologists suspect that similar events in the past may have left an impression on local culture that is still felt in traditional customs (Le Guern, Shanklin, and Tebor, 1992; Ladbury, 1996).

STRESS AS AN ADDITIONAL COMPLICATION

The psychosocial impacts of stress itself are increasingly being recognized, certain aspects of which are particularly applicable to environmental hazards. Conditions such as "sick building syndrome," which were (and sometimes still are) dismissed as mass hysteria (Bauer et al., 1992), can reveal a reluctance on the part of the authorities to acknowledge that psychological impacts of any sort are "real." The assumption is that they are not based on anything quantifiable, and will simply "go away" if people can only change their attitude.

Some researchers, such as Ooi and Goh (1997), suggest that even if poor workplace air quality cannot account for all observed symptoms, work-related psychological stress can be a significant contributor to health problems. Hayes (1999) takes the view that stress can have significant physical repercussions, since psychology and physiology are linked by endocrine responses, and by the immune system.

Havenaar and van den Brink (1997) do not find firm evidence for the stress of toxicological disasters having an effect on physical or psychiatric morbidity, but argue that the threat of toxic exposure can have major impacts on subjective health. Havenaar and co-workers (2003) suggest that most of the broader health complaints in the region surrounding Chernobyl were stress-related.

In addition to the stress people may be experiencing about a specific threat (e.g., toxic chemicals, radiation, or a biological contagion), the other stresses related to the event would be an extra burden (Gee and Payne-Sturges, 2004). In the case of the WTC collapse, the possibility of further terrorist attacks, and for some the loss of workplaces, colleagues, or family, and displacement from their homes, created even more strain. (Indeed, soon after 9/11 came the anthrax contamination scare, and further disruption and uncertainty. That particular case has not yet been resolved.)

Other MPREs have been associated with the prospect of losing one's job—for example, the damage done by the Exxon Valdez oil spill to the local fishing industry (Palinkas, Downs, Petterson, and Russell, 1993). In the case of aboriginal communities, the repercussions could include the loss of traditional lands and culture. Palinkas and colleagues (1993) report an increase in generalized anxiety, even post-traumatic stress, following the spill. The Aral Sea is another example of an ongoing disaster which has strong psychosocial dimensions, as communities have lost their livelihood and fallen into a downward spiral of poverty and disease (Crighton, Elliott, van der Meer, Small, and Upshur, 2003a,b)

MITIGATING FACTORS

There are a number of characteristics that tend to decrease the level of stress during and after a mass pollutant release event.

1) *Effective knowledge.* A clear understanding of the situation, and/or the kinds of precautions that would be necessary, would not only increase safety but also give individuals confidence that they would be able to make it through. An example would be the awareness that boiling bacteria-contaminated water would help them avoid getting sick. Princeembury (1992a) notes that after Three Mile Island, the respondents who had a greater level of understanding about the technological issues also had fewer psychological symptoms.

2) *Experts on the scene.* The presence or quick deployment of authorities, without delay, would reassure people that the situation was well in hand.

3) *Choice of reasonable options.* If people have some latitude for decision-making (e.g., deciding whether or not to leave or, if evacuation is mandatory, having some leeway over where to go), that would allow them to feel somewhat in control of their own fate.

4) *Trust in experts and authority.* If those who are in charge, and giving advice, appear to know what they are doing and are making reasonable decisions, this makes the threat appear more manageable. The appearance of openness and transparency would also increase the level of trust (Princeembury, 1992b).

However, these could be the very factors which are in doubt, depending on the circumstances:

1) People may not be aware of which precautions to take, or be unwilling to follow them, for various reasons. For example, almost 80% of the WTC rescue workers surveyed did not wear appropriate safety gear (Levin et al., 2004), even though there were early media reports of asbestos in the air at Ground Zero (e.g., Cook and Robertson, 2001).

2) After an emergency, there may be a delay before trained experts and their equipment can reach the affected area, by which time people may have unwittingly become contaminated. Also, as Mitchell (2002) notes regarding the example of arsenic in the groundwater, even scientists may be uncertain of the potential long-term hazards.

3) Regarding the choice of options—especially in the case of airborne pollutants, residents may not be able to evacuate before the cloud reaches them. For neighbourhoods adjacent to Anniston Army Depot in the state of Alabama: "people who live within 6 miles of the incinerator have been issued protective plastic hoods, portable air filters, duct tape and plastic and told to prepare a 'safe room' in their homes," in case of an accidental release of sarin or nerve gas (Copeland, 2003). Widespread skepticism has been expressed about the effectiveness of these measures, and the warning system currently in place. The residents' response to this loss of control has been fatalism, frustration, and in some cases, anger.

4) Accusations of unfairness, concealment, or incompetence are common in these situations. Referring to the perceived cover-up of responsibility for past dioxin contamination at Gagetown, one resident argued that "The government is too big and too crooked" (Morris, 2005). Government and military officials were criticized for carelessness over Love Canal ("Love Canal probe 'botched,'" 1991). Controversy has also surrounded the WTC clean-up, with accusations that the EPA underestimated the danger and failed to warn people at Ground Zero to take adequate precautions (Schneider, 2002). It was later discovered that the vacuum trucks deployed to clean the air did not have the proper filters to remove potentially dangerous fine particles (Bazinet, 2002) and, in fact, may have worsened the situation by blowing more of the particles into the atmosphere.

Regarding 4), suspicion about the official version of things is evident when looking at the schism between government sources and alternative media, concerning such issues as Agent Orange and Gulf War Syndrome, as to what is causing the problem. This degree of suspicion can also influence whether people are willing to listen to official advice, for example, on evacuation or other precautions. It is part of the psychosocial impact of these types of events. Goldsteen and co-workers (1992) note that mistrust of the authorities was linked to perceptions of danger, and to levels of distress, in the Three Mile Island case. Rahu (2003) writes that, after the Chernobyl accident, apprehension and misconceptions about what was going on were widespread—and not helped by ongoing government secrecy. In the absence of information, any health problems, even if they were actually unrelated, were blamed on the accident.

In addition, when people are feeling powerless and manipulated, not only are frustration levels high, with the potential for violence, but vulnerability to exploitation, or wild speculation increases. At present, after major disasters the proliferation of conspiracy theories on the Internet or in casual conversation is inevitable. Under these conditions, psychological and physiological impacts of stress would not be addressed, and might become more severe.

Wilkinson (2005), with regards to heart disease, argues that the ongoing "stress of disrespect" experienced by marginalized populations may end up being more of a health issue than poor nutrition. Cleeland (2005), reporting on a forum organized by the National Institute for Occupational Safety and Health, mentions anecdotal evidence, collected from Norway, that the spread of a rumour that a town's major employer might be closing was observed to raise the blood pressure of the entire community.

On the positive side, however, if a sense of powerlessness has major psychosocial impacts in MPRE situations, there is also the hope that some of this could be addressed with more public involvement. Walton (2004) describes the opposition to sour gas wells in Alberta—the residents feel they are being excluded from decision-making. As with other environmental management issues, being allowed to take an active role in creating development rules or emergency plans could result in increased community participation, and more workable strategies (Mitchell, 2002).

PERCEPTION AND THE MEDIA

"Ignorance is Bliss"—Missouri bumper sticker commenting on Times Beach contamination caused by contractor Russell Bliss

Media coverage of mass pollution release events is important: it reflects public consciousness, and also shapes it. Given the ability of news networks to offer 24-hour live coverage of these kinds of stories, it is not surprising that events such as Three Mile Island, the WTC collapse, and the flooding of New Orleans would have a psychological impact even on those who were not actually in the contamination zone for those events.

This poses an interesting quandary for those who report on MPREs, study them, or engage in environmental activism or litigation. Would any of these activities, aimed at raising awareness, end up creating more stress for the affected population? Greve and co-authors (2005) report that pending lawsuits appear to increase the emotional effects of a toxic release event. Could a forecast of widespread post-traumatic stress disorder, as was made by Herman and colleagues (2002) after 9/11, be a self-fulfilling prophecy?

It is likely that these possibilities would have to be weighed for each different circumstance. There are probably many environmental hazards, such as severe ground-level ozone or contaminated drinking water, where the benefits of advising people to take adequate precautions would outweigh any potential negative psychosocial impacts of the warning itself. Any information that would help avoid careless, possibly fatal accidents (e.g., the mishandling of dangerous chemicals) would make the situation safer, without causing unnecessary apprehension. In that case, ignorance would definitely not be bliss.

Conclusion

Past incidents involving the mass release of pollutants demonstrate that chemical contaminants can have physical effects on the mucous membranes, and on the respiratory and circulatory systems. Research into these is complicated by situations such as anomalous symptoms, which do not match with the amount, or even type, of contaminants being released. There is mounting evidence for psychosocial effects that are associated with sociological and cultural risk factors, in addition to the environmental contaminants themselves. The relationships between environmental perception and health, and particularly the psychosocial factors contributing to mental and physical illness, require more investigation. There is reason to suspect that stress, as it relates to short- and long-term environmental hazards, can have significant health impacts. Existing research highlights the importance of factors such as availability of reliable information, degree of public involvement, and the efficiency and transparency of the official response to problems.

If anything, the examples in the preceding sections have shown that there is no substitute for public education and participation in these kinds of circumstances, together with an open approach that acknowledges mistakes and makes a commitment to learn from them. Mitchell (2002) admits that this more adaptive style of management can be challenging, and that there are situations that may be too dangerous, fragile, or urgent to allow trial-and-error experimentation. But the conditions that make societies vulnerable to MPREs also tend to intensify stress, increase suspicion, and hamper the ability of the public and the authorities to respond to crises: by comparison, anything that encourages trust and effectiveness would be a more hopeful alternative.

REFERENCES

Bauer, R.M., Greve, K.W., Besch, E.L., Schramke, C.J., Crouch, J., Hicks, A., Ware, M.R., and Lyles, W.B. (1992). The role of psychological factors in the report of building-related symptoms in sick building syndrome. *Journal of Consulting Clinical Psychology*, 60(2), 213-219.

Bazinet, K.R. (2002). WTC trucks had wrong dust filters. *New York Daily News*, August 14, 2002. http://www.nydailynews.com/news/story/11015p-10416c.html.

Bickerstaff, K. (2004). Risk perception research: Socio-cultural perspectives on the public experience of air pollution. *Environment International*, 30(6), 827-840.

Bowie, C., Hill, A., and Murray, V. (1998). The effect of a lindane and mercury polluting incident on the health of a community: The Somerton health survey. *Public Health*, 112(4), 249-255.

Bowler, R.M., Mergler, D., Huel, G., and Cone, J.E. (1994). Psychological, psychosocial, and psychophysiological sequelae in a community affected by a railroad chemical disaster. *Journal of Traumatic Stress*, 7(4), 601-624.

Brody, S.D., Peck, B.M., and Highfield, W.E. (2004). Examining localized patterns of air quality perception in Texas: A spatial and statistical analysis. *Risk Analysis*, 24(6), 1561-1574.

Brook, R.D., Brook, J.R., Urch, B., Vincent, R., Rajagopalan, S., and Silverman, F. (2002). Inhalation of fine particulate air pollution and ozone causes acute arterial vasoconstriction in healthy adults. *Circulation*, 105(13), 1534-153.

Browning, K.A., Alam, R.J., Ballard, S.P., Barnes, R.T.H., Bennetts, D.A., Maryon, R.J., Mason, P.J., McKenna, D.S., Mitchell, J.F.B., Senior, C.A., Slingo, A., and Smith, F.B. (1992). Environmental effects from burning oil wells in the Gulf. *Weather*, 47(6), 201-212.

Bryant, E. (2004). *Natural hazards* (2nd ed.). New York: Cambridge University Press.

Carson, R. (1962). *Silent Spring*. Boston: Houghton Mifflin.

Charlton, R. (1988). PCB's: The reality. *The Ottawa Citizen*, 31 October, A9.

Chattopadhyay, P.K., Som, B., and Mukhopadhyay, P. (1995). Air pollution and health hazards in human subject: Physiological and self-report indices. *Journal of Environmental Psychology*, 15(4), 327-331.

Cleary, P.D., and Houts, P.S. (1984). The psychological impact of the Three-Mile-Island incident. *Journal of Human Stress*, 10(1), 28-34.

Cleeland, N. (2005). Job stress hits workers' cardiovascular health. *Los Angeles Times*, April 3.

Cook, G., and Robertson, T. (2001). Asbestos dust poses threat to rescue crews. *Boston Globe*, September 14, A23.

Copeland, L. (2003). Alabamians fear chemical disaster. *USA Today*, August 18.

Crighton, E.J., Elliott, S.J., van der Meer, S., Small, I., and Upshur, R. (2003a). Impacts of an environmental disaster on psychosocial health and well-being in Karakalpakstan. *Social Science & Medicine*, 56(3), 551-567.

Crighton, E.J., Elliott, S.J., Upshur, R., van der Meer, J., and Small, I. (2003b). The Aral Sea disaster and self-rated health. *Health & Place*, 9(2), 73-82.

Dayal, H.H., Baranowski, T., Li, Y.H., and Morris, R. (1994). Hazardous chemicals—Psychological dimensions of the health sequelae of a community exposure in Texas. *Journal of Epidemiology and Community Health*, 48(6), 560-568.

Dhara, V.R., and Dhara, R. (2002). The Union Carbide disaster in Bhopal: A review of health effects. *Archives of Environmental Health*, 57(5), 391-404.

Dohrenwend, B.P. (1983). Psychological implications of nuclear accidents—The case of Three-Mile-Island. *Bulletin of the New York Academy of Medicine*, 59(10), 1060-1076.

Eggleston, P.A., Buckley, T.J., Breysse, P.N., Wills-Karp, M., Kleeberger, S.R., and Jaakkola, J.K.K. (1999). The environment and asthma in US inner cities. *Environmental Health Perspectives*, 107, 439-450.

Elliott, S.J., Taylor, S.M., Walter, S., Steib, D., Frank, J., and Eyles, J. (1993). Modeling psychosocial effects of exposure to solid-waste facilities. *Social Science & Medicine*, 37(6), 791-807.

Fagan, J., Galea, S., Ahern, J., Bonner, S., and Vlahov, D. (2002). Self-reported increase in asthma severity after the September 11 attacks on the World Trade Center—Manhattan, New York, 2001. *Journal of the American Medical Association*, 288(12), 1466-1467.

Foster, H. (2003). *What really causes schizophrenia*. Victoria, BC: Trafford.

Foster, R.P. (2002). The long-term mental health effects of nuclear trauma in recent Russian immigrants in the United States. *American Journal of Orthopsychiatry*, 72(4), 492-504.

Gee, G.C., and Payne-Sturges, D.C. (2004). Environmental health disparities: A framework integrating psychosocial and environmental concepts. *Environmental Health Perspectives*, 112(17), 1645-1653.

Ginzburg, H.M. (1993). The psychological consequences of the Chernobyl accident: Findings from the International Atomic Energy Agency study. *Public Health Reports*, 108(2), 184-192.

Goldsteen, R.L, Goldsteen, K., and Schorr, J.K. (1992). Trust and its relationship to psychological distress—The case of Three Mile Island. *Political Psychology*, 13(4), 693-707.

Greve, K.W., Bianchini, K.J., Doane, B.M., Love, J.M., and Stickle, T.R. (2005). Psychological evaluation of the emotional effects of a community toxic exposure. *Journal of Occupational and Environmental Medicine*, 47(1), 51-59.

Havenaar, J.M., and van den Brink, W. (1997). Psychological factors affecting health after toxicological disasters. *Clinical Psychology Review*, 17(4), 359-574.

Havenaar, J.M., deWilde, E.J., van den Bout, J., Drozzt-Sjoberg, B.M., and van den Brink, W. (2003). Perception of risk and subjective health among victims of the Chernobyl disaster. *Social Science & Medicine*, 56(3), 569-572.

Hayes, M. (1999). "Man, disease and environmental associations": From medical geography to health inequities. *Progress in Human Geography*, 23(2), 289-296.

Herman, D., Felton, C., and Susser, E. (2002). Mental health needs in New York state following the September 11th attacks. *Journal of Urban Health—Bulletin of the New York Academy of Medicine*, 79(3), 322-331.

Huppe, M., and Janke, W. (1994). The nuclear plant accident in Chernobyl experience by men and women of different ages—Empirical study in the years 1986-1991. *Anxiety, Stress and Coping*, 7(4), 339-355.

Jacobs, S.V., Evans, G.W., Catalano, R., and Dooley, D. (1984). Air pollution and depressive symptomatology—Exploratory analyses of intervening psychosocial factors. *Population and Environment*, 7(4), 260-272.

Kimes, D., Levine, E., Timmins, S., Weiss, S.R., Bollinger, M.E., and Blaisdell, C. (2004). Temporal dynamics of emergency department and hospital admissions of pediatric asthmatics. *Environmental Research*, 94(1), 7-17.

Ladbury, R. (1996). Model sheds light on a tragedy and a new type of eruption. *Physics Today*, 49(5), 20-22.

Le Guern, F., Shanklin, E., and Tebor, S. (1992). Witness accounts of the catastrophic event of August 1986 at Lake Nyos (Cameroon). *Journal of Volcanology and Geothermal Research*, 51(1-2), 171-184.

Levin, S.M., Herbert, R., Moline, J.M., Todd, A.C., Stevenson, L., Landsbergis, P., Jiang, S., Skloot, G., Baron, S., and Enright, P. (2004). Physical health status of World Trade Center rescue and recovery workers and volunteers – New York City, July 2002-August 2004. *Journal of the American Medical Association*, 292, 1811-1813.

Love Canal probe 'botched'. *Calgary Herald*, May 15, 1991, D17.

Luginaah, I.N., Taylor, S.M., Elliott, S.J., and Eyles, J.D. (2000). A longitudinal study of the health impacts of a petroleum refinery. *Social Science & Medicine*, 50(7-8), 1155-1166.

Luginaah, I.N., Taylor, S.M., Elliott, S.J., and Eyles, J.D. (2002a). Community reappraisal of the perceived health effects of a petroleum refinery. *Social Science & Medicine*, 55(1), 47-61.

Luginaah, I.N., Taylor, S.M., Elliott, S.J., and Eyles, J.D. (2002b). Community responses and coping strategies in the vicinity of a petroleum refinery in Oakville, Ontario. *Health & Place*, 8(3), 177-190.

Masjedi, M.R., Jamaati, H.R., Dokouhaki, P., Ahmadzadeh, Z., Taheri, S.A., Bigdeli, M., Izadi, S., Rostamian, A., Aagin, K., and Ghavam, S.M. (2003). The effects of air pollution on acute respiratory conditions. *Respirology*, 8(2), 213-230.

Matas, R. (2005). Strahl stricken with lung cancer at the age of 48. *The Globe and Mail*, 23 August 2005, S1-2.

McKinney, K., Benson, S., Lempert, A., Singal, M., Wallingford, K., and Snyder, E. (2002). Occupational exposures to air contaminants at the World Trade Center disaster site—New York, September-October, 2001. *Journal of the American Medical Association*, 287(24), 3201-3202.

Melnik, T.A., Baker, C.T., Adams, M.L., O'Dowd, K., Mokdad, A.J., Murphy, W., Giles, W.H., and Bales, V.S. (2002). Psychological and emotional effects of the September 11 attacks on the World Trade Center—Connecticut, New Jersey, and New York, 2001. *Journal of the American Medical Association*, 288(12), 1467-1468.

Mitchell, B. (2002). Resource and Environmental Management (2nd ed.). Harlow, UK: Pearson Education Ltd.

Morris, C. (2005). Ottawa won't rubber-stamp N.B. claims for Agent Orange compensation. *Canadian Press*, August 15, 2005.

Ooi, P.L., and Goh, K.T. (1997). Sick building syndrome: An emerging stress-related disorder? *International Journal of Epidemiology*, 26(6), 1243-1249.

Palinkas, L.A., Downs, M.A., Petterson, J.S., and Russell, J. (1993). Social, cultural, and psychological impacts of the Exxon Valdez oil spill. *Human Organization*, 52(1), 1-13.

Pongracic, J., and Evans, R. (2001). Environmental and socioeconomic risk factors in asthma. *Immunology and Allergy Clinics of North America*, 21(3), 413.

Porteous, J.D. (1996). *Environmental aesthetics: Ideas, politics and planning*. London: Brunner-Routledge.

Prezant, D.J., Weiden, W., Banauch, G.I., McGuinness, G., Rom, W.N., Aldrich, T.K., and Kelly, K.J. (2002). Cough and bronchial responsiveness in firefighters at the World Trade Center site. *New England Journal of Medicine*, 347(11), 806-815.

Princeembury, S. (1988). Psychological symptoms of residents in the aftermath of the Three Mile Island nuclear accident and restart. *Journal of Social Psychology*, 128(6), 779-790.

Princeembury, S. (1992a). Information attributes as related to psychological symptoms and perceived control among information seekers in the aftermath of technological disaster. *Journal of Applied Social Psychology*, 22(14), 1148-1159.

Princeembury, S. 1992b. Psychological symptoms as related to cognitive appraisals and demographic differences among information seekers in the aftermath of technological disaster at Three Mile Island. *Journal of Applied Social Psychology*, 22(1), 38-54.

Rachman, S. (2004). Fear of contamination. *Behaviour Research and Therapy*, 42(11), 1227-1255.

Rahu, M. (2003). Health effects of the Chernobyl accident: Fears, rumours and the truth. *European Journal of Cancer*, 39(3), 295-299.

Reid, B. (1986). Mercury poisoning again. *The Whig-Standard*, Kingston, ON, April 21, 1986.

Rotko, T., Oglesby, L., Kunzli, N., Carrer, P., Nieuwenhuijsen, M.J., and Jantunen, M. (2002). Determinants of perceived air pollution annoyance and association between annoyance scores and air pollution (PM 2.5, NO2) concentrations in the European EXPOLIS study. *Atmospheric Environment*, 36(29), 4593-4602.

Ruback, R.B., and Pandey, J. (2002). Mental distress and physical symptoms in the slums of New Delhi: The role of individual, household, and neighborhood factors. *Journal of Applied Social Psychology*, 32(11), 2296-2320.

Schachter, H. (1990). Chernobyl's afterglow. *The Whig-Standard*, Kingston, ON, May 7, 1990.

Schauer, A., and Dornow, R. (2001). Mental disorders and environmental control. *Gesundheitswesen*, 63(2), 79-84.

Schell, L.M., and Denham, M. (2003). Environmental pollution in urban environments and human biology. *Annual Review of Anthropology*, 32, 111-134.

Schmidt, W. (1990). Missourians battle over burying a toxic ghost town; Times Beach, evacuated in '83, is national symbol like Love Canal. *The Gazette*, Montreal, June 23, 1990.

Schneider, A. (2002). NYC under an asbestos cloud. *Seattle Post-Intelligencer*, January 14, 2002.

Sellers, C. (2003). September 11 and the history of hazard. *Journal of the History of Medicine and Allied Sciences*, 58(4), 449-458.

Shaw, H. (1999). Largest evacuation in Canada was 20 years ago. *Tribune*, Welland, ON, November 10, 1999.

Smith, K. (1996). *Environmental hazards: Assessing risk and reducing disaster* (2nd ed.). London: Routledge.

United States Government Accountability Office (2004). Testimony before the Subcommittee on National Security, Emerging Threats, and International Relations, Committee on Government Reform, House of Representatives. September 11. Health Effects in the Aftermath of the World Trade Center Attack. Statement of Janet Heinrich, Direct, Health Care – Public Health Issues. GAO-04-1068T. *http://www.gao.gov/htext/d041068t.html* (accessed February 28, 2007).

Wakefield, S.E.L., Elliott, S.J., Cole, D.C., and Eyles, J.D. (2001). Environmental risk and (re)action: Air quality, health, and civic involvement in an urban industrial neighbourhood. *Health & Place*, 7(3), 163-177.

Walton, D. (2004). Plans to drill gas wells near Calgary raise fears. *The Globe and Mail*, 12 April, A1, A5.

Wilkinson, R. (2005). *The impact of inequality: How to make sick societies healthier*. New York: New Press.

Wolfe, J., Proctor, S.P., Erickson, D.J., and Hu, H. (2002). Risk factors for multisymptom illness in US army veterans of the Gulf War. *Journal of Occupational and Environmental Medicine*, 44(3), 271-281.

Under the Weather: The Biometeorology of Mental Health Status

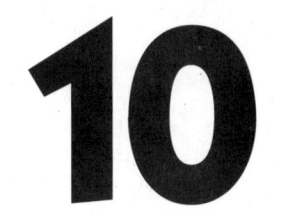

Lisa Kadonaga
Department of Geography, University of Victoria

James A. LeClair
Department of Geography, Nipissing University

INTRODUCTION

Weather got you down?

The connection between weather and climate and our emotional well-being appears to be well-entrenched in the English language—consider that both prevailing atmospheric conditions and one's mood might be characterized as 'foul,' 'miserable,' or 'gloomy.' We might find ourselves 'in a fog,' or suffering from 'the doldrums.' We may describe someone as having a 'sunny' disposition, characterize another's temper as 'stormy,' or their emotional state as 'changing with the wind.'

The belief in a causal link between weather and climate and health status has a long pedigree, going back at least to Hippocrates' oft-cited work, *On Airs, Waters, and Places*, written in 400BCE:

> Whoever wishes to investigate medicine properly, should proceed thus: in the first place to consider the seasons of the year, and what effects each of them produces for they are not at all alike, but differ much from themselves in regard to their changes. Then the winds, the hot and the cold, especially such as are common to all countries, and then such as are peculiar to each locality (translated by Adams, 1849).

Numerous attempts to identify and explain seasonal patterns in mood and behaviour have been made (Ennis and McConville, 2003). Psychiatric admissions and suicide rates, for example, exhibit a distinct seasonality, with an apparent spring-summer peak and winter trough (Kim et al., 2004; Papadopoulos et al., 2005). Likewise, Ohtani and coworkers (2006) report August and December peaks for panic disorder symptoms.

Through the late 1980s and into the 1990s, increasing interest was shown in the potential mental health impacts of environmental stressors such as temperature (Sundstrom, Bell, Busby, and Asmus, 1996). In terms of both public recognition and theoretical mechanisms, however, the best-known of these is undoubtedly Seasonal Affective Disorder (SAD), and its relationship to annual variations in sunlight received at the earth's surface.

In this chapter, we consider the research evidence linking a number of weather- and climate-related factors to psychological well-being. Specifically, attention is paid to the role of seasonal and other cyclical effects, as well as the potential impact of variations in temperature, humidity, wind, barometric pressure, and air quality. Finally, we reflect on what role climate change may play in ameliorating—or exacerbating—the weather- and climate-related effects discussed.

SUNLIGHT AND SEASONAL AFFECTIVE DISORDER

Early in the 20th century, scientists generally dismissed the idea that seasonal changes in sunlight duration and intensity affected humans, although photoperiod changes were known to influence the behaviour of other organisms (Peters, 1994). Colloquial reports of 'winter blues' or 'cabin fever,' rather than being considered to have a possible medical basis, were generally attributed to other factors, such as restlessness or boredom, exacerbated by the restriction of social activities during inclement winter weather. Not until a landmark study by Rosenthal and colleagues (1984) did the topic of seasonal depression gain official standing, along with the name Seasonal Affective Disorder, or SAD.

In the intervening decades, there have been many attempts to document the prevalence of SAD, and to investigate the underlying physiological and psychological causes of the condition. Assessments of the percentage of the population afflicted have been carried out in many regions, including Sweden (Chotai, Smedh, Johansson, Nilsson, and Adolfsson, 2004; Rastad, Ulfberg, and Sjoden, 2006), the US (Agumadu et al., 2004), Japan (Imai, Kayukawa, Ohta, Li, and Nakagawa, 2003) and Australia (Morrissey, Raggatt, James, and Rogers, 1996; Murray, 2004). Within these populations, SAD appears to be more prevalent in females than in males (Peters, 1994; Magnusson and Boivin, 2003).

Rather than being an 'either/or' situation, SAD appears to occur along a continuum. In addition to the chronic sufferers, there is a much larger group who experience less severe symptoms of the condition (Morrissey, Raggatt, James, and Rogers, 1996, Chotai et al., 2004). These individuals undergo mood changes which are significant, and affect quality of life, but not so acutely that they would be considered to suffer from full-blown SAD (Peters, 1994). Researchers now recognize the existence of summer and winter variants of Seasonal Affective Disorder (Fieve, 1989), with the winter type being more widespread (Imai et al., 2003; Agumadu et al., 2004; Maeno et al., 2005)—at least in temperate latitudes. Morrissey and coworkers (1996) present evidence that, in the tropics, the ratio may be reversed: their research in a northern Australian town found that 9% of respondents reported summer SAD, compared with 1.7% for the winter type.

Two types of SAD sufferers have been identified: those experiencing recurrent depression and those in a bipolar state, wherein depression alternates with euphoria during other seasons (Peters, 1994). Peters also notes that feelings of dread or panic may occur during sub-seasonal weather fluctuations (such as several continuous days of cloudy weather), or during the lead-up to the winter season, as nights lengthen; a situation made more noticeable after the end of daylight savings time in the autumn.

The prevalence of this condition appears to increase with latitude: some sources claim that in excess of 10% of people in the vicinity of the 49th parallel are affected; others suggest that the actual prevalence in the population may be less than half that. However, once those manifesting less severe 'winter blues' are included, the proportion rises to at least 12%—and possibly as high as 25% —in Canada and the US border states (Peters, 1994).

The causal mechanisms underlying Seasonal Affective Disorder are not completely understood, but appear to involve neurotransmitters such as serotonin (Magnusson and Boivin, 2003; Sher et al., 2005). It has been suggested that there may be an anatomical factor present in some individuals which impairs neurotransmission, and hence enhances susceptibility to SAD. Based on a higher occurrence of myopia among SAD patients, for example, it has been proposed that, in such individuals, not enough light reaches the photoreceptors and travels along the optic nerve to stimulate the hypothalamus (Peters, 1994). An alternate hypothesis suggests that disruptions to the circadian system, such as through developmental alcohol exposure, may make people more susceptible to seasonal mood disorders such as SAD, and also to non-seasonal ones like depression and bipolar symptoms (Sher, 2004).

Papadoupoulous and coworkers (2005) take a different approach to the study of how sunlight affects mental health. Pointing to the early summertime peak in suicide rates, they propose a lag-and-duration effect wherein exposure to intense sunshine has an antidepressant effect that may actually improve motivation before influencing mood. This may result in a temporary increase in suicide risk for up to 4 days.

Although the exact processes have not yet been conclusively described, investigations into the origins of SAD have led to more research into photosensitivity and the possible ramifications of light and other electromagnetic radiation for human health. Aboulnaga (2006), for example, suggests that the blockage of particular light wavelengths (as may occur with new varieties of energy-saving architectural glass) could adversely affect the mood and overall mental health of people who live and work in those buildings.

Work is also being undertaken on the pineal gland and the function of the melatonin it produces (Macchi and Bruce, 2004). Other researchers are trying to understand what, if any, relationship exists between SAD-linked depression and other psychological disorders (Kim et al., 2004; Michalak et al, 2004; Ibrahim, Strempel, and Tschernitschek, 2005; Sher et al., 2005).

As well, sociobiological theories of SAD have been posited, the suggestion being that SAD may have conveyed a possible reproductive advantage on prehistoric humans (Eagles, 2004; Davis and Levitan, 2005). Eagles (2004) proposes an 'attenuated hibernation' model, wherein the minor hypomania experienced by some winter SAD sufferers in the spring and summer could increase reproductive success, at least for mid-latitude regions. Women would be more likely to conceive during the summer, and give birth the following spring—in theory, this would be at a time when the weather was becoming milder, and more food was becoming available, as the growing season progressed. Eagles also suggests that the winter depression symptoms of SAD may be beneficial to pregnancies, and to female-mate pair-bonding, both of which would tend to increase pregnancy survivability for women and their offspring. Davis and Levitan (2005) broaden the evolutionary advantages of SAD to include energy conservation in general, pointing out that lethargy and weight gain would be taking place at a season when the food supply was low.

The growing willingness to view Seasonal Affective Disorder as a *bona fide* medical condition was helped by the fact that the treatment of SAD using exposure to artificial light is highly effective (Rosenthal et al., 1984; Magnusson and Boivin, 2003; Levitan, 2005): Fieve (1989) notes that the response to light, whether natural or artificial, is rapid. The simplicity and straightforwardness of things such as 'bright light' therapy, when compared with a pharmacological approach, likely contributed to the acceptance of SAD in popular culture. Within a few years of Rosenthal and colleagues' (1984) paper, the condition was being discussed in popular science and mainstream periodicals.

TEMPERATURE EFFECTS

While both summer and winter SAD have been recognized, most of the existing body of research has focused on the more common winter variant. There is increasing interest, however, in summer (the so-called 'reverse') SAD (Fieve, 1989). In this case, the environmental triggers for seasonal affect are thought to be related to heat and humidity rather than photoperiod (Peters, 1994). Summer SAD patients "have been treated by manipulating both temperature and light conditions during different seasons of the year" (Fieve, 1989, p. 89), presumably by controlling indoor illumination, heating, and air conditioning.

There appear to be some differences in the affected population: summer SAD tends to be found in an older cohort (over-30s), compared to winter SAD sufferers who can be in their 20s or younger (Peters, 1994). In addition, men seem to be more prone to summer SAD, and the symptoms (depression, agitation, insomnia, loss of appetite, lack of energy, nominal sex drive) are more consistent with other depressive disorders than with winter SAD (Peters, 1994). Peters also warns that suicide risk appears higher for summer SAD. As well, some individuals appear to suffer from both winter and summer depression. This is rare, however, and winter-only SAD is more prevalent by far.

Although Chotai and co-workers (2004) report that women, in particular, seem to be emotionally-responsive to changes in temperature (that is, negative to short/cold days, and positive to long/hot days), Garvey and coworkers (1988) do not find that extremely cold winter temperatures are a significant factor in depressive symptomatology.

High temperatures have, however, been observed as a risk factor for depressive episodes in people affected by bipolar disorders. Shapira and colleagues (2004) note a significant correlation between mean maximum monthly temperatures and admission rates for bipolar (as opposed to unipolar) patients. In addition, Maes and co-workers (1994) report that violent suicide is significantly and positively correlated, not only with temperature and amount of sunlight, but with temperature increases over a number of weeks.

For some time there has been anecdotal evidence that summer hot spells can have a negative effect on mood in the general population: the experience of frustration when a workplace or residential building's air conditioning system breaks down, for example, is widespread. Keller and colleagues (2005) provide some psychological research to confirm a relationship between hot summer weather and deterioration in mood. Of particular interest are studies carried out in schools and offices, where aggressive behaviour, restlessness, low morale, and difficulty concentrating have been linked with uncomfortably warm temperatures (Auliciems, 1977; Arnetz, Berg, and Arnetz, 1997; Lundin, 1999).

THE ROLE OF RELATIVE HUMIDITY AND WEATHER VARIABILITY

Although it is often said that hot, humid conditions are much more unpleasant than a 'dry heat,' the research evidence for a link between high relative humidity and diminished mental health is, at best, ambiguous. Peters (1994) notes that heat and humidity are implicated in both the onset of summer SAD, and a decline in mood in the general population during the June-August months for the northern hemisphere. Likewise, Persinger (1975) attempts to match self-evaluated mood report with weather variables such as temperature, barometric pressure, relative humidity, duration of sunlight, and wind speed. Although based on a very small sample (n=10), the results obtained reveal a weak yet statistically significant correlation between 'lower' moods and higher relative humidity in the preceding 48 hour period. A significant positive relationship is also observed between relative humidity and suicide among the elderly (Salib, 1997). Salib and Sharp (2002), on the other hand, report a significant *inverse* relationship between hospital admissions for affective disorders and relative humidity values during the previous week.

The equivocal nature of the humidity-mental health link apparent in these results may be due to the confounding effects of related variables—consider that relative humidity is related to temperature, precipitation, and the passing of weather fronts—the impact of lag effects, and even the outcome variables considered (mortality measures versus treatment-seeking behaviours, for example). This question of possible cumulative effects is addressed by Maes and coworkers (1992), who suggest that a combination of present and recent-past conditions explain mood changes better than present environmental conditions alone, although the sample size employed is even smaller than that of Persinger. In a later study, Maes and colleagues (1994) note that violent suicide is correlated with rising temperatures occurring over several weeks, not just with ambient temperature and day length. In the same study, violent suicide appears to have a negative relationship with relative humidity (in contrast with temperature and sunlight hours, both of which exhibited a significant positive correlation).

Some research points to an apparent sensitivity to weather conditions among those people with a diagnosed psychological disorder. Barnston (1988), for example, compares students and crisis intervention service clients. Students and crisis callers with 'mild' problems are reported to have been more stressed in unstable, cloudy, warm, and humid conditions, and less so in clear, dry, cool conditions. However, these reactions were opposite for crisis service clients with more severe problems.

In a study by North and co-workers (1998), homeless people in general, and males in particular, appear more vulnerable to the apparent mood-altering effects of daily weather conditions. The researchers, studying the diagnosis of mental illness in homeless men and women, report that women in the sample do not show significant correlations between weather variables and psychiatric diagnoses. However, among the men, lifetime diagnoses of major depression and lifetime drug use disorder are both associated with precipitation and colder temperatures on the interviewing day. Diagnoses of both current depression and lifetime anti-social personality disorder are associated with precipitation. The authors comment, however, that these data are insufficient to reveal whether it is primarily the reporting of the information in the interviews which is being affected by the weather, or the actual occurrence of the disorders themselves.

Such gender discrepancies could be due to a number of factors. North and colleagues (1998) claim that previous work was not specifically geared to identify gender differences, instead combining male and female cases for analysis. Another possible explanation is that in the study sample the women were being allowed to stay in the homeless shelters all day, while the men were more exposed to inclement weather since they were required to leave and not allowed back in until the evening. The authors emphasize that diagnoses of lifetime disorders are evidently not due to the weather conditions on a single day, focusing instead on the possibility that the correlation between cold, wet weather and major depression could simply indicate the vulnerability of those without housing to increased misery, hardship, and stress, which may trigger mental illness. If this is the case, a significant number of clinically-depressed homeless people may not be responsive to treatments developed for other, 'biological' types of depression. Instead they may (and according to the authors, do) show improvement when the stressors themselves are addressed—namely, by addressing their need for housing, a cheaper and more effective solution than misapplied psychiatric treatment (North et al., 1998).

WIND AND AIR PRESSURE CHANGES

In many cultural traditions, winds are linked with human history, health, and fortune. Reflective of this, Watson (1984) attempts to describe the influence of a wide range of atmospheric phenomena on human culture. Connections between wind speed and/or direction, and human moods, for example, have been alluded to in the humanistic literature (see Golinski, 2001, for instance), with some attempts at more scientific investigation. An early study by Auliciems (1977) reports that, among his student sample, aggression increased with windiness, even when the children were indoors.

Wind, frontal systems, and barometric pressure have not been the focus of as much scientific research as the other climate-related variables discussed, such as temperature (e.g., Cohn and Rotton, 2000; Hipp, Bauer, Curran, and Bollen, 2004) and sunshine (Hirshleifer and Shumway, 2003; Goetzmann and Zhu, 2005). However, there are a few research topics that have consistently attracted attention, such as proposed connections between locally-famous winds like California's Santa Ana and crime patterns within the affected region (Miller, 1968). The Santa Ana has also been implicated in physiological ailments, such as asthma (Corbett, 1996), while frontal systems and pressure changes in general have been blamed for migraines (Watson, 1984).

Other specific wind patterns, like the Chamsin of the Near East (Gilbert, 1973) and the Chinooks of the Rockies, have been investigated. Rose, Verhoef, and Ramcharan (1995) identify 'Chinook sensitivity' in specific subgroups, such as those with a history of chronic health problems or mood disorders.

AIR QUALITY ISSUES

In the realm of workplace health and safety, 'sick building syndrome' is an ongoing concern. The health problems characteristic of this syndrome may be due to the presence of airborne contaminants (such as volatile organic compounds from carpeting and adhesives, tobacco smoke, and vehicle exhaust), and to poor air circulation and hypoxia, even without the presence of hazardous chemicals. Respiratory ailments, irritation of the mucous membranes, and headaches have all been found to contribute to distraction, discomfort, anxiety, and ongoing stress (Arnetz, Berg, and Arnetz, 1997; Lundin, 1999; Kimmel et al., 2000). Worries about long term exposure to these conditions have prompted such measures as banning smoking and fragrances from the workplace.

Other atmospheric components that have been studied, aside from chemical contaminants, are positively- and negatively-charged ions. Higher levels of positively-charged ions are believed to be associated with not just headaches, but depression and irritability through increased brain serotonin levels (Gilbert, 1973; Fornof and Gilbert, 1988). The results of experiments have been mixed: tests by Albrechtsen and co-workers (1978) on human subjects do not show significant effects after exposure to both positive and negative atmospheric ions, and the authors suggest that the general population may not be sensitive to these conditions. Inbar and colleagues (1982), using a slightly larger sample size, report some improvements in cardiovascular and thermoregulatory variables during exertion in a hot, dry environment (around 40°C and 25% relative humidity). Fornof and Gilbert (1988) consider elementary school children who had already been identified as environmentally sensitive, and find that negative air ionization appears to improve their attention span and classroom performance.

Although the science is not conclusive, and many other factors such as existing stressors and illnesses appear to be involved in making individuals susceptible to changes in air ionization (Fornof and Gilbert, 1988), electronic 'ionizing units' for the home or office have been marketed commercially for a number of years, often combined with filtration units to screen out contaminants such as airborne pollen, spores, and dust.

SEASONALITY AND CYCLICAL EFFECTS

There has been speculation about the possible role of environmental conditions at or before the time of birth, and whether susceptibility to mental illness could be affected. Various researchers have noted an apparent pattern in season of birth and the diagnosis of schizophrenia later in life. A range of studies carried out in different countries have shown an apparent winter-spring peak in birth seasonality for schizophrenia-related and bipolar disorders (Torrey, Miller, Rawlings, and Yolken, 1997), although some authors have found it statistically insignificant (Fouskakis et al., 2004). Possible explanations for this pattern include seasonal effects of particular genes, pregnancy and birth complications, environmental contaminants, temperature and other climatic factors, shifts in diet/nutrition, and even infectious pathogens such as viruses (Torrey et al., 1997; Kinney et al., 2000). Kinney and colleagues (2000) propose that the seasonality of births among those with schizophrenia might be due to a combination of conditions, with environmental factors affecting winter births, and genetics playing a more critical role for schizophrenics born in the milder spring and fall seasons. By contrast, Fouskakis and co-workers (2004) report no seasonal effects on fetal growth, and while there appears to be an increased risk of schizophrenia for winter births in their sample, they do not consider it significant. Apparent birth seasonality has also been observed for suicide [May] (Salib, 2002), autism [March], and major depression [March-May] (Torrey et al., 1997).

Going beyond seasonal patterns, McGrath, Selten, and Chant (2002) report an apparent negative association between decreasing long term (inter-annual) trends in hours of bright sunshine, and increasing schizophrenia birth rates among males (but not females). They note that diagnosed schizophrenics of both sexes who were born during low-sunshine intervals had earlier ages of first registration (a proxy for age of onset of the disorder). The authors were unable to offer an explanation for the gender differences, but suggest that easier transmission of unspecified pathogens in crowded indoor settings, during rainy weather, might be something that could affect individuals when they were still in the pre/perinatal phase. Alternatively, a decrease in bright sunshine might be connected with lower ultraviolet (UV) radiation levels, altering human immune response in such a way as to affect fetuses and newborns. A further possibility is that decreasing UV could affect perinatal vitamin D availability, which is suspected to influence fetal brain development.

Another cyclical effect is suggested by Davis and Lowell (2004). They point to higher ultraviolet radiation exposure during the peaks of some 11-year solar cycles, and speculate that this could lead to an increased incidence of mutation-induced neurochemical abnormalities in temperate and subtropical regions between the equator and the poles—areas that experience the most variability in UV levels.

CLIMATE CHANGE

Over the past decade, a substantial amount of work has been done on the potential impacts of global warming on human health. While the physical health implications of global warming are now routinely discussed in impact assessments (e.g., Watson, Zinyowera, and Moss, 1998) and policy documents (e.g., US Department of State, 2002 and Health Canada, 2003), mental and psychosocial impacts remain relatively understudied.

Since photoperiod is the trigger for the winter type of SAD (Fieve, 1989; Peters, 1994), increasing temperatures would not likely ameliorate this, without some indirect effect, such as a shift in atmospheric circulation patterns that reduced cloud cover in the temperate or polar latitudes, where the population tends to be the most vulnerable. In fact, according to the Intergovernmental Panel on Climate Change, cloud cover and annual precipitation has increased in the past few decades, possibly connected with rising global temperatures (IPCC, 2001). A Canadian federal study forecasts more precipitation in the fall and winter months, for the Yukon and BC respectively, due to global warming;

all other factors being equal, this would imply less sunlight during those months of the year (Environment Canada, 2004). Milder winter temperatures could, however, induce more people to go outdoors, increasing their exposure to natural light (albeit the reduced solar intensity of winter days).

Although the temperature changes expected with global climate change would not affect the planet's axial tilt, which is the main cause of the seasonal cycle associated with winter SAD, the potential impact of rising temperatures poses a particular concern for summer SAD. Researchers have suggested that an increasing frequency and severity of heat waves (US Department of State, 2002) and periods of high humidity are a likely outcome of global warming (IPCC, 2001)—the same factors which, as suggested previously, have been linked to summer SAD (Peters, 1994). Temperate areas that normally experience only a few days each year over 30°C would have many more. For many Canadian cities, the average number of hot days could nearly triple, totalling almost 2 weeks per year for Victoria and Calgary, and 35 days or more for cities such as Winnipeg, London, and Fredericton (Hengeveld, 1991). Urban populations would be particularly vulnerable, as they remain warm at night, and offer little relief from daytime heat (US Department of State, 2002).

While Shindell and Raso (1997) downplay the psychosocial impacts of global warming, they do suggest that local differences in social, political, and economic conditions will ultimately affect responses. In fact, the vulnerability of some areas to natural disasters has already been demonstrated by events such as the Chicago heat wave of 1995. Klinenberg (2002a) examines how community characteristics contributed to the death toll in Chicago's inner city. In a later interview, he notes that social isolation, abandonment by private and public services, and the lack of official understanding created "hazardous social conditions that are always present but difficult to perceive...everyday disasters" (Klinenberg, 2002b). This example not only foreshadows what happened during the Hurricane Katrina disaster in New Orleans but it also suggests that the same conditions could hamper diagnosis and treatment of ailments such as summer SAD, on an individual scale. Isolated sufferers unwilling or unable to seek help would find these obstacles difficult to surmount. This is of particular concern since, as noted earlier, the risk of suicide appears to be higher for summer SAD than for its winter variant (Peters, 1994).

While it is not known how many people who presently manifest borderline summer SAD might experience more severe symptoms with increasing temperatures, anecdotal evidence and some supporting research (such as Morrissey et al., 1996 and Peters, 1994) suggest that a substantial proportion of the population already experiences emotional (and physical) discomfort during hot, humid weather. If such conditions become more frequent and severe, lethargy, nausea, and increased sensitivity to respiratory problems and migraine headaches could have a significant impact on both physical and psychosocial well-being, with potential negative health effects for individuals, families, and entire communities.

Conclusion

When it comes to our mental health, can we really find ourselves 'under the weather'? Although in many cases the evidence for weather- and climate-related effects on psychological well-being is fragmentary and equivocal (with the notable exception of SAD), such explanations are at least worthy of further consideration and research attention. Although physical environmental conditions are only one category of factors that can influence mental health, there are some environmental variables that research has revealed as having significant implications for mood and overall psychological well-being.

Seasonal patterns for various psychological disorders, such as depression and schizophrenia, have been documented and efforts are underway to uncover possible mechanisms that could account for them, such as the relationship between seasonality, ultraviolet radiation, and biological variables like immune response and vitamin D availability.

Seasonal Affective Disorder (SAD), which gained clinical acceptance in the mid-1980s, is probably the most widely recognized and best understood of these environmentally-triggered illnesses. In the intervening two decades, numerous researchers have mapped its prevalence, and undertaken to investigate the underlying physiological and sociobiological causes of the disorder. In addition to those who are chronically afflicted with SAD, there are many individuals who experience less severe symptoms that affect their quality of life. Summer and winter variants of SAD have been identified, with the winter type being more widespread, at least in temperate latitudes. While winter SAD is activated by decreased levels of sunlight, 'reverse' or summer SAD is believed to be connected with heat and humidity. These findings have had significant implications for the successful treatment of this condition.

For other disorders, environmental relationships are more complicated. An apparent winter-spring peak in birth seasonality has been observed for schizophrenia and bipolar disorders, and while there are no universally-accepted explanations yet, a variety of hypotheses have been proposed. Also, longtime anecdotal associations between environmental factors, such as temperature or the occurrence of seasonal winds like California's Santa Ana, and violent crime rates have been shown to involve many more socio-cultural variables.

As we enter a period when profound global environmental changes are unfolding, there is increasing interest from scientists and policymakers in assessing the potential impacts of such changes on human health. In addition to physical factors, for example from storms, heat stress, and new or more widespread pathogens, it seems apparent that mental and psychosocial effects should also be considered in order to plan for future health care delivery.

REFERENCES

Aboulnaga, M.M. (2006). Towards green buildings: glass as a building element – the use and miuse in the Gulf region. *Renewable Energy*, 31(5), 631-653.

Adams, F. (Translator) (1849). *On Airs, Waters, and Places*. The complete text of this work is available online at "The Internet Classics Archive." Retrieved November 1, 2006 from http://classics.mit.edu/Hippocrates/airwatpl.html.

Agumadu, C.O., Yousufi, S.M., Malik, L.S., Nguyen, M.C.T., Jackson, M.A., Soleymani, K., Thrower, C.M., Peterman, M.J., Walters, G.W., Niemtzoff, M.J., Bartko, J.J., and Postolache, T.T. (2004). Seasonal variation in mood in African-American college students in the Washington, DC metropolitan area. *American Journal of Psychiatry*, 161(6), 1084-1089.

Albrechtsen, O., Clausen, V., Christensen, F.G., Gensen, J.G., and Moller, T. (1978). The influence of small atmospheric ions on human well-being and mental performance. *International Journal of Biometeorology*, 22(4), 249-262.

Arnetz, B.B., Berg, M., and Arnetz, J. (1997). Mental strain and physical symptoms among employees in modern offices. *Archives of Environmental Health*, 52(1), 63-67.

Auliciems, A. (1978). Mood dependency on low intensity atmospheric variability. *International Journal of Biometeorology*, 22(1), 20-32

Barnston, A.G. (1988). The effect of weather on mood, productivity, and frequency of emotional crisis in a temperate continental climate. *International Journal of Biometeorology*, 32, 134-143.

Chotai, J., Smedh, K., Johansson, C., Nilsson, L.G., and Adolfsson, R. (2004). An epidemiological study on gender differences in self-reported seasonal changes in mood and behaviour in a general population of northern Sweden. *Nordic Journal of Psychiatry*, 58(6), 429-437.

Cohn, E.G., and Rotton, J. (2000). Weather, seasonal trends and property crimes in Minneapolis, 1987-1988. A moderator-variable time-series analysis of routine activities. *Journal of Environmental Psychology*, 20(3), 257-272.

Corbett, S.W. (1996). Asthma exacerbations during Santa Ana winds in southern California. *Wilderness and Environmental Medicine*, 7(4), 304-311.

Davis, C., and Levitan, R.D. (2005). Seasonality and seasonal affective disorder (SAD): An evolutionary viewpoint tied to energy conservation and reproductive cycles. *Journal of Affective Disorders*, 87(1), 3-10.

Davis, G.E., and Lowell, W.E. (2004). Chaotic solar cycles modulate the incidence and severity of mental illness. *Medical Hypotheses*, 62(2), 207-214.

Eagles, J.M. (2004). Seasonal affective disorder: A vestigial evolutionary advantage? *Medical Hypotheses*, 63(5), 767-772.

Ennis, E., and McConville, C. (2003). Personality traits associated with seasonal disturbances in mood and behavior. *Current Psychology*, 22(4), 326-338.

Environment Canada (2004). Canada Country Study (summary). http://climatechange.gc.ca/english/publications/ccs. Updated 2004-08-20.

Fieve, R. (1989). *Moodswing (2nd ed.)*. New York: William Morrow and Company.

Fornof, K.T., and Gilbert, G.O. (1988). Stress and physiological, behavioral and performance patterns of children under varied air ion levels. *International Journal of Biometeorology*, 32, 260-270.

Fouskaskis, D., Gunnell, D., Rasmussen, F., Tynelius, P., Sipos, A., and Harrison, G. (2004). Is the season of birth association with psychosis due to seasonal variations in foetal growth or other related explosures? A cohort study. *Acta Psychiatrica Scandinavica*, 109(4), 259-263.

Garvey, M.J., Goodes, M., Furlong, C. and Tollefson, G.D. (1988). Does cold winter weather produce depressive symptoms? *International Journal of Biometeorology*, 32, 144-146.

Gilbert, G.O. (1973). Effect of negative air ions upon emotionality and brain serotonin levels in isolated rats. *International Journal of Meteorology*, 17(3), 267-275.

Goetzmann, W.N., and Zhu, N. (2005). Rain or shine: Where is the weather effect? *European Financial Management*, 11(5), 559-578.

Golinski, J. (2001). "Exquisite atmography": Theories of the world and experiences of the weather in a diary of 1703. *British Journal for the History of Science*, 34(121), 149-171.

Health Canada (2003). Canada's health concerns from climate change and variability. Retrieved November 1, 2006 from *http://www.hc-sc.gc.ca/ewh-semt/climat/health_table-tableau_sante_e.html*.

Hengeveld, H. (1991). *Understanding Atmospheric Change. SOE Report 91-2.* Ottawa: Environment Canada.

Hipp, J.R., Bauer, D.J., Curran, P.J., and Bollen, K.A. (2004). Crimes of opportunity or crimes of emotion? Testing two explanations of seasonal change in crime. *Social Forces*, 82(4), 1333-1372.

Hirshleifer, D., and Shumway, T. (2003). Good day sunshine: Stock returns and the weather. *Journal of Finance*, 58(3), 1009-1032.

Ibrahim, Z.G., Strempel, J., and Tschernitschek, H. (2005). The effects of seasonal changes on temporomandibular disorders. *Cranio—The Journal of Craniomandibular Practice*, 23(1), 67-73.

Imai, M., Kayukawa, Y., Ohta, T., Li, L., and Nakagawa, T. (2003). Cross-regional survey of seasonal affective disorders in adults and high school students in Japan. *Journal of Affective Disorders*, 77(2), 127-133.

Inbar, O., Rotstein, A., Dlin, R., Dotan, R., and Sulman, F.G. (1982). The effects of negative air ions on various physiological functions during work in a hot environment. *International Journal of Biometeorology*, 26(2), 153-163.

Intergovernmental Panel on Climate Change (2001). *Climate Change 2001: Synthesis Report*, eds. Robert Watson and the Core Writing Team. Cambridge: Cambridge University Press.

IPCC (2001). Climate Change 2001: Synthesis Report. R.T. Watson and the Core Writing Team (Eds.). Cambridge University Press.

Keller, M.C., Frederickson, B.L., Ybarra, O., Cote, S., Johnson, K., Mikels, J., Conway, A., and Wager, T. (2005). A warm heart and a clear head—The contingent effects of weather on mood and cognition. *Psychological Science*, 16(9), 724-731.

Kim, C.D., Lesage, A.D., Seguin, M., Chawky, N., Vanier, C., Lipp, O., and Tureki, G. (2004). Seasonal differences in psychopathology of male suicide completers. *Comprehensive Psychiatry*, 45(5), 333-339.

Kimmell, R., Dartsch, P.C., Hildenbrand, S., Wodarz, R., and Schmahl, F.W. (2000). Pupils' and teachers' health disorders after renovation of classrooms in a primary school. *Gesundheitswesen*, 62(12), 660-664.

Kinney, D.K., Jacobsen, B., Jansson, L., Faber, B., Gramer, S.J., and Suozzo, M. (2000). Winter birth and biological family history in adopted families. *Schizophrenia Research*, 44(2), 95-103.

Klinenberg, E. (2002a). *Heat wave: A social autopsy of disaster in Chicago.* Chicago: University of Chicago Press.

Klinenberg, E. (2002b). Dying alone: An interview with Eric Klinenberg. Retrieved November 1, 2006 from *http://www.press.uchicago.edu/Misc/Chicago/443213in.html*.

Levitan, R.D. (2005). What is the optimal implementation of bright light therapy for seasonal affective disorder (SAD)? *Journal of Psychiatry and Neuroscience*, 30(1), 72-72.

Lundin, L. (1999). Allergic and non-allergic students' perception of the same high school environment. *Indoor Air—International Journal of Indoor Air Quality and Climate*, 9(2), 92-102.

Macchi, M.M., and Bruce, J.N. (2004). Human pineal physiology and functional significance of melatonin. *Frontiers in Neuroendocrinology*, 25(3-4), 177-195.

Maeno, N., Kusunoki, K., Kitajima, T., Iwata, N., Ono, Y., Hashimoto, S., Imai, M., Li, L., Kayukawa, Y., Ohta, T., and Ozaki, N. (2005). Personality of seasonal affective disorder analyzed by Tri-Dimensional Personality Questionnaire. *Journal of Affective Disorders*, 85(3), 267-273.

Maes, M., De Meyer, F., Peeters, D., Meltzer, H., Cosyns, P., and Schotte, C. (1992). Seasonal variation and meteotropism in various self-rated psychological and physiological features of a normal couple. *International Journal of Biometeorology*, 36, 195-200.

Maes, M., De Meyer, F., Thompson, P., Peeters, D., and Cosyns, P. (1994). Synchronized annual rhythms in violent suicide rate, ambient temperature and the light-dark span. *Acta Psychiatrica Scandinavica*, 90(5), 391-396.

Magnusson, A., and Boivin, D. (2003). Seasonal affective disorder: An overview. *Chronobiology International*, 20(2), 189-207.

McGrath, J., Selten, J.P., and Chant, D. (2002). Long-term trends in sunshine duration and its association with schizophrenia birth rates and age at first registration—Data from Australia and the Netherlands. *Schizophrenia Research*, 54(3), 199-212.

Michalak, E.E., Tam, E.M., Manjunath, C.V, Solomons, K., Leavitt, A.J., Levitan, R., Enns, M., Morehouse, R., Yatham, L.N., and Lam, R.W. (2004). Generic and health-related quality of life in patients with seasonal and nonseasonal depression. *Psychiatry Research*, 128(3), 245-251.

Miller, W.H. (1968). Santa Ana winds and crime. *Professional Geographer*, 20(1), 23-27.

Morrissey, S.A., Raggatt, P.T.F., James, B., and Rogers, J. (1996). Seasonal affective disorder: Some epidemiological findings from a tropical climate. *Australian and New Zealand Journal of Psychiatry*, 30(5), 579-586.

Murray, G. (2004). How common is seasonal affective disorder in temperate Australia? A comparison of BDI and SPAQ estimates. *Journal of Affective Disorders*, 81(1), 23-28.

North, C.S., Pollio, D.E., Thompson, S.J., Spitznagel, E.L., and Smith, E.M. (1998). The association of psychiatric diagnosis with weather conditions in a large urban homeless sample. *Social Psychiatry and Psychiatric Epidemiology*, 33(5), 206-210.

Ohtani, T., Kaiya, H., Utsumi, T., Inoue, K., Kato, N., and Sasaki, T. (2006). Sensitivity to seasonal changes in panic disorder patients. *Psychiatry and Clinical Neurosciences*, 60(3), 379-383.

Papadopoulos, F.C., Frangakis, C.E., Skalkidou, A., Petridou, E., Stevens, R.G., and Trichopous, D. (2005). Exploring lag and duration effect of sunshine in triggering suicide. *Journal of Affective Disorders*, 88(3), 287-297.

Persinger, M.A. (1975). Lag responses in mood reports to changes in the weather matrix. *International Journal of Biometeorology*, 19(2), 108-114.

Peters, C.E. (1994). *Fight the winter blues, don't be SAD: Your guide to conquering seasonal affective disorder*. Calgary: Script Publishing.

Rastad, C., Ulfberg, J., and Sjoden, P.O. (2006). High prevalence of self-reported depressive mood during the winter season among Swedish senior high school students. *Journal of the American Academy of Child and Adolescent Psychiatry*, 45(2), 231-238.

Rose, M.S., Verhoef, M.J., and Ramcharan, S. (1995). The relationship between chinook conditions and women's illness-related behaviours. *International Journal of Biometeorology*, 38, 156-160.

Rosenthal, N.E., Sack, D.A., Gillin, J.C., Lewy, A.J., Goodwin, F.K., Davenport, Y., Mueller, P.S., Newsome, D.A., and Wehr, T.A. (1984). Seasonal Affective Disorder: A description of the syndrome and preliminary findings with light therapy. *Archives of General Psychiatry*, 41, 72-80.

Salib, E. (1997). Elderly suicide and weather conditions: Is there a link? *International Journal of Geriatric Psychiatry*, 12(9), 937-941.

Salib, E. (2002). Month of birth and suicide: An exploratory study. *International Journal of Psychiatry in Clinical Practice*, 6(1), 39-44.

Salib, E., and Sharp, N. (2002). Relative humidity and affective disorders. *International Journal of Psychiatry in Clinical Practice*, 6(3), 147-153.

Shapira, A., Shiloh, R., Potchter, O., Hermesh, H., Popper, M., and Weizman, A. (2004). Admission rates of bipolar depressed patients increase during spring/summer and correlate with maximal environmental temperature. *Bipolar Disorders*, 6(1), 90-93.

Sher, L. (2004). Etiology, pathogensis, and treatment of seasonal and non-seasonal mood disorders: Possible role of circadian rhythm abnormalities related to developmental alcohol exposure. *Medical Hypotheses*, 62(5), 797-801.

Sher, L., Oquendo, M.A., Galfalvy, H.C., Zalsman, G., Cooper, T.B., and Mann, J.J. (2005). Higher cortisol levels in spring and fall in patients with major depression. *Progress in Neuro-Psychopharmacology and Biological Psychiatry*, 29(4), 529-534.

Shindell, S., and Raso, M. (1997). *Global Climate Change and Human Health*. New York: American Council on Science and Health. Retrieved November 1, 2006 from http://www.acsh.org/publications/pubID.868/pub_detail.asp. Posted 1997-10-01.

Sundstrom, E., Bell, P.A., Busby, P.L., and Asmus, C. (1996). Environmental Psychology 1989-1994. *Annual Review of Psychology*, 47, 485-512.

Torrey, E.F., Miller, J., Rawlings, R., and Yolken, R.H. (1997). Seasonality of births in schizophrenia and bipolar disorder: A review of the literature. *Schizophrenia Research*, 28(1), 1-38.

United States Department of State (2002). *United States Climate Action Report 2002. Chapter 6: Impacts and Adaptation*. Washington DC: US Department of State. Retrieved November 1, 2006 from http://www.usgcrp.gov/usgcrp/Library/thirdnatcom/chapter6toc.htm.

Watson, L. (1984). *Heaven's breath: A natural history of the wind*. London: Hodder & Stoughton, Ltd.

Watson, R.T., Zinyowera, M.C., and Moss, R.H. (1998). *The regional impacts of climate change. An assessment of vulnerability*. Cambridge: Cambridge University Press.

Plate 7 Electric Storm (NOAA Photo Library, NOAA Central Library) ▶

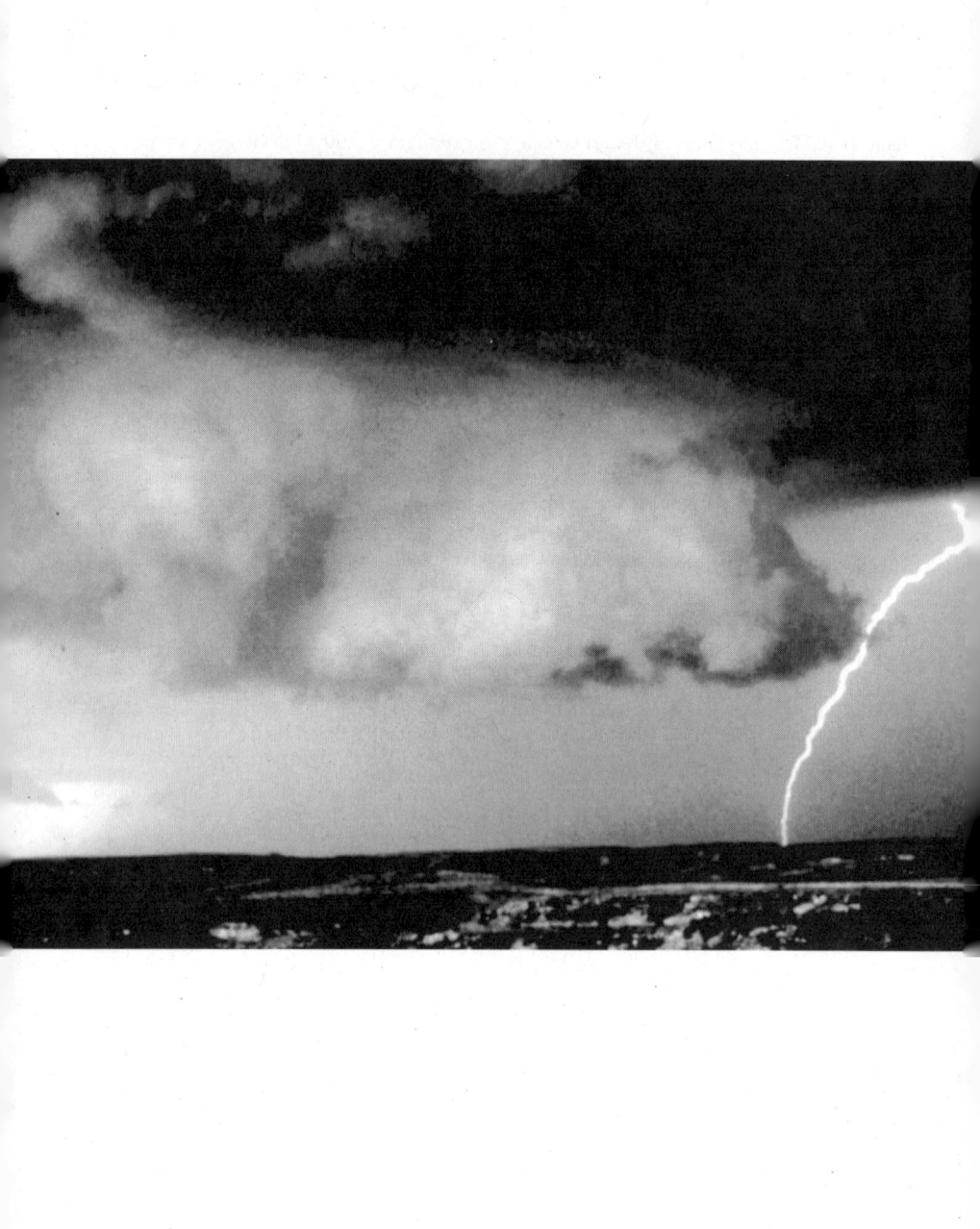

Developing a Research-Policy Partnership to Improve Children's Mental Health in British Columbia

Charlotte Waddell and Cody A. Shepherd
Children's Health Policy Centre, Faculty of Health Sciences, Simon Fraser University

Jayne Barker
Child and Youth Mental Health, Ministry of Children and Family Development

INTRODUCTION

Our research-policy partnership was motivated by a complex public health problem of mutual concern. Mental health, or social and emotional well-being, is crucial for children to thrive. Yet many Canadian children experience mental disorders, the causes and consequences of which impede their development. Mental disorders in childhood frequently persist, causing ongoing distress and disability in adulthood. Given the prevalence and the potential lifelong impact, mental disorders are arguably the leading health problems that Canadian children face after infancy. In response, public policy in most jurisdictions across Canada has traditionally emphasized "downstream" specialized treatment services for children with disorders. However, these services have only ever reached a small minority of the children who have disorders. Meanwhile, there has been little investment in "upstream" approaches such as early child development (ECD) or prevention programs with a focus on mental health, which have the potential to promote health and reduce the number of children who go on to develop disorders.

As researchers and as policy-makers, we were concerned that the status quo was insufficient to improve children's mental health in the population. Even increasing specialized treatment investments would not address the need to intervene earlier, before disorders became established. Instead, we believed that a comprehensive public health strategy was needed: promoting healthy development for all children; preventing disorders in children at risk; providing effective treatment for children with disorders; and monitoring outcomes for all children.

Children's mental health is one of the most important investments society can make, but creating a new strategy to improve the situation requires more than action by policy-makers. Researchers also need to contribute. Motivated by our common commitment to improving children's mental health in the population, we have therefore engaged in a long-term research-policy partnership in BC. Here, we discuss the problem that motivated our partnership, the process of developing a partnership to address the problem, the challenges that we encountered during the process, and the sustainability of our partnership. Throughout, we interpret our experience with reference to research literature in the interdisciplinary fields of children's mental health and "knowledge transfer." We conclude that, despite the challenges, research-policy partnerships can mutually benefit researchers *and* policy-makers who are committed to addressing problems of mutual concern. More importantly, such partnerships may be an innovative and necessary way of addressing complex public health problems such as children's mental health.

MOTIVATION FOR THE PARTNERSHIP

Mental health, or social and emotional well-being, is fundamental to healthy child development, yet at any given time an estimated 14% of children (over 100,000 in BC and over 800,000 in Canada) experience mental disorders that cause significant symptoms and impair their functioning in multiple domains (Waddell, McEwan, Shepherd, Offord, and Hua, 2005). The causes and consequences of these disorders impede children's development and prevent them from thriving. Mental disorders in childhood frequently persist, causing ongoing distress and disability in adulthood, at considerable cost to society (Costello, Mustillo, Erkanli, Keeler, and Angold, 2003; Kim-Cohen et al., 2003; Kessler et al., 2005). In 2001, the direct and indirect costs attributable to mental disorders in Canada were estimated to exceed $14 billion (Stephens and Joubert, 2001). Given the prevalence and the persistence throughout the lifespan, mental disorders are arguably the leading health problems that Canadian children face after infancy.

Table 11.1 presents prevalence estimates for specific mental disorders from recent cross-sectional surveys of representative community samples in Canada, the US, and Britain, plus estimates of the number of children affected in BC and Canada (Waddell, Offord, Shepherd, Hua, and McEwan, 2002; Waddell et al., 2005). Anxiety, attention, conduct, and depressive disorders are the most common in children. Disorders such as autism and schizophrenia are less common but more disabling. Most children with a mental disorder have at least one additional concurrent mental disorder compounding their distress (Waddell et al., 2002). Notably, these prevalence estimates include only those children with significant symptoms *and* significant impairments in functioning and therefore meet generally accepted diagnostic criteria (American Psychiatric Association,

Table 11.1 Prevalence of children's mental disorders and population affected in British Columbia and Canada

			British Columbia		Canada	
Disorder	Estimated Prevalence (%)[a]	Age Range (Years)	Estimated Population[b]	Estimated Population Affected[c]	Estimated Population[b]	Estimated Population Affected[c]
Any Anxiety Disorder	6.4	5–17	657,300	42,100	5,286,900	338,400
Attention-Deficit/ Hyperactivity Disorder	4.8	4–17	700,100	33,600	5,642,600	270,800
Conduct Disorder	4.2	4–17	700,100	29,400	5,642,600	237,000
Any Depressive Disorder	3.5	5–17	657,300	23,000	5,286,900	185,000
Substance Abuse	0.8	9–17	473,200	3,800	3,777,700	30,200
Pervasive Developmental Disorders	0.3	5–15	548,600	1,600	4,454,500	13,400
Obsessive-Compulsive Disorder	0.2	5–15	548,600	1,100	4,454,500	8,900
Any Eating Disorder	0.1	5–15	548,600	500	4,454,500	4,500
Tourette's Disorder	0.1	5–15	548,600	500	4,454,500	4,500
Schizophrenia	0.1	9–13	256,400	300	2,088,200	2,100
Bipolar Disorder	<0.1	9–13	256,400	<300	2,088,200	<2,100
Any Disorder	**14.3**	**4–17**	**700,100**	**100,100**	**5,642,600**	**806,900**

[a]For references to original studies and for methods use to pool prevalence rates, see Waddell et al., 2002
[b]Population estimates for children in each age range drawn from Statistics Canada, 2004
[c]Estimated prevalence multiplied by estimated population

2000). As many as 20% of children may be affected if milder mental health problems are also counted (National Institute of Mental Health [NIMH], 2001).

Public policy for children's mental health in most jurisdictions across Canada has traditionally emphasized downstream healthcare investments in specialized treatment services for individuals with disorders. However, of the 14% of children who *have* established mental disorders, only 25% have typically received such healthcare services (Waddell et al., 2005). The prevalence of children's mental disorders has greatly exceeded specialized treatment capacity. Given the number of children affected and the limited reach of treatment services, it has become increasingly evident that such services alone cannot meet the needs of children who have disorders, let alone the needs of all children in the population (Offord, Kraemer, Kazdin, Jensen, and Harrington, 1998). Investing more in the status quo is also not a feasible option. Even if the resources were available, simply increasing specialized treatment services downstream would not address the need to intervene upstream, to promote health and prevent disorders before they became established.

Looking upstream, ECD has been widely recognized in Canada and elsewhere as a determinant of the health of populations (Willms, 2002). Numerous ECD programs have been funded in provinces and territories across Canada in recent years (Government of Canada, 2005). However, few ECD programs have focused specifically on mental health or produced demonstrable improvements in children's mental health outcomes (Waddell, McEwan, Peters, Hua, and Garland, 2006). Prevention programs also have considerable upstream potential to lower the number of children in need by reducing early symptoms and subsequent diagnoses of disorders (Andrews and Wilkinson, 2002). For example, school-based cognitive-behavioural training (CBT) can reduce symptoms and diagnoses of anxiety and depression, while parent training with high-risk families can reduce symptoms and diagnoses of conduct disorder (Waddell, Shepherd, Hua, Garland, Peters, and McEwan, 2006). The World Health Organization (WHO) has suggested that prevention is the *only* sustainable approach for reducing the impact of mental disorders (WHO, 2004). Historically, however, few prevention programs in Canada have focused on children's mental health (Waddell, McEwan et al., 2006). Prevention has also been a low priority on the public policy agenda overall. BC has devoted less than 3% of health spending to prevention (Select Standing Committee on Health [SSCH], 2004). Across Canada, public health (including prevention) has never accounted for more than 5.5% of total health expenditures (Canadian Institute for Health Information, 2005).

Looking downstream, the most pressing concern has been access to *effective* treatments. For example, CBT is a highly effective treatment for anxiety and depression, as is parent training for conduct disorder (Chorpita et al., 2002), yet these treatments have not been widely available. Instead, ineffective treatments have persisted, such as unproven psychotherapies or antidepressant medications with unfavourable balances between risks and benefits (NIMH,

2001; Garland, 2004). Historically, the organization of treatment services has also been problematic in children's mental health, exacerbating the problem of access to effective treatments. Policy-makers are beginning to realize the potential of new service models to extend the reach of scarce specialist resources, for example, by redeploying specialists to consult to primary healthcare and schools where many more children may be seen. However, such models have not been widely implemented (or evaluated) in Canada (Waddell et al., 2005). Services have also not been well coordinated across the many sectors that share responsibility for children's mental health, including public health, ECD, primary and acute healthcare, education, youth justice, and child protection (Waddell, Lavis et al., 2005). Meanwhile, attempts to monitor children's mental health in several provinces have been restricted to the outputs and outcomes of treatment services (Barwick, Boydell, Cunningham, and Ferguson, 2004). There has been no systematic monitoring of children's mental health outcomes in the population. Population monitoring is necessary given the small proportion of children, of even those *with* mental disorders, who have received treatment services.

Despite the prevalence of mental disorders in children and the potential impact of these disorders across a lifespan, and despite widespread acknowledgement of the importance of children's development for the health of populations, children's mental health has never figured highly on the Canadian health policy agenda. If mental health has been one of the "orphan children" of health and healthcare (Romanow, 2002, p. 178), then children's mental health has been the "orphan's orphan" (Kirby and Keon, 2006, p. 155). As researchers and as policy-makers, we became convinced that maintaining the status quo would not meet the mental health needs of all children in the population. Only a "radical" strategy would suffice. We believed that such a strategy should be comprehensive and should reflect both upstream (health) and downstream (healthcare) perspectives: promoting the healthy development of all children; preventing disorders in children at risk; providing effective treatment for children with disorders; and monitoring outcomes for all children (Waddell et al., 2005). Figure 11.1 depicts this strategy.

DEVELOPING THE PARTNERSHIP

Our partnership was motivated by a common commitment to improving children's mental health in the population. From the outset, we believed that more policy-making should be informed by research evidence and that more research should be relevant to policy-making. By developing a research-policy partnership, we hoped to raise children's mental health on the public policy agenda, to promote a comprehensive strategy for improving children's mental health, and to increase upstream investments. Encouraging "evidence-based" policy and practice has been an ongoing, underlying objective of our partnership.

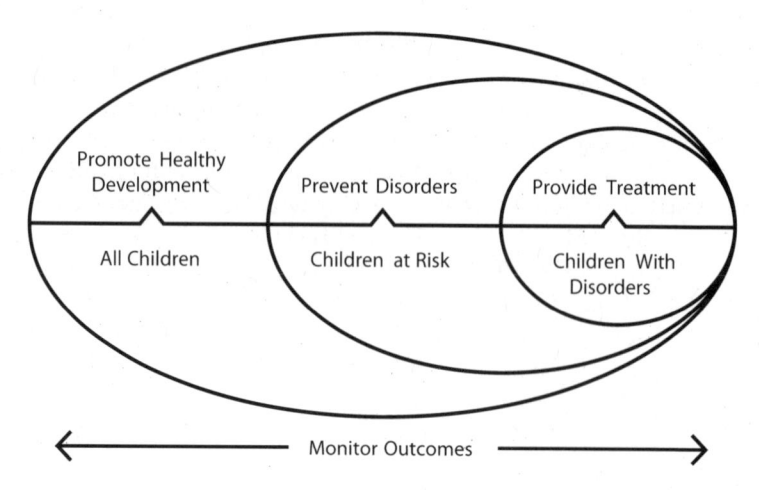

Figure 11.1 Public health strategy to improve children's mental health

The partnership had its origins when a new provincial Ministry for Children and Family Development (MCFD) was formed in 1996 to better coordinate children's programs and services including mental health, youth justice, child protection, and ECD. (The Ministry of Health retained responsibility for public health and primary and specialized healthcare for children, while the Ministry of Education retained responsibility for school-based services.) In previous ministries, higher-profile programs such as adult mental health had often eclipsed children's mental health. However, in the new ministry children's mental health was rapidly eclipsed by child protection. In response to the concerns expressed by practitioners and community leaders, MCFD decided to strengthen its commitment to children's mental health and embarked on a planning process to address the concerns.

The ministry first conducted province-wide consultations to gather the perspectives of children, families, practitioners, and community leaders. The ministry then approached the University of British Columbia (UBC) seeking to build children's mental health policy capacity in the university. A university faculty position was established and a qualified faculty member recruited to develop and lead a research team jointly funded by government and research funding agencies. A formal consulting role was simultaneously established and the new faculty member was appointed as Provincial Child Psychiatrist for Child and Youth Mental Health within MCFD. At the same time, MCFD recruited a new provincial Executive Director to assume leadership of Child and Youth Mental Health. A formal research-policy partnership was established in early 2001.

Initially, the university research team prepared reviews of the best currently available research evidence to support MCFD's planning process. Researchers also began regular consultations with MCFD on applying the research evidence. MCFD then incorporated both the research evidence and results of the earlier province-wide consultations to produce a comprehensive plan to improve children's mental health. With a change of government in 2001, a new Premier and a new Minister signalled strong support for children's mental health. Provincial Cabinet subsequently approved the *Child and Youth Mental Health Plan for British Columbia* (the *Plan*), the first of its kind in Canada (Ministry of Children and Family Development [MCFD], 2003; Province of British Columbia, 2003). Approval of the *Plan* was followed by announcements for practitioners and community leaders and by news coverage in provincial media.

The *Plan* has firmly placed children's mental health on the public policy agenda in BC, as evidenced not only by political support, but also by widespread support from practitioners and community leaders. Now being implemented by MCFD over 5 years from 2003 through 2008, the *Plan* has already fundamentally changed the nature and delivery of mental health services for children in BC: by explicitly encouraging evidence-based policy and practice; by emphasizing both upstream and downstream approaches for the first time; and by coordinating services across different sectors and ministries. Consistent with a public health strategy, the *Plan* is based on a comprehensive framework for improving children's mental health: providing treatment and support, reducing risk, and building capacity, with performance monitoring underlying each part of the framework (MCFD, 2003). Figure 11.2 depicts this framework.

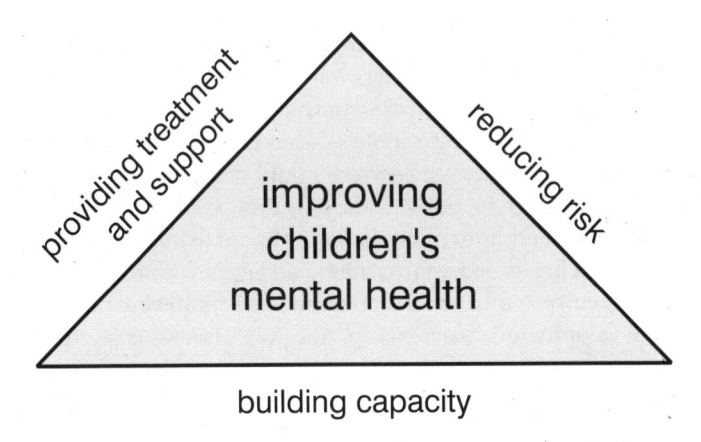

Figure 11.2 Framework of the *Child and Youth Mental Health Plan for BC*

Encouraging evidence-based policy and practice through MCFD's *Plan* remains an ongoing objective of our research-policy partnership. To meet this objective, the university research team has provided ongoing knowledge transfer services to policy-makers in the form of reviews of the best currently available research evidence on a variety of prevention and treatment topics. Reviews have been communicated through a website dedicated to children's mental health, as well as through regular consultations and education sessions with policy-makers, practitioners, and community leaders. The university has also sponsored province-wide practitioner education sessions and community demonstration and evaluation projects in partnership with the ministry, with funding through the *Plan*.

In early 2006, the research team relocated to the new Faculty of Health Sciences at Simon Fraser University (SFU), which has a mandate to integrate research and policy for population and public health. The partnership continues between MCFD and the new Children's Health Policy Centre (CHPC) in the Faculty of Health Sciences, with long term funding from SFU, MCFD, and research funding agencies. At SFU, there is explicit recognition of the value of research-policy partnerships in the form of tenure and promotion incentives for policy engagement, as well as university infrastructure support for CHPC.

CHALLENGES FOR THE PARTNERSHIP

Since initiating the partnership, both researchers and policy-makers have benefited. Ministry support has enabled CHPC to establish an innovative scholarly program to conduct research on the policy process *and* research to inform policy-making, with a focus on children's mental health. The partnership has served as a laboratory for studying the dynamic interaction between the research process and the policy process. The partnership has also provided unusual opportunities for researchers to constructively influence policy. For MCFD, having research partners based in the university has raised the profile and credibility of children's mental health in government and across the province. Researchers were often able to advocate for children's mental health at the political level when civil servants could not, helping to maintain children's mental health on the public policy agenda. CHPC's research, consultation, and education activities have also contributed to building support for the *Plan* and for evidence-based approaches at all levels within MCFD. However, despite the benefits, we have also encountered significant challenges in the process of developing our partnership. We now discuss these challenges and our approaches to addressing them.

Limits to the Research Evidence

At a minimum, policy-makers needed three kinds of research evidence pertinent to planning for children's mental health: on the prevalence of disorders; on effective means to prevent and treat disorders; and on the cost-effectiveness of various intervention options. CHPC was committed to systematically identifying and reviewing the best currently available research evidence to inform policy-making. However, the applicability of much of the available research was limited. The epidemiology literature yielded high-quality cross-sectional surveys that reported prevalence rates for various disorders, but the diversity of samples and survey methodologies meant that substantial interpretation was necessary to provide disorder-specific prevalence estimates applicable to the population of children in BC. Similarly, the child psychology and psychiatry literature yielded numerous high-quality randomized-controlled trials (RCTs) of prevention and treatment interventions for various disorders. However, these studies typically focused on intervention *efficacy* in populations outside of BC. For example, programs for the prevention of conduct disorder, such as prenatal nurse home visitation and preschool childhood education, were well-researched in the US (Waddell, Hua et al., 2006). However, US children have had access to significantly fewer baseline health, education, and social services compared to BC children such that the *effectiveness* of these programs in local settings was unknown. Meanwhile, little research on *cost-effectiveness* was identified.

We addressed these challenges in several ways. CHPC invested special effort in conducting thorough but pragmatic research reviews and interpreting findings through a local policy lens. For example, researchers prepared a review of the best available epidemiologic studies relevant to BC children, then tailored interpretations to BC and Canadian policy audiences. This review produced estimates of the number of children affected by mental disorders that were directly incorporated in the *Plan* and subsequently quoted by the Premier (MCFD, 2003; Province of BC, 2003). Similarly thorough reviews were completed on a dozen prevention and treatment topics. MCFD then convened ad hoc "expert" committees to specifically apply the findings to local program and service needs. In some cases, this process led directly to the implementation of new programs based on the research evidence. For example, a school-based CBT program for the prevention of anxiety was implemented across the province, following recommendations from the research team and endorsement by a local expert committee. The research team has also pursued peer-reviewed research funding to address gaps in the literature, and has encouraged other researchers to undertake more policy-relevant studies (Waddell et al., 2005). The lack of applicable research has remained frustrating for policy-makers, though, because conducting these new studies will take considerable time.

Limits to the Use of Research Evidence in Policy-Making

In some instances, there *was* applicable research evidence, but for political reasons policy-makers did not or could not fully apply it. For example, the CHPC's reviews suggested that new prevention programming should be a major focus of the *Plan*. However, the provincial government had competing priorities, including simultaneous reductions in tax revenues and program expenditures. The ensuing climate of fiscal restraint was not conducive to new investments. Children's mental health treatment services had also been chronically under-funded compared to higher-profile programs within MCFD. When new funding *was* allocated to children's mental health as a result of the

Plan, policy-makers were eager to protect these funds from being diffused across a broad array of social programs, some of which could have contributed to prevention. At the same time, some practitioners were advocating for further investment in specialized treatment services, such as increased hospital capacity, potentially impinging on new funding available for prevention programs. As a result of these competing influences, while the *Plan* supported risk reduction and capacity building, new prevention investments were mainly directed toward one school-based CBT program for anxiety disorders. Early childhood programs for preventing conduct disorder remain a consideration for the future.

In response to these challenges, researchers continued to promote the research evidence on prevention with policy-makers, practitioners, and community leaders. Researchers encouraged evidence-based prevention initiatives that had particularly strong support among all stakeholders, such as school-based CBT for anxiety disorders. Independent peer-reviewed research funding was also obtained to conduct a full systematic review and a survey on the state of Canadian prevention programming. Emerging findings were shared with the ministry and with others working in public and population health in the province. Independent research funding was essential to enable researchers to pursue a prevention agenda without directly challenging decisions at the political level. This approach in turn assisted amenable policy-makers to gradually build support for prevention ideas within government and without. As a result, prevention investments grew to comprise 15% of *Plan* expenditures, a considerable achievement given that BC has typically devoted only 3% of overall health spending to prevention (SSCH, 2004).

Constraints in Research Organizations

Universities impose significant organizational constraints on researchers who wish to engage with policy-makers. While the climate is changing, tenure and promotion criteria still favour peer-reviewed publications and grants to the exclusion of almost all other activities, including policy engagement. Scientific impact is what "counts." Time spent consulting with policy-makers or producing policy-relevant publications detracts from doing what counts. Meanwhile, policy impact is not measured. In CHPC's case, the research reviews produced for government were rigorous, perhaps overly so by policy standards. The reviews also had considerable policy impact, particularly when combined with consultation to assist policy-makers with interpretation, and education to assist practitioners with application. Yet these reviews did not meet academic publication standards without substantial revisions, which time constraints often precluded. Alternatively, when publications were prepared for academic journals first, journal editors typically requested embargoes during peer-review, a process that could take many months. This lengthy process frustrated policy-makers who needed immediate access to research findings, and frustrated researchers who were obliged to rewrite academic publications for policy audiences regardless. Consequently, for researchers, policy engagement was often academically unproductive and therefore risky from a career perspective.

In CHPC's case, several factors mitigated these constraints. For researchers, having policy experience before working in the university engendered respect and appreciation for the demands and standards of the policy process. For policy-makers, undertaking doctoral studies while working in the Ministry enhanced respect and appreciation for the demands and standards of the research process. For researchers, it was also crucial to negotiate careful boundaries in the partnership to protect time to develop an independent research agenda, to obtain peer-reviewed research funding, and to prepare academic publications. Being interdependent but not dependent on government was necessary for maintaining credibility in the academic community, and for maintaining "arm's length" ability to constructively critique public policy when needed. MCFD's infrastructure funding was also valuable. This funding provided for resources otherwise difficult to obtain from universities or peer-reviewed research funding agencies, such as professional staff to manage administration, finances, and communications. It was also essential to have ongoing encouragement from senior academic colleagues who explicitly understood the costs yet nevertheless supported policy engagement.

Constraints in Policy Organizations

Policy-makers also encountered significant organizational constraints on research engagement. A climate of fiscal restraint generated internal pressure to limit investments in research-related activities. There were always urgent competing demands on policy-makers' time and funds. This issue was exacerbated by frequent changes of senior leadership within MCFD, which meant that the research-policy partnership was continually vulnerable and constantly had to be justified. Fragmentation was another significant constraint. In BC, despite recent coordinating efforts, children's mental health remained divided across multiple sectors (health and education in addition to MCFD), levels within government (provincial and regional), and different disciplines (psychology, social work, nursing, medicine, and others). Overcoming this fragmentation was a prerequisite to obtaining buy-in for the evidence-based approach that underlay the *Plan* and the partnership. The *Plan* appealed to a presumably shared concern for improving children's outcomes by way of basing policy and practice on the best currently available research evidence on "what works." However, obtaining buy-in was often arduous for policy-makers leading the *Plan* because evidence-based approaches had to be separately marketed with every sector, level, and discipline. Resistance became apparent when new evidence-based approaches challenged established policies and practices. Research receptivity had to be nurtured.

To manage these constraints, it was essential to have a tenacious commitment to the idea of using research evidence to inform policy-making. The *Plan* focused MCFD's efforts by raising awareness of children's mental health and explicitly encouraging use of research evidence as a way to improve outcomes for children. For example, province-wide training sessions were held with practitioners who were unfamiliar with effective treatments such as CBT. Through training and exposure to the potential applications, more practitioners began to include CBT in their prevention and treatment repertoires. MCFD was also fortunate to have support for children's mental health at the political level. With the change of government in 2001, a new commitment was made to mental health in BC, including increased resources for children's mental health despite widespread cutbacks across government. The Premier also spoke publicly about his family's experience with suicide. His candour brought needed public and media support. This political context was critical in establishing support for the *Plan* and its evidence-based approach. When needed, researchers also communicated directly with politicians, senior civil servants, practitioners, community leaders, and the media to convey messages from the research evidence in support of children's mental health and the *Plan*.

SUSTAINING THE PARTNERSHIP

The challenges that we encountered in the process of developing a research-policy partnership were not trivial. As we tried to address these challenges, we often turned to the emerging literature in the field of knowledge transfer for suggestions on how to make research-policy partnerships sustainable.

Health researchers have long advocated the use of more research evidence in policy-making. Generally, researchers have taken the "producer push" approach, arguing that policy-makers *should* use more research evidence (Davies, Nutley, and Smith, 2001). Encouraging evidence-based *clinical* policy was the priority for much of the last decade. Numerous research-practice "gaps" were documented and interventions were developed to bridge the gaps, albeit with limited success (Grol and Grimshaw, 2003). This research was helpful in articulating the difficulties in engaging practitioners, but it was not directly applicable to our situation. For example, most studies have focused on changing physicians' behaviour. There was little to guide us in the interdisciplinary territory of children's mental health (Waddell and Godderis, 2005).

More recently, attention has turned to research use by politicians and civil servants involved in *legislative* and *administrative* policy. Much work has focused on the presumed "cultural" differences that arise when researchers and policy-makers work in isolation from one another. Personal contacts, timely communications, and policy relevance have all been proposed as means to increase use of research evidence in policy-making (Innvaer, Vist, Trommald, and Oxman, 2002; Hanney, Gonzalez-Block, Buxton, and Kogan, 2003). Numerous case studies now document researchers' (more and less successful) experiences interacting with policy-makers (e.g., Jacobson, Butterill, and Goering, 2005; Kothari, Birch, and Charles, 2005). Methods such as systematic reviews and tailored syntheses have also been recommended for conveying bodies of high-quality research evidence to policy-makers (Lavis, Posada, Haines, and Osei, 2004). We implemented these suggestions. While helpful, however, these suggestions did not directly address some of the specific challenges we faced in sustaining our partnership, such as dealing with limits to the research evidence, or dealing with the constraints in our respective organizations.

Policy-makers have argued that researchers must appreciate the competing influences on the policy process, including institutional constraints, stakeholder interests, and the role of ideas more generally (Lavis et al., 2002). In children's mental health, research evidence *is* valued and used by policy-makers, but as just one source of ideas among many in a dynamic environment (Waddell et al., 2005). These broader perspectives on the policy process helped us interpret our partnership experiences *and* prompted us to reflect upon the research process, which less knowledge transfer literature has explored. For those based in universities, organizational disincentives still create daunting barriers to engaging with policy-makers, barriers that researchers themselves largely define and perpetuate (Jacobson, Butterill, and Goering, 2004). Research funding agencies have started to create helpful incentives for research-policy engagement (Lomas, 2000). Universities are also starting to recognize policy impact, along with usual tenure and promotion criteria (Goering, Butterill, Jacobson, and Sturtevant, 2003; Lavis, Ross, McLeod, and Gildiner, 2003). We have been fortunate to have necessary supports within our university environment, making our partnership sustainable. However, more innovations in universities would help make policy engagement sustainable for others too, particularly researchers early in their careers.

As the knowledge transfer literature suggests, overcoming cultural differences, understanding the competing influences on the policy process, and creating new incentives within research organizations are all prerequisites for research-policy engagement. However, beyond these prerequisites, a fundamentally different way of thinking is necessary if research-policy partnerships are to be sustained. Both researchers and policy-makers must adopt a relational perspective, an openness to *mutual* influence in the spirit of meaningful collaboration (Denis and Lomas, 2003). We concur with those who conceive of evidence-based policy-making as "a social process, not a technical task" (Lomas, 2004, p. 288). We also accept the definition of policy-making as "making and implementing collective ethical judgments" (Greenhalgh and Russell, 2006, p. 35). In keeping with this definition, our partnership enabled us to advance children's mental health in a way not possible had we worked apart.

Conclusion

Not all researchers can engage in policy partnerships, and not all researchers should. The production of curiosity-driven knowledge will always be central to the university's mandate, and even policy-minded researchers must constantly balance academic rigour with policy relevance. Similarly, not all policy-makers can or should engage in research partnerships. Some policy problems are not amenable to the solutions that researchers have to offer. But where there is openness to mutual influence, research-policy partnerships are worth pursuing because the learning they involve is so mutually enriching. Five years later, we agree that the benefits of our partnership have outweighed the challenges. Consequently, our partnership appears to be sustainable. More importantly, sustainability matters, because partnerships such as ours may be an innovative and necessary way of addressing complex public health problems such as children's mental health. We encourage others to engage as we have.

Acknowledgements

We are grateful for the enthusiastic support of our colleagues at the Children's Health Policy Centre in the Faculty of Health Sciences, Simon Fraser University, and at Child and Youth Mental Health in the Ministry of Children and Family Development, British Columbia. Michael Hayes and Alan Markwart provided particular encouragement within our respective research and policy organizations. Jonathan Lomas and George McLauchlin made formative intellectual contributions to our ideas about integrating research and policy. We appreciated the opportunity to present our ideas at a Canadian Health Services Research Foundation workshop in 2004. Finally, we are grateful to Leslie Foster for the invitation to contribute to this volume.

References

American Psychiatric Association (2000). *Diagnostic and statistical manual of mental disorders: DSM-IV-TR* (4th ed.). Washington: American Psychiatric Association.

Andrews, G., and Wilkinson, D.D. (2002). The prevention of mental disorders in young people. *Medical Journal of Australia*, 177 Suppl, S97-S100.

Barwick, M., Boydell, K.M., Cunningham, C.E., and Ferguson, H.B. (2004). Overview of Ontario's screening and outcome measurement initiative in children's mental health. *Canadian Child & Adolescent Psychiatry Review*, 13(4), 105-109.

Canadian Institute for Health Information (2005). *National health expenditure trends 1975-2005*. Ottawa: Canadian Institute for Health Information.

Chorpita, B.F., Yim, L.M., Donkervoet, J.C., Arensdorf, A., Amundsen, M.J., McGee,C., Serrano, A., Yates, A., Burns, J., and Morelli, P. (2002). Toward large-scale implementation of empirically supported treatments for children: A review and observations by the Hawaii Empirical Basis to Services Task Force. *Clinical Psychology: Science & Practice,* 9(2), 165-190.

Costello, E.J., Mustillo, S., Erkanli, A., Keeler, G., and Angold, A. (2003). Prevalence and development of psychiatric disorders in childhood and adolescence. *Archives of General Psychiatry,* 60(8), 837-844.

Davies, H.T.O., Nutley, S.M., and Smith, P.C. (Eds.) (2001). *What works? Evidence-based policy and practice in public services.* Bristol, UK: The Policy Press.

Denis, J.-L., and Lomas, J. (2003). Convergent evolution: The academic and policy roots of collaborative research. *Journal of Health Services Research and Policy,* 8 Suppl 2, 1-6.

Garland, E.J. (2004). Facing the evidence: Antidepressant treatment in children and adolescents. *Canadian Medical Association Journal,* 170(4), 489-491.

Goering, P., Butterill, D., Jacobson, N., and Sturtevant, D. (2003). Linkage and exchange at the organizational level: A model of collaboration between research and policy. *Journal of Health Services Research and Policy,* 8(Suppl. 2), 14-19.

Government of Canada (2005). *Early childhood development activities and expenditures.* Ottawa: Social Development Canada, Public Health Agency of Canada, and Indian and Northern Affairs Canada.

Greenhalgh, T., and Russell, J. (2006). Reframing evidence synthesis as rhetorical action in the policy making drama. *Healthcare Policy,* 1(2), 34-42.

Grol, R., and Grimshaw, J. (2003). From best evidence to best practice: Effective implementation of change in patients' care. *Lancet,* 362(9391), 1225-1230.

Hanney, S.R., Gonzalez-Block, M.A., Buxton, M.J., and Kogan, M. (2003). The utilisation of health research in policy-making: Concepts, examples and methods of assessment. *Health Research Policy and Systems,* 1(2), 1-28.

Innvaer, S., Vist, G., Trommald, M., and Oxman, A. (2002). Health policy-makers' perception of their use of evidence: A systematic review. *Journal of Health Services Research & Policy,* 7(4), 239-244.

Jacobson, N., Butterill, D., and Goering, P. (2004). Organizational factors that influence university-based researchers' engagement in knowledge transfer activities. *Science Communication,* 25(3), 246-259.

Jacobson, N., Butterill, D., and Goering, P. (2005). Consulting as a strategy for knowledge transfer. *Milbank Quarterly,* 83(2), 299-321.

Kessler, R.C., Berglund, P., Demler, O., Jin, R., Merikangas, K.R., and Walters, E.E. (2005). Lifetime prevalence and age-of-onset distributions of DSM-IV disorders in the National Comorbidity Survey Replication. *Archives of General Psychiatry,* 62(6), 593-602.

Kim-Cohen, J., Caspi, A., Moffitt, T.E., Harrington, H., Milne, B.J., and Poulton, R. (2003). Prior juvenile diagnoses in adults with mental disorder: Developmental follow-back of a prospective-longitudinal cohort. *Archives of General Psychiatry,* 60(7), 709-717.

Kirby, M.J.L., and Keon, W.J. (2006). *Out of the shadows at last: Transforming mental health, mental illness and addiction services in Canada.* Ottawa: The Standing Senate Committee on Social Affairs, Science and Technology.

Kothari, A., Birch, S., and Charles, C. (2005). "Interaction" and research utilisation in health policies and programs: Does it work? *Health Policy,* 71(1), 117-125.

Lavis, J.N., Posada, F.B., Haines, A., and Osei, E. (2004). Use of research to inform public policy-making. *Lancet,* 364(9445), 1615-1621.

Lavis, J.N., Ross, S.E., Hurley, J.E., Hohenadel, D.M., Stoddart, G.L., Woodward, C.A., and Abelson, J. (2002). Examining the role of health services research in public policymaking. *Milbank Quarterly,* 80(1), 125-154.

Lavis, J., Ross, S., McLeod, C., and Gildiner, A. (2003). Measuring the impact of health research. *Journal of Health Services Research & Policy*, 8(3), 165-170.

Lomas, J. (2000). Using 'linkage and exchange' to move research into policy at a Canadian foundation. *Health Affairs*, 19(3), 236-240.

Lomas, J. (2004). Postscript: Understanding evidence-based decision-making – or, why keyboards are irrational. In L. Lemieux-Charles and F. Champagne (Eds.), *Using knowledge and evidence in health care: Multidisciplinary perspectives* (pp. 281-289). Toronto: University of Toronto Press.

Ministry of Children and Family Development (2003). *Child and youth mental health plan for British Columbia*. Retrieved September 1, 2004, from http://www.mcf.gov.bc.ca/mental_health/mh_publications/cymh_plan.pdf.

National Institute of Mental Health (2001). *Blueprint for change: Research on child and adolescent mental health*. Washington, DC: National Institute of Mental Health.

Offord, D.R., Kraemer H.C., Kazdin A.E., Jensen P.S., and Harrington R. (1998). Lowering the burden of suffering from child psychiatric disorder: Trade-offs among clinical, targeted and universal interventions. *Journal of the American Academy of Child and Adolescent Psychiatry*, 37(7), 686-94.

Province of British Columbia (2003). *Transcript of the open cabinet meeting: February 7, 2003*. Retrieved September 1, 2004 from http://www.prov.gov.bc.ca/prem/down/tran/open_cabinet_meeting_february_7_2003.htm

Romanow, R.J. (2002). *Building on values: The future of health care in Canada: final report*. Ottawa: Commission on the Future of Health Care in Canada.

Select Standing Committee on Health (2004). *The path to health and wellness: Making British Columbians healthier by 2010*. Victoria, BC: Legislative Assembly of British Columbia.

Statistics Canada (2004). Table 051-0001: Estimates of population, by age group and sex, Canada, provinces and territories, annual [Data file]. Available from E-STAT website, *http://www.statcan.ca/english/estat/licence.htm*

Stephens, T., and Joubert, N. (2001). The economic burden of mental health problems in Canada. *Chronic Diseases in Canada*, 22(1), 18-23.

Waddell, C., and Godderis, R. (2005). Rethinking evidence-based practice for children's mental health. *Evidence Based Mental Health*, 8(3), 60-62.

Waddell, C., Hua, J.M., Garland, O., Peters, R., and McEwan, K. (in press). Preventing mental disorders in children: A systematic review to inform policy-making in Canada. *Canadian Journal of Public Health*.

Waddell, C., Lavis, J.N., Abelson, J., Lomas, J., Shepherd, C.A., Bird-Gayson, T., Giacomini, M., and Offord, D.R. (2005). Research use in children's mental health policy in Canada: Maintaining vigilance amid ambiguity. *Social Sciece & Medicine*, 61, 1649-1657.

Waddell, C., McEwan, K., Peters, R., Hua, J.M., and Garland, O. (in press). Preventing mental disorders is a public health priority. *Canadian Journal of Public Health*.

Waddell, C., McEwan, K., Shepherd, C.A., Offord, D.R., and Hua, J.M. (2005). A public health strategy to improve the mental health of Canadian children. *Canadian Journal of Psychiatry*, 50(4), 226-233.

Waddell, C., Offord, D.R., Shepherd, C.A., Hua, J.M, and McEwan, K. (2002). Child psychiatric epidemiology and Canadian public policy-making: The state of the science and the art of the possible. *Canadian Journal of Psychiatry*, 47(9), 825-832.

Willms, J.D. (2002). *Vulnerable children*. Edmonton, AB: University of Alberta Press.

World Health Organization (2004). *Prevention of mental disorders: Effective interventions and policy options: Summary report*. Geneva: WHO Department of Mental Health and Substance Abuse.

An Educational Response to Mental Health Issues in the Classroom

12

Darlene Brackenreed, Ron Common, Lorraine Frost, Warnie Richardson, and Paula Barber
Faculty of Education, Nipissing University

INTRODUCTION

Although teachers form the 'frontline' in the mental health field, they receive little or no training or support in dealing with child and adolescent mental health issues (Evans, 1999). While schools have increasingly become the *de facto* mental health service system for many children and adolescents (Burns et al., 1995), student services professionals continue to search for models of intervention that go beyond existing systems of service delivery; such systems having been criticized as fragmented, limited, and narrowly focused (Adelman and Taylor, 2000; Adler and Gardner, 1994; Knitzer, Steinberg, and Fleisch, 1990).

Educational reform, occurring in response to external criticism of the education system, has focused mainly on improving academic instruction and performance, and on the management of schools. However, a key area of concern for many professionals working with young people is school mental health, and the delivery of services intended to address barriers to learning for all students, not just those in special education (Brener, Martindale, and Weist, 2001). Adelman and Taylor (2000) advocate the inclusion of health, mental health, family problems, environmental factors, and other barriers to academic success as a component of school reform.

Highlighting the magnitude of the mental health issue in schools, the 2001 Ontario Student Drug Use Survey (OSDUS) Mental Health and Well-being Report (Centre for Addiction and Mental Health, 2001)—part of the longest on-going school survey of adolescents in Canada—reports that:

- 1 in 10 students has low self-esteem, and one in 20 is at high risk for depression.
- 34% feel constantly under stress, and 27% report that they lose sleep over worry.
- 1 in 10 seriously considered attempting suicide in the preceding 12 month period.

- 1 in 10 report visiting a mental health professional in the past year, and 2% are on medication for depression.
- 1 in 7 report being involved in three or more delinquent acts during the past 12 months.
- 8% had a problem with gambling during the past year.

As freestanding mental health services are increasingly closed or downsized, individuals with mental health problems are frequently integrated into their communities, with teachers often constituting the primary source of intervention for those affected. As a result, teachers require additional information and skills in order to undertake successful interactions with children and youth who either have a mental health problem themselves, or are living with a family member who does.

In this chapter, we report the results of a study undertaken in order to assess the skill and informational needs of teaching professionals as they relate to working with children and youth with mental health problems. As well, we examine the creation and implementation of a Bachelor's-level option course on mental health issues currently offered to students attending the Faculty of Education at Nipissing University, North Bay, Ontario.

THE STUDY

With financial assistance received from the Northeast Mental Health Task Force and the Ministry of Health and Long-term Care, we undertook a two-stage needs assessment. In the first stage of the research, a survey was developed to identify the mental health-related challenges that teachers report facing in their day-to-day practice. Teachers were asked to respond to a total of 42 items using a five-point Likert scale indicating their level of agreement with statements about mental health issues, and about working with students with mental health problems. Items in the questionnaire addressed topics relating to self-perceived abilities in managing mental health-related classroom issues, the stress and stigmatization associated with such problems, the availability of support services in the community, and their perception of the adequacy of the professional development opportunities available to them.

Questionnaires were mailed to a total of 800 teachers in the northeastern region of Ontario. Survey packages included a stamped, self-addressed envelope within which they could return their anonymous responses.

Phase Two of the study consisted of interviews with mental health professionals practicing in Northeastern Ontario. All agencies identified as providing mental health services in the area were invited to nominate a representative of their organization to participate in the study. Those who agreed to participate were provided with a copy of the interview questions in advance, in order to allow reflection on their responses to the questions prior to participation.

Respondents were interviewed at a date and time of their choosing, either in person or over the telephone, and their responses were audio-taped with permission. The 12 questions that constituted the interview focused on the agency with which they worked, their role within that organization, the clientele they served, and what they thought were the key skills and knowledge bases teachers would require in order to successfully work with students with mental health problems.

Results of the Study: Phase One

The survey returns yielded a response rate of 22%, which is considered acceptable in educational research (Gay and Airaisian, 2001). Analysis of the responses (shown in detail in Appendix A) yielded useful information for an assessment of the professional development needs of teachers with respect to mental health issues. General trends in the data obtained are discussed in the paragraphs that follow.

The survey results suggest that teachers do not feel as though they are part of a multi-disciplinary team when it comes to their interactions with students with mental health concerns. They report a high level of contact with students experiencing mental health issues, and many have referred their students to other agencies for help. Most, however, feel that they do not receive adequate support or feedback regarding diagnosis or programming. As well, while they feel informed about mental health problems, they are not confident in their own ability to deal with these issues; the vast majority report needing more professional preparation in this area.

Teachers appear to be sympathetic to the needs of students with mental health issues, agreeing there is stigma attached to mental illness, that this stigma is a barrier to accessing help, and that advocacy on behalf of those individuals is required. Indeed, most teachers report that advocacy is part of their professional role. However, they were divided on the idea that the regular classroom was the 'least restrictive setting' for students with mental health concerns.

With regard to the day-to-day management of these students, teachers were concerned about the administration of medications, how to handle a crisis situation, and how to access services. Fewer than half of the teachers who responded indicate that they are uncomfortable with persons with mental illness, but the majority believe that services for such persons are not adequate, both in the school and in the community at-large. The teachers also report that services outside urban centres are more difficult to obtain, and that minority group members with mental health needs are less well-served. Transitions from mental health facilities to school settings were identified as requiring attention, and mental health promotion and illness prevention programs were identified as inadequate. Teachers were aware that families of persons with mental health concerns may experience significant problems.

Teachers do not feel that they have the information essential for the early identification of mental health problems, but they are willing to access supports on behalf of their students and to advocate for their right to equitable services in the educational system. It would appear that the vital component for this delivery of service is to provide teachers in all school boards with information on the different resources available in their community and how to access them.

RESULTS OF THE STUDY: PHASE TWO

The mental health professionals interviewed in the second phase of this study felt that teachers need to be aware of the basic symptoms of mental health problems, and the stigma associated with these symptoms. In addition, they expressed a belief that teachers had a responsibility to research the specific mental illness affecting the students under their charge. Teachers were also seen as a crucial link to support services available in the broader community to themselves, their students, and their students' families.

With respect to what the educational system needs to do for students and families affected by mental health issues, the professionals in question were asked to identify areas for individual, family, and educational support. In the area of individual supports, promoting healthy living and providing service and teacher training were the most frequent responses. Family supports identified were the need for increased communication among students, parents, teachers, and the school, and collectively working to dispel the myths and stigma surrounding mental illness. Responses regarding educational supports included the development of instructional adaptations for students experiencing mental health concerns, and providing a general education for teachers that promotes early intervention as the central philosophical tenet. An apparent theme in the responses received concerning individual, family, and educational supports was the need to develop an inventory of services available in the teacher's community that could be accessed on an as-needed basis.

Significantly, the sample of mental health professionals unanimously expressed a profound concern with the negative stigma associated with mental illness. As a follow-up to this question of the existence of stigma, the mental health professionals were asked to identify an effective strategy to address the problem. The most frequent response to this question was an identification of the need for provision of educational opportunities, wherein all issues related to mental illness or mental disorders could be studied.

Overall, the mental health professionals interviewed expressed a belief that persons experiencing or recovering from mental illness need to be placed back into the communities from which they came, highlighting once again the need for teachers to be capable of coping with the needs of these students in order to provide them with quality educational experiences.

DISCUSSION

Through the analysis of the interview responses, we learned that mental health professionals do not have a clear understanding of the roles, responsibilities, and constraints of teachers. The realities of teaching in a busy classroom, with 20 to 33 or more students, precludes the ability to spend individual time with a student who is experiencing difficulties for the purpose of assessment or providing interventions. Associated with this idea is the limited amount of time teachers have to devote to researching the mental health issues of an individual student. Placing these demands on the classroom teacher overextends a professional who is dealing with a vast array of abilities in an inclusive classroom. Teachers are empathic, but they also are clear that they need support from the mental health community in order to meet these demands.

Increased communication between all stakeholders may be enhanced through the education of teachers in the basics of mental health. Informed teachers will be better able to make instructional accommodations to meet the social and learning needs of their students. As well, enhanced dialogue and professional development would be of mutual benefit to educators and mental health professionals, allowing teachers to become the link to resources that the mental health professionals identified as essential.

OUTCOME OF THE STUDY

As a direct outcome of this study, Nipissing University's Faculty of Education developed and offered a new course on educating students with mental health issues. This new option course, offered at the Bachelor of Education level, has had enrolments exceeding 60 students since its inception.

Communication among stakeholders is enhanced when they have a mutual understanding of the issues. To enhance understanding, topics in the course include key terms, characteristics, and early indicators of mental health problems, all with the aim of enhancing the ability of teachers to recognize symptoms in their students' behaviours, and to more effectively communicate with mental health professionals and other interested parties.

To address the concern of access to services reported in the study, teachers build a portfolio of mental health resources in their home communities. This increases awareness among teachers of the services available to them in their role as student advocate, facilitating access to such services when required.

The issue of stigma is addressed in the coursework, and strategies for dealing with such negative perceptions are stressed. The behaviour of the teacher as a role model is explored through self-evaluation of their values and beliefs regarding the continuum of mental health and the incidence and prevalence of different disorders. Empathy and understanding are built through presentations by individuals with mental health concerns, parents of affected students, and professionals in the mental health community. Pedagogical approaches are presented and discussed in areas such as resiliency, mental health issues in diverse populations, conflict resolution, and crisis interventions.

The success of this course may best be expressed by the student who wrote "this is the most valuable course I have taken this year, or perhaps that I have ever taken. All teachers should take this course." Many students returning from practice teaching tell of incidents that had occurred in their schools, but which they felt better prepared to deal with as a result of the content of this course. As another student more specifically put it:

> I don't have to make the diagnosis, but because I now have some information at my disposal, I can sure ask some questions and certainly demand some answers. In some instances, to manage and control may not be enough. It may be bigger than that and I can certainly help move the whole thing forward.

These general comments, when combined with the preliminary results of an ongoing 3 year study that examines the educational concerns of the truly inclusive high school classroom, would tend to suggest that very small amounts of in-service education would significantly alleviate overall feelings of incompetence or helplessness surrounding mental health-related issues (Richardson and Brackenreed, 2006). With reference to this view, general feedback from the Northeastern Ontario Mental Health Task Force has been overwhelmingly positive, and our partnership with them has continued. Guest speakers from the mental health community have travelled from all parts of the Province of Ontario, often at their own expense, eagerly accepting the opportunity to talk to teachers.

Over the last 15 years, the philosophical educational approach to dealing with "special needs" students, particularly in North America and Europe, has been one of full inclusion or integration (Amado, 1993; Hinz, 1996; Lipsky and Garner, 1997; Ainscow, 1999). Consequently, teachers are being called upon in ever increasing numbers to deal with areas of exceptionality, of which they have, at best, limited understanding.

To summarize, our initial study clearly suggests that there is both a need and a desire to better prepare educators to deal with myriad issues whose genesis is exclusively within the field of mental health. As a consequence, Nipissing University responded with the creation and implementation of a course designed to prepare educators for their dealings with mental health issues in their classrooms. Given that the number of student teachers who selected this course far exceeded the university's expectations, and that the general feedback from the first cohort of student teachers to have successfully completed the course has been overwhelmingly positive, it would seem that serious consideration should be given to making the course mandatory, and that similar courses should be offered as part of the curriculum in all faculties of Education.

REFERENCES

Adelman, H., and Taylor, L. (2000). Mental health in schools and system restructuring. *Clinical Psychology Review*, 19, 137-163.

Adler, L., and Gardner, S. (Eds.) (1994). *The politics of linking schools and social services*. Washington: Falmer Press.

Ainscow, M. (1999). *Understanding the development of inclusive schools*. London: Falmer Press.

Amado, A. (1993). *Friendships and community connections between people with and without developmental disabilities*. Baltimore: Paul H. Brookes.

Brener, N., Martindale, J., and Weist, M. (2001). Mental health and social services: Results from the school health policies and programs study. *Journal of School Health*, 71(7), 305-313.

Burns, B., Costello, E., Angold, A., Tweed, D., Stangl, D., Farmer, E., and Erkanli, A. (1995). Children's mental health service use across service sectors. *Health Affairs*, 14(3), 147-159.

Centre for Addiction and Mental Health (2001). *The 2001 OSDUS mental health and well-being report*. Toronto: Ontario Student Drug Use Survey.

Evans, S. (1999). Mental health services in schools: Utilization, effectiveness and consent. *Clinical Psychology Review*, 19, 165-178.

Gay, L., and Airasian, P. (2000). *Educational research: Competencies for analysis and application (6th Ed.)* Upper Saddle River: Prentice Hall.

Hinz, A. (1996). Inclusive education in Germany: The example of Hamburg. *European Electronic Journal on Inclusive Education in Europe*, 1.

Knitzer, J., Steinberg, Z., and Fleisch, B. (1990). *At the schoolhouse door*. New York: Bank Street College of Education.

Lipsky, S.K., and Gartner, A. (1997). *Inclusion and school reform: Transforming America's classrooms*. Baltimore: Paul H. Brookes.

Richardson, W., and Brackenreed, D. (2006). [The educational concerns of the truly inclusive high school classroom]. Unpublished raw data.

Appendix A   Mental health issues questionnaire

Bolded numbers indicate the percentage (rounded) of respondents selecting each option.

1. I have taught students who had a diagnosis of a type of mental illness.
Disagree **12**   *Tend to Disagree* **5**   *Tend to Agree* **12**   *Agree* **55**   *Unsure* **16**

2. I have taught students who appeared to have mental health needs that I felt ill-equipped to deal with.
Disagree **3**   *Tend to Disagree* **8**   *Tend to Agree* **22**   *Agree* **63**   *Unsure* **4**

3. I have referred students to a guidance counsellor or resource teacher due to inappropriate or unusual behaviour.
Disagree **17**   *Tend to Disagree* **2**   *Tend to Agree* **10**   *Agree* **68**   *Unsure* **3**

4. I feel that I have supports from the mental health community in dealing with the mental health issues of my students.
Disagree **16**   *Tend to Disagree* **26**   *Tend to Agree* **26**   *Agree* **10**   *Unsure* **22**

5. I have received helpful feedback from referrals made for students with mental health issues.
Disagree **18**   *Tend to Disagree* **33**   *Tend to Agree* **16**   *Agree* **14**   *Unsure* **19**

6. I understand mental health issues and concerns.
Disagree **10**   *Tend to Disagree* **28**   *Tend to Agree* **35**   *Agree* **22**   *Unsure* **5**

7. I feel confident in dealing with students who demonstrate symptoms of mental illness.
Disagree **23**   *Tend to Disagree* **40**   *Tend to Agree* **22**   *Agree* **10**   *Unsure* **5**

8. I would like to receive training in the area of mental health.
Disagree **1**   *Tend to Disagree* **4**   *Tend to Agree* **21**   *Agree* **71**   *Unsure* **3**

9. I believe that training for teachers in the area of mental health is needed.
Disagree **2**   *Tend to Disagree* **1**   *Tend to Agree* **15**   *Agree* **81**   *Unsure* **1**

10. I am aware of the services and supports that are available to students and their families in the area of mental health.
Disagree **15**   *Tend to Disagree* **37**   *Tend to Agree* **28**   *Agree* **17**   *Unsure* **3**

11. I know how to effectively connect students and their families to community supports for mental health.
Disagree **21**   *Tend to Disagree* **35**   *Tend to Agree* **31**   *Agree* **9**   *Unsure* **4**

12. I feel that there is a negative stigma attached to the area of mental illness.
Disagree **1**   *Tend to Disagree* **3**   *Tend to Agree* **23**   *Agree* **72**   *Unsure* **1**

13. I believe that advocacy is needed to address the stigma of mental illness.
    Disagree 1   *Tend to Disagree 0*   *Tend to Agree 18*   *Agree 77*   *Unsure 4*

14. Addressing the stigma of mental illness would be of benefit to teachers and should be part of our role.
    Disagree 5   *Tend to Disagree 10*   *Tend to Agree 27*   *Agree 55*   *Unsure 3*

15. I believe that the stigma attached to mental illness prevents individuals from seeking help.
    Disagree 0   *Tend to Disagree 5*   *Tend to Agree 25*   *Agree 67*   *Unsure 3*

16. I believe that my students have access to the services which best meet their mental health needs.
    Disagree 28   *Tend to Disagree 42*   *Tend to Agree 12*   *Agree 2*   *Unsure 16*

17. I understand the roles and responsibilities of the persons in the mental health care field.
    Disagree 15   *Tend to Disagree 35*   *Tend to Agree 29*   *Agree 8*   *Unsure 13*

18. I believe that the management of student medications is well laid-out and administered.
    Disagree 24   *Tend to Disagree 25*   *Tend to Agree 20*   *Agree 17*   *Unsure 14*

19. I have been contacted by a mental health care professional for feedback regarding a student's behaviour at school.
    Disagree 43   *Tend to Disagree 16*   *Tend to Agree 16*   *Agree 16*   *Unsure 9*

20. I have been contacted by a mental health care professional regarding a student's response to medication.
    Disagree 61   *Tend to Disagree 16*   *Tend to Agree 6*   *Agree 9*   *Unsure 8*

21. I am aware of programs that are available to students and their families to address mental health issues and concerns.
    Disagree 25   *Tend to Disagree 36*   *Tend to Agree 28*   *Agree 9*   *Unsure 2*

22. I feel that I am an informed, contributing member of a multi-disciplinary team approach to the mental health care needs of my students.
    Disagree 25   *Tend to Disagree 41*   *Tend to Agree 21*   *Agree 7*   *Unsure 6*

23. I feel well-prepared to handle a crisis situation should one occur.
    Disagree 21   *Tend to Disagree 38*   *Tend to Agree 23*   *Agree 13*   *Unsure 5*

24. I feel confident that I can contact the appropriate team member(s) in a crisis situation.
    Disagree 14   *Tend to Disagree 33*   *Tend to Agree 28*   *Agree 17*   *Unsure 8*

25. I feel that I would benefit from training in the area of crisis intervention.
Disagree 0   Tend to Disagree 0   Tend to Agree 20   Agree 78   Unsure 2

26. I am well-educated in recognizing the signs and symptoms of mental illness.
Disagree 21   Tend to Disagree 39   Tend to Agree 30   Agree 5   Unsure 5

27. Persons demonstrating signs and symptoms of mental illness cause me to feel uncomfortable.
Disagree 20   Tend to Disagree 37   Tend to Agree 28   Agree 10   Unsure 5

28. The sharing of, and access to, client information within the confines of consent and confidentiality is adequate for my role as the teacher of a student with mental illness.
Disagree 10   Tend to Disagree 22   Tend to Agree 23   Agree 28   Unsure 17

29. I believe that all persons with mental health issues are currently receiving the services and supports they require.
Disagree 55   Tend to Disagree 35   Tend to Agree 2   Agree 0   Unsure 10

30. I believe that we have appropriate educational programming for students with mental health issues.
Disagree 48   Tend to Disagree 39   Tend to Agree 1   Agree 2   Unsure 10

31. I believe that the school system should play a role in the education of students about mental health.
Disagree 2   Tend to Disagree 3   Tend to Agree 36   Agree 54   Unsure 5

32. I understand that students may refuse treatment as a part of the symptoms of their disease.
Disagree 0   Tend to Disagree 6   Tend to Agree 22   Agree 55   Unsure 17

33. In my opinion, students in our community receive the same level of services as students in larger centers.
Disagree 42   Tend to Disagree 31   Tend to Agree 2   Agree 3   Unsure 22

34. Transitions from a mental health facility to a school setting is effective, with adequate sharing of information and supports in place.
Disagree 21   Tend to Disagree 26   Tend to Agree 16   Agree 5   Unsure 32

35. I understand which students are most appropriate for specialized mental health services and how referrals are made.
Disagree 29   Tend to Disagree 35   Tend to Agree 11   Agree 5   Unsure 20

36. We have adequate mental illness prevention and promotion programs in place.
Disagree 35   Tend to Disagree 39   Tend to Agree 5   Agree 0   Unsure 21

An Educational Response to Mental Health Issues in the Classroom

37. The provision of direct services is in partnership with and appropriate to ethno-racial communities.
Disagree **19**   *Tend to Disagree* **16**   *Tend to Agree* **8**   *Agree* **1**   *Unsure* **56**

38. Students with mental health concerns have adequate school and social experiences to provide them with support to practice social skills and receive feedback and support.
Disagree **33**   *Tend to Disagree* **39**   *Tend to Agree* **7**   *Agree* **1**   *Unsure* **20**

39. Students with mental health issues and concerns have adequate side-by-side support and coaching.
Disagree **34**   *Tend to Disagree* **41**   *Tend to Agree* **4**   *Agree* **0**   *Unsure* **21**

40. I understand the stress on the family of a student with mental illness.
Disagree **4**   *Tend to Disagree* **13**   *Tend to Agree* **31**   *Agree* **48**   *Unsure* **4**

41. I believe that public school is the least restrictive environment for students with mental health concerns.
Disagree **13**   *Tend to Disagree* **17**   *Tend to Agree* **19**   *Agree* **10**   *Unsure* **41**

42. I believe that we have adequate expertise among our teaching staff to deal with issues and concerns of the mental well-being of our students.
Disagree **38**   *Tend to Disagree* **43**   *Tend to Agree* **6**   *Agree* **4**   *Unsure* **9**

Plate 8 "Sitting, waiting" (J. LeClair) ▶

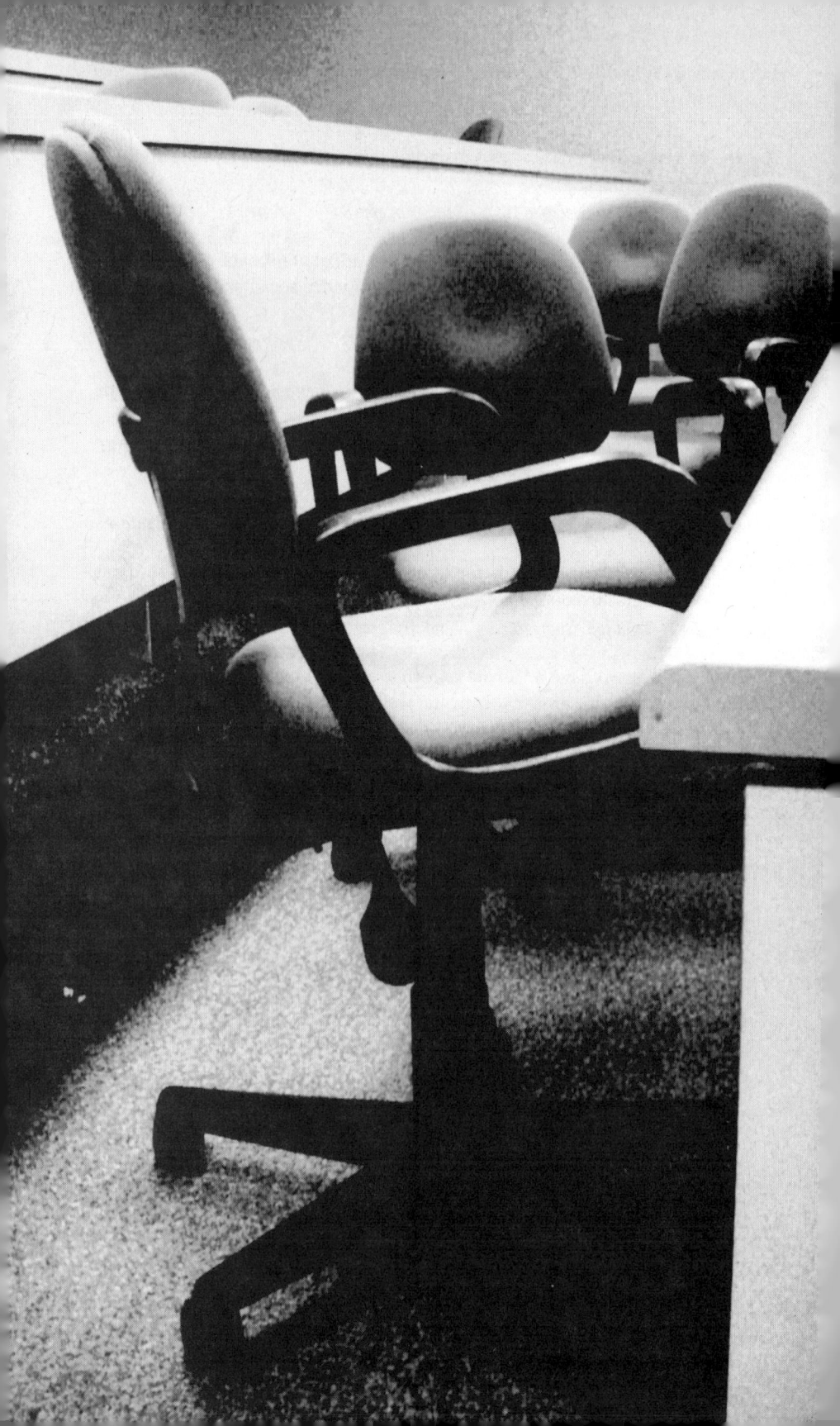

Teacher Stress and Stigma in Northern Ontario

Kristen Ferguson, Lorraine Frost, Kristian Kirkwood
Faculty of Education, Nipissing University

David Hall
Department of Sociology, Criminal Justice & Social Welfare, Nipissing University

INTRODUCTION

As a normal part of life, stress is caused by a variety of everyday situations and experiences. Depending on its situation and degree, stress can be a positive or negative force in one's life. As Selye (1976) suggests, some stress—referred to as eustress—can be motivating. Stress can, however, be dangerous if it becomes overwhelming (Cedoline, 1982). What is colloquially referred to as being 'stressed out' occurs when the dangerous or harmful aspects of stress begin to negatively affect an individual's day-to-day functioning. Stress responses are far from universal, as individuals differ both in terms of what they perceive as stressful, and in their reaction to having 'too much stress' (Canadian Mental Health Association, n.d.a).

Occupational stress, or job stress, is the result of situations related to the workplace that disrupt or enhance the mental or physical condition of the worker (Cedoline, 1982). Individuals spend hours each day at work and, according to Wilson and co-workers (2000), their mental health is directly linked to work climates. It is important to note that, while occupational stress is caused by work, its impacts can become manifest both in work and social life, and at any time in the future (Cedoline, 1982). Wilson and co-workers (2000) report that depression and stress disorders at work are driving disability rates higher, and represent more than 30% of all disabilities recorded at three of Canada's best-known corporations. In Canada, 1.4 million workers—10% of the working population—suffer from depression (Wilson, Joffe, Wilkerson, and Bastable, 2000). In addition, Wilson and co-workers (2000) suggest that ignoring stress and depression in the workplace produces an army of 'walking wounded;' that is, a workforce that is partly disabled, and increasingly unproductive.

Teachers are exposed to occupational stress, as are all professionals. Kyriacou (2001) defines teacher stress as "the experience by a teacher of unpleasant, negative emotions, such as anger, anxiety, tension, frustration, or depression, resulting from some aspect of their work as a teacher" (p. 28). In an early study on teacher stress, Kyriacou and Sutcliffe (1978) report that 19.9% of English teachers rate their jobs as very to extremely stressful. Borg and Riding (1991) identify even higher stress levels in Maltese teachers, with 33.6% of them rating their jobs as either very or extremely stressful. Likewise, a study of New Zealand intermediate teachers by Manthei and Gilmore (1996) finds that 26.1% of teachers feel that teaching is very or extremely stressful.

De Heus and Diekstra (1999), in a survey of employees in various occupations in the Netherlands, report that teachers have higher burnout scores than any other human service profession. Furthermore, teachers demonstrate more emotional exhaustion and reduced personal accomplishment than individuals in all other social professions.

Canadian teachers appear to be experiencing similar levels of stress. According to the Canadian Teachers' Federation (2001), 6 out of 10 teachers surveyed find that their job is more stressful than it was in the recent past. The Global Business and Economic Roundtable on Addiction and Mental Health, in researching data from the Ontario Teachers' Insurance Plan, reports that the rate of stress-related long-term disability among Ontario teachers is one-third higher than for other professionals. Furthermore, the research reveals that depression and other mental disorders are the leading source of prescription drug use and long-term disability among teachers in the province (Harvey, 2004).

According to the Canadian Mental Health Association (n.d.b), stigma is a "mark of shame or discredit." The perceived stigma surrounding stress appears in some of the qualitative research done on teacher stress (Brown, Ralph, and Brember, 2002; Troman, 2000; Younghusband, Garlie, and Church, 2003). For many teachers, the result of stress appears to be 'suffering in silence.' For some, acknowledging one's stress becomes associated with personal weakness and professional incompetence, comparable to being a failure or a bad teacher (Dunham, 1992; Troman, 2000; Younghusband et al., 2003). The perceived stigma of stress can fill a teacher with feelings of despair and failure, and impair their ability to cope (Brown, Ralph, and Brember, 2002). Teachers often hesitate to acknowledge their own stress: participants in a study by Younghusband and co-workers (2003) note that teacher stress is 'taboo,' and that little professional development in the areas of stress or stress management is available to them.

In this chapter, we consider results from a study of teacher stress, and the perception of stigma associated with such stress, among Northern Ontario teachers. Specifically, we assess the prevalence of stress and the perception of stigma in the target population, and identify demographic and job-related factors that are associated with an increased risk for experiencing these mental health-related issues.

METHOD

Instrument

Data concerning teacher stress and stigma were derived using a self-report questionnaire developed from a review of previous research, including that of Kyriacou and Sutcliffe (1978), Fimian (1984), Borg and Riding (1991), Manthei and Gilmore (1996), and the British Columbia Teachers' Federation (cited in Edudata, n.d.). This method of instrument development increases the validity and reliability of the questionnaire, as it was patterned on existing instruments using response formats and instructions that have already been tested (Slavin, 1984). A focus group of teachers, including both males and females, and from a variety of teaching backgrounds, pre-tested the questionnaire. Changes and modifications of the instrument were made using the feedback from the focus group.

The resulting questionnaire consists of eight sections dealing with various aspects of teacher stress, as well as socio-demographic information. Sections on self-reported stress, the stigma of teacher stress, and the demographic information are reported and discussed in this chapter:

- Respondents were asked to rate their stress levels through the question, "In general, how stressful do you find being a teacher?" on a 5-point scale of *not at all stressful, mildly stressful, moderately stressful, very stressful,* and *extremely stressful.*

- Another section of the questionnaire asked teachers to: "Please indicate how often you discuss stress with the following people" on a 5-point scale of *never, rarely, sometimes, often,* and *always.*

- A specific question addressed the perceived stigma of teacher stress, asking teachers, "Do you think that there is a stigma associated with having stress and being a teacher?" Respondents rated this item on a 5-point scale of *no stigma, mild stigma, moderate stigma, much stigma,* and *extreme stigma.*

- The demographics sections asked respondents questions concerning their sex, age, years of experience in teaching, grade level, and current assignment. Respondents were asked to select one answer for each question; however, if a respondent selected more than one answer, the first answer selected was recorded.

Study Sample

The sample for the study was taken from the entire population of teachers from Northern Ontario enrolled in additional qualification courses through Nipissing University, North Bay, Ontario, during the winter session of 2005. Northern Ontario teachers were identified from their home postal codes using the data base in Nipissing University's Registrar's Office. Northern Ontario postal codes start with the letter "P," and include the following areas: northeastern Ontario, starting at Honey Harbour in the south; James Bay; and northwestern Ontario, to the Manitoba and the US borders. This large geographic area covers nine English-language public district school boards, nine English-language Catholic district school boards, two French-language public district school boards, and four French-language Catholic district school boards, as well as many band-controlled First Nations schools (Ministry of Education, n.d.).

Research undertaken by the Faculty of Education at Nipissing University suggests that the majority of teachers in northeastern Ontario are actively involved in formal learning: more than 70% of teachers have taken one or more formal courses or workshops within the preceding 12 to 48 months. In addition, 91% of teacher respondents in northeastern Ontario indicate that they have completed 51 to 300 hours of formal courses and/or workshops over a 4 year period (Wideman, 2005). Therefore, contacting those enrolled in additional qualification courses is an appropriate sampling procedure for surveying a wide range of teachers in the region.

Survey questionnaires were mailed to the 566 teachers living within the region who had also enrolled in an additional qualification course at Nipissing University during the defined study period. In order to ensure the privacy and confidentiality of the teachers in question, questionnaire packages were addressed and mailed to the home residence by an employee from the Registrar's Office at Nipissing University. Teachers completed the questionnaires and returned them to the researchers in the self-addressed, postage-paid envelope provided. In order to encourage a high response rate, a reminder notice was subsequently mailed to the subjects. A total of 274 questionnaires were completed and returned, a response rate of 48%.

Data Analysis

Analyses of survey data were completed using logistic regression analysis. This flexible technique enables researchers to predict a categorical outcome such as high stress/low stress from a set of potential predictor variables which can be continuous or categorical, or a mix of the two. As well, unlike linear regression techniques, logistic regression analysis makes no assumptions about the distributions, linear relations, or variances of the predictor variables.

The first set of binary logistic regression analyses (Model One and Model Two) used teacher stress as the dependent (outcome) variable, and the following predictor variables:

- grade level currently taught
- age of respondent[1]
- sex of respondent
- position (full- or part-time)
- current assignment (elementary or secondary)
- others with whom the respondent discusses stress

For Model Two, another factor, a continuous variable corresponding to the reported perception of stigma around teacher stress, is included as a predictor.

In order to provide a dichotomous outcome variable for the logistic regression analyses, responses to the stress-related survey question were recoded as a dummy variable: teachers reporting that they find being a teacher *very stressful* or *extremely stressful* are effect-coded (i.e., assigned a value of 1), and teachers who find being a teacher *moderately, mildly,* or *not at all stressful* are the reference category (assigned a value of 0). Similarly, the categorical predictor variables were recoded as dummy co-variates with females, full-time positions, and currently working in elementary school assignments serving as the respective reference groups for the categorical predictor variables included in the models. The remaining predictor variables (grade level, age, others with whom the respondent discusses stress, and perceived stigma associated with stress) are assumed to be continuous variables, and entered into the regression models without recoding.

The second series of binary logistic regression models (Model Three and Model Four) were conducted on respondent perceptions of the stigma associated with teacher stress as the dependent (outcome) variable. For these models, the outcome of perceptions of stigma was recoded into a dummy variable with teachers who indicated that they felt *much* or *extreme stigma* effect-coded (i.e., assigned a value of 1), and those who felt *moderate, mild,* or *no stigma* attached to the stress of teaching serving as the reference category (i.e., assigned a value of 0). The predictor variables for Model Three and Model Four were the same as those used for Models One and Two. For Model Four, one additional factor, a continuous variable corresponding to the reported level of stress associated with teaching, is also included as a predictor.

As with Model One and Model Two, the categorical predictor variables were recoded into dummy co-variates with females, full-time positions, and currently working in elementary school assignments serving as the reference groups for the categorical predictors in the models. Likewise, grade level, age, others with whom the respondent discusses stress, and reported level of teacher stress were assumed to be continuous variables, and entered in the regression models without recoding.

RESULTS

Self-Reported Stress, Talking About Stress, and Perceived Stigma of Stress

In response to the question, "In general, how stressful do you find being a teacher?" 24.8% of respondents rated being a teacher *very stressful*, and 3.2% rated it as *extremely stressful*. While 48.4% found teaching to be *moderately stressful*, 22.0% rated teaching to be *mildly stressful* and 1.6% said it was *not at all stressful*.

Respondents were also asked to rate how frequently they discussed stress with other teachers, their principal, their friends, their family, their doctor, and other people, on a scale of *never, rarely, sometimes, often,* and *always*. Teachers in the study sample most frequently spoke with their family about stress (49.1% of respondents reporting that they *often* to *always* speak with family), followed by 40.3% of respondents who stated that they *often* to *always* speak with other teachers about stress. The percentages of those respondents who *often* to *always* discuss stress include: 36.4% that speak to other people, 34% that discuss it with their friends, 5.8% that speak to their doctor, and 3.7% that discuss stress with their principal. While many respondents state that they discuss stress with a variety of people, many other respondents indicate that they *never* to *rarely* discuss stress. A large number of respondents, 46%, state that they *never* discuss stress with their doctors, and 34.2% state that they *rarely* do so. As well, 68.8% indicate that they *rarely* or *never* discuss stress with their principals

Finally, respondents were asked to respond to the question "Do you think there is a stigma associated with having stress and being a teacher?" on a scale of *no stigma, mild stigma, moderate stigma, much stigma,* and *extreme stigma*. There was *much stigma* associated with teacher stress according to 25.1% of respondents, while 3.0% indicated that they believed there to be *extreme stigma*. *Moderate stigma* was reported by 42.2% of respondents, 21.3% reported *mild stigma*, and *no stigma* was indicated by only 8.4% of respondents.

Modelling Teacher Stress

Binary logistic regression was used to model teacher stress because, for the purposes of this research, the dependent or outcome variable was coded as dichotomous, with two categories indicating if respondents found being a teacher highly (negatively) stressful or not (low stress/eustress). In this case, logistic regression analysis determines which predictor variables are most strongly associated with the probability of high stress levels among the respondent teachers. For our purposes, the most relevant statistics generated in the logistic regression models are the exponentiated beta coefficients, which are reproduced in Table 13.1 (for stress) and Table 13.2 (for stigma).

These coefficients measure how a change in the value of a predictor variable increases or decreases the probability of a teacher indicating that they find teaching to be highly (or negatively) stressful. For example, coefficients close to a value of 1 show that the probability of the outcome (a high teaching stress level) does not materially change as the values of a predictor variable change. On the other hand, coefficients greater than 1 reflect an increase in the probability of the outcome as values of a predictor variable change. Finally, coefficients less than 1 indicate that a predictor reduces the probability of being in the negative stress group as values of that predictor variable change. In addition, the coefficients capture the effect of each predictor variable in the

Teacher Stress and Stigma in Northern Ontario

Table 13.1 Binary logistic regression models of teacher stress: Ontario, 2005 (exponentiated beta coefficients)

Independent Variables	Negative Stress vs. Low Stress/Eustress Model 1 (Stigma Excluded)	Negative Stress vs. Low Stress/Eustress Model 2 (Stigma Included)
Grade Level	1.550**	1.606**
Age	1.620**	1.744**
Gender: Male	1.473	1.458
Female*		
Position: Part-time/Occasional	0.191**	0.191**
Full-time*		
Current Assignment: Secondary	0.096**	0.113**
Other	0.105**	0.102**
Elementary*		
Discuss Stress: Doctor	1.971**	1.924**
Principal	0.797	0.912
Family	1.345	1.375**
Other teachers	1.838**	1.620**
Stigma	—	1.487**
Intercept	-6.843**	-8.280**
Chi-Square	64.311**	65.206**
Nagelkerke R Square	0.339	0.355
*Reference category	** p < 0.05	** p < 0.05

Table 13.2 Binary logistic regression models of teacher stigma associated with stress: Ontario, 2005 (exponentiated beta coefficients)

Independent Variables	High Stigma vs. Low Stigma Model 3 (Stress Excluded)	High Stigma vs. Low Stigma Model 4 (Stress Included)
Grade Level	0.974	0.925
Age	0.883	0.827
Gender: Male	1.393	1.644
Female*		
Position: Part-time/Occasional	1.144	1.469
Full-time*		
Current Assignment: Secondary	0.837	1.311
Other	1.318	1.300
Elementary*		
Discuss Stress: Doctor	1.654**	1.300
Principal	0.744	0.736
Family	1.080	0.944
Other teachers	1.541**	1.381
Stress	—	3.055**
Intercept	-2.743**	-4.914**
Chi-Square	18.200**	35.789**
Nagelkerke R Square	0.100	0.207
*Reference category	** p < 0.05	** p < 0.05

model while statistically controlling for, or holding constant, the effects of all the other predictor variables in the model.

Model One, which excludes the variable measuring stigma associated with teacher stress, shows that grade level, age, position, current assignment, and discussing stress with doctors or discussing stress with other teachers are all statistically and substantively significant predictors of negative stress in educators. In particular, the exponentiated beta coefficient for grade level (beta = 1.55) shows that, net of the other predictors in the model, every one unit increase in grade level increases the probability of experiencing high or negative stress by 55%. Furthermore, each increment in age measured on the survey (e.g., from under 25 years, to 25-34 years, to 35-40 years, and so on) increases the odds of finding teaching highly stressful by 62% (beta = 1.62).

On the other hand, part-time/occasional teachers (beta = 0.191) are almost 80% less likely to experience high stress when compared to our reference group of full-time teachers. Other predictors that significantly diminish the probability of experiencing negative teaching stress include teaching in a secondary classroom (beta = 0.096) or 'other' classroom (beta = 0.105), both of which lower the odds of being in the high stress group by around 90% when compared to the reference category of teaching in an elementary classroom.

Finally, respondents who discussed stress with their doctors, or with other teachers, are much more likely to be in the outcome group. Indeed, every one unit increment in the frequency of such discussions (never→rarely→sometimes→often→always) with one's doctor is associated with a near doubling of the probability (beta = 1.971) of being in the high stress group. Similarly, every one unit increase in the frequency of discussions with other teachers increases the odds of being in the negative stress outcome group by at least 80% (beta = 1.838).

Model Two, which incorporates a measure of perceived stigma of teacher stress, yields a stronger predictive model of teacher stress than does Model One. As with the first model, predictors such as teaching on a part-time or occasional basis, and working in a secondary school or 'other' assignment materially reduce the probability of negative stress when compared to their respective reference groups (full-time positions and elementary school assignments). Also, increases in grade level, age, and frequency of discussions about stress with doctors or with other teachers all significantly increase the probability of negative stress. With stigma included in Model Two, however, discussions about stress with your family are significantly associated with a higher probability of being in the outcome category. Moreover, stigma is also a major risk factor, as each increment in respondent perceptions of the stigma associated with teacher stress (no stigma→mild stigma→moderate stigma→much stigma→extreme stigma) increases the probability of experiencing negative stress by nearly 50% (beta = 1.487).

Clearly, the analysis of teacher stress in Model Two is superior to that in Model One. The addition of stigma not only adds a salient predictor of the outcome variable, but captures a statistically significant effect between increased discussions with family and negative stress in teachers. It is also worth noting that the gender of respondents and frequency of discussions about stress with principals have no statistically significant association with our outcome variable. In other words, the teacher's gender and the frequency of teacher interactions with principals regarding job-related stress do not predict if a teacher is experiencing high stress.

Modelling the Perceived Stigma of Teacher Stress

For the binary regression models concerned with predicting perceived stigma (Model Three and Model Four), the dependent variable was again coded with two categories indicating if respondents think that there is a high stigma associated with teacher stress or not. Shifting our attention to these models, the results of which are summarized in Table 13.2, it is evident that background variables are generally poor at predicting the outcome variable of high stigma. For example, Model Three, which excludes teacher stress levels, uncovers only two statistically significant predictors of respondent perceptions of stigma. Specifically, increments in the frequency of discussions about stress with their doctor (beta = 1.654) and other teachers (beta = 1.541) increase the probability of educators being in the high-stigma outcome category by at least 65% and 54% respectively. Model Four, which includes stress as a predictor, turns out to be a better model even though it yields only one statistically significant predictor; that is, stress. Importantly, each one unit increment in teacher stress (not at all stressful→mildly stressful→moderately stressful→very stressful→extremely stressful) is associated with a three-fold increase (beta = 3.055) in the likelihood of being in the high-stigma outcome group. This finding suggests that educators experiencing the highest amount of negative job-related stress may also be reluctant to seek support or help from others in dealing with the stress because of the stigma that they attach to teacher stress. It also raises the possibility of a feedback relationship between negative stress and high stigma.

DISCUSSION

With 28% of respondents indicating that they find teaching *very stressful* to *extremely stressful*, it is evident that some teachers in Northern Ontario experience high levels of occupational stress, and that this stress could be a destructive force in their lives. For the 48.4% who found teaching *moderately stressful*, the reported stress may be eustress, and hence a motivating force in their job performance. In comparison with the existing body of research, the results of this study suggest that teachers in Northern Ontario experience levels of stress comparable to, and in some cases higher than, teachers in other countries.

This study illuminated some significant predictors of stress based on the demographics of the respondents. First, age was an important stress predictor: as a teacher increased in age, the likelihood of her/him experiencing negative stress increased dramatically. A possible explanation for this finding is that teachers may be in different stages in their professional lives and must deal with educational change, in addition to the possibility of having different issues to deal with outside of the workplace, such as family obligations, which younger teachers may not yet have. It is also interesting to note that elementary school teachers were much more likely to experience negative stress than secondary teachers. Issues such as working conditions and preparation time differ between the two levels of teaching and further research is required to investigate the discrepancies of stress levels between the two panels. Finally, position was an important predictor for experiencing stress. As might be hypothesized, full-time teachers were much more likely to experience negative stress than part-time or occasional teachers. Being a full-time teacher usually involves a different workload than part-time or occasional teaching; for example, occasional teachers do not have to complete report cards as do full-time teachers.

As far as the present authors are aware, no other quantitative research studies about the stigma of teacher stress have been undertaken. Therefore, the data presented in this chapter offer unique insight into the relationship between the experience of occupational stress among teachers and their perception of the stigma attached to such stress.

Over 28% of those participating in this study indicate that they believe there is *much* or *extreme* stigma attached to teacher stress, a finding that is reflective of previous qualitative research suggesting the existence of such stigma (see Brown et al., 2002; Troman, 2000; Younghusband et al., 2003). It is interesting to note that this is approximately the same percentage of respondents (28.0%) who stated that they found teaching to be *very* to *extremely* stressful. A clear relationship emerged between perceived stigma of teacher stress and experiencing negative stress. Simply put, those respondents who indicated that they perceive a stigma associated with teacher stress had an increased probability of experiencing negative stress.

High percentages of respondents state that they *often* to *always* discuss stress with their family, other teachers, other people, and their friends. In fact, respondents who discuss stress with their doctors and other teachers are much more likely to experience negative stress. Despite the fact that such a high proportion of respondents state that they find teaching to be *very* to *extremely* stressful, only 5.8% *often* to *always* speak to their doctor and 3.7% *often* to *always* speak to their principal. Most respondents, 46.0%, *never* speak to their doctor, and 34.2% indicate that they *rarely* do. Given the obvious mental health-related implications of high levels of occupational stress, it is troubling that those experiencing it are relatively unlikely to broach the subject with their primary health care provider. Indeed, the results obtained in this study suggest that if teachers tend to discuss stress, they will discuss it with a variety of people. However, if teachers do not tend to discuss stress, they will not likely discuss it with anyone. There appears to be little middle ground. In addition, it is disconcerting that the frequency of discussing stress with one's doctor or other teachers increases the probability of a teacher perceiving high levels of stress-related stigma. This reinforces the idea that for many teachers, there is shame in discussing stress with colleagues, and even with one's health care provider.

The fact that 69.2% of respondents *never* to *rarely* discuss stress with their principals is consistent with previous qualitative research undertaken by Troman (2000), wherein some teachers report having difficulty discussing stress with principals. Younghusband and colleagues (2003) suggest that the apparent reluctance of teachers to discuss stress with their superiors may be due to a fear that they will be perceived as weak, or as a failure. In this regard, the perceived stigma of teacher stress may be interpreted as a threat to one's professional credibility or advancement. Furthermore, results from the binary logistic regression modelling suggest that as levels of stress increase, so too does the perception of stigma. As a result, it would seem plausible to suggest that those experiencing the highest levels of occupational stress—that is, those whose mental well-being are at greatest risk—are the least likely to feel comfort in seeking the help of others.

Limitations of the Study

The characteristics of the sample may have introduced a bias into the results obtained. There is a clear gender imbalance in the sample: males made up only 17.6% of the sample. While women outnumber men in the teaching profession, the ratio of men to women in this study does not represent the ratio in Northern Ontario. As well, a large number of teachers represent a younger age bracket, as 43.3% of the respondents were under the age of 34. Newer teachers also make up the majority of respondents, with 35.3% having 0 to 4 years experience and 30.1% having 4 to 9 years experience. Secondary teachers accounted for only 16.1% of the respondents, and as such are also underrepresented in the sample. It is unclear how such biases may have influenced the results obtained.

Furthermore, the population from which the sample was drawn includes all teachers from Northern Ontario enrolled in winter 2005 additional qualification courses at Nipissing University. While, as noted earlier, 70.58% of teachers in northeastern Ontario took one or more formal courses or workshops in the last 12 to 48 months, it is plausible that certain demographic subgroups may be more likely to take additional qualification courses, and that those teachers experiencing the highest levels of occupational stress may be less likely to enroll.

Due to the varying nature of a teacher's job, other limitations to the study are related to time and history threats. A teacher's current assignment, school, class, principal, and other related factors can change from year to year and, as a result, so can their stress levels. As well, current situations occurring in a teacher's personal or working life may affect how he or she responds to the questionnaire. For example, the stress factor "split grade classrooms" had a very high standard deviation (1.377). Having a split grade classroom might have been very stressful if respondents were in that situation when the questionnaire was distributed; however, if respondents did not teach in a split grade at the time, it would cause less or little stress. However, the nature of teaching is that it continually changes. Due to the high return rate and sample size, the wide variation of different situations should be distributed across the sample.

In addition, the nature of stress itself creates some limitations because stress is subjective to the individual (Brown et al., 2002). Stress is different for everyone, so it is somewhat problematic trying to compare different teachers and to identify their stress levels. Because stress is unique to each individual, a self-report questionnaire proved to be an appropriate tool to measure stress.

Suggestions for Future Research

The findings of this research raise a number of questions that highlight areas worthy of further consideration by researchers. Further research involving the demographic characteristics of teachers, and their links to levels of self-reported stress, are required. What is the cause of these varying levels of stress from individual to individual? Some existing research in this area offers insight into the psychological variables of teachers and their impact on teacher stress. Perceptions of self-concept (Friedman and Farber, 1992) and perfectionism in teachers (Flett, Hewitt, and Hallett, 1995), for example, are shown to have an effect on teachers' levels of stress. In addition, Wilhelm, Dewhurst-Savellis, and Parker (2000) report that teachers enter the profession with a variety of preconceived ideas about teaching, and that these ideas influence a teacher's decision to leave or stay in the teaching profession: "those who felt more positive about teaching were prepared to tolerate more stressors in the first few years" (p. 303). Hence, studies of the impact of personality type, among other psychological factors, seem justified.

The finding that teachers appear more reluctant to discuss stress with school administrators highlights the need to identify school-based factors which cause stress, strategies for reducing stress among teachers, and how to remove the stigma associated with such stress. Litrell and Billingsley (1994) and Starnaman and Miller (1992) suggest that school principals play a key role in reducing teacher stress. An avenue for future research would involve considering the role of principals' leadership styles in relation to stress levels and perceptions of stigma among teachers in their schools. Furthermore, attention might be given to school culture—the importance of which is highlighted in the chapter by Miller—and the collegial relationships among teachers.

While this study investigated teacher stress and the perceived stigma of teacher stress solely in Northern Ontario, it would be worthwhile to compare the results obtained for teachers in Northern Ontario with those working elsewhere in Ontario and throughout Canada. Indeed, it may be particularly useful to undertake such comparative analyses between schools located in urban versus rural areas, and in the core versus the periphery. One of few such studies, conducted by Abel and Sewell (1999), compares stress and burnout in rural and urban secondary school teachers. Teachers in Northern Ontario have very different working conditions and situations compared to those in Southern Ontario and other core regions of the country. It is clearly of importance to understand the ways in which the geographical and jurisdictional contexts of teachers in various parts of Canada impact upon working conditions, and the stressors experienced as a result.

Conclusion

This study reveals that occupational stress is relatively common among teachers in Northern Ontario, with more than one quarter of the teachers surveyed reporting that their job is either very or extremely stressful. For many teachers there is a perception of stigma surrounding teacher stress and, perhaps as a result, they appear generally reluctant to discuss their stress. In spite of the implications of living with unhealthy levels of stress, over 80% of those surveyed rarely or never speak to their doctors about stress.

As Wilson and co-workers (2000) suggest, stress and depression create a compromised workforce. As a consequence, the cost of teacher stress seems clear with respect to the mental heath of the individuals with whom our children spend many hours each day. Parents entrust their children with teachers that they assume are stable and healthy, and able to provide positive learning environments. A 'stressed out' teacher might negatively affect student learning and achievement. Less widely considered, however, are the implications for the mental health and well-being of children in their care if, as Brackenreed and colleagues suggest in Chapter 12, teachers form the 'front line' in the provision of mental health services for children.

Clearly, it is in the interests of both the teaching profession and society at large to recognize and address the problem of occupational stress and its stigma among teachers. Teachers need to be educated about the nature and symptoms of stress, and the resources available to them to manage stress, through workshops and open discussions within their schools. Given the perception of stigma, such open acknowledgment of the existence of job stress among teachers may go a long way toward removing some of the shame and discredit associated with it.

Endnote

[1] It is worth noting that preliminary screening of potential predictors found that the variables 'age' and 'years of experience in teaching' were highly correlated. Accordingly, 'years of experience in teaching' was excluded from further analysis, while 'age' was used in all of the models.

References

Abel, M.H., and Sewell, J. (1999). Stress and burnout in rural and urban secondary school teachers. *Journal of Educational Research*, 92(5), 287-293.

Borg, M.G., and Riding, R.J. (1991). Occupational stress and satisfaction in teaching. *British Educational Research Journal*,17(3), 263-281.

Canadian Mental Health Association (n.d.a). Coping with stress. Retrieved July 7, 2004 from http://www.cmha.ca/english/coping_with_stress/

Canadian Mental Health Association (n.d.b). Stigma: An overriding concern. Retrieved July 19, 2004 from http://www.cmha.ca/english/research/camimh/call_for_action/stigma.htm

Canadian Teachers' Federation (2001). Canadian Teachers' Federation June 2001 workplace survey. Retrieved July 7, 2004 from http://www.ctf-fce.ca/en/press/2001/Workplc.htm

Cedoline, A.J. (1982). *Job burnout in public education: Symptoms, causes and survival skills*. New York: Teachers College Press.

de Heus, P., and Diekstra, R.F.W. (1999). Do teachers burn out more easily? A comparison of teachers with other social professions on work stress and burnout symptoms. In R. Vandenberghe and A.M. Huberman (Eds.), *Understanding and preventing teacher burnout: A sourcebook of international research and practice* (pp. 269-284). Cambridge: Cambridge University Press.

Dunham, J. (1992). *Stress in teaching* (2nd ed.). London: Routledge.

Fimian, M.J. (1984). The development of an instrument to measure occupational stress in teachers: The teacher stress inventory. *Journal of Occupational Psychology*, 57(4), 277-293.

Flett, G.L., Hewitt, P.L., and Hallett, C.J. (1995). Perfectionism and job stress in teachers. *Canadian Journal of School Psychology*, 11(1), 32-42.

Friedman, I.A., and Farber, B.A. (1992). Professional self-concept as a predictor of teacher burnout. *Journal of Educational Research*, 86(1), 28-35.

Harvey, R. (2004, April 30). Depression haunts teachers. *The Toronto Star*. Retrieved July 7, 2004 from the Canadian Newsstand database.

Kyriacou, C., and Sutcliffe, J. (1978). Teacher stress: Prevalence, sources, and symptoms. *British Journal of Educational Psychology*, 48, 159-167.

Kyriacou, C. (2001). Teacher stress: Directions for future research. *Educational Review*, 53(1), 127-35. Retrieved July 5, 2004 from the Academic Search Premier database.

Litrell, P.C.,and Billingsley, B.S. (1994). The effects of principal support on special education and general educators' stress, job satisfaction, school commitment, health, and intent to stay in teaching. *Remedial & Special Education*, 15(5), 297-310.

Manthei, R., and Gilmore, A. (1996). Teacher stress in intermediate schools. *Educational Research*, 28, 3-19.

Ministry of Education (n.d.). School board profiles. Retrieved October 30, 2005 from http://esip.edu.gov.on.ca/english/default.asp

Selye, H. (1976). *The stress of life* (Rev. ed.). New York: McGraw-Hill.

Slavin, R.E. (1984). *Research methods in education: A practical guide*. New Jersey: Prentice-Hall.

Starnaman, S.M., and Miller, K.I. (1992). A test of a causal model of communication and burnout in the teaching profession. *Communication Education*, 41(1), 40-55.

Troman, G. (2000). Teacher stress in a low trust society. *British Journal of Sociology of Education*, 21(3), 331-354.

Wilhelm, K., Dewhurst-Savellis, J., and Parker, G. (2000). Teacher stress? An analysis of why teachers leave and why they stay. *Teachers & Teaching*, 6(3), 291-304.

Wideman, R. (2005). *Personal Communication*. Associate Dean, Faculty of Education, Nipissing University, North Bay, Ontario.

Wilson, M., Joffe, R.T., Wilkerson, B., and Bastable, C. (2000). The unheralded business crisis in Canada: Depression at work: An information paper for business, incorporating 12 steps to a business plan to defeat depression. Retrieved August 14, 2005 from http://www.mental healthroundtable.ca/aug_round_pdfs/Roundtable%20report_Jul20.pdf

Younghusband, L., Garlie, N., and Church, E. (2003). High school teacher stress in Newfoundland Canada: A work in progress. Paper presented at the Hawaii International Conference on Education, January 7-10, 2003. Retrieved July 8, 2004 from http://www.hiceducation.org/Edu_Proceedings/Lynda%20Younghusband.pdf

Plate 9 "Jailhouse Perspective" (R. LeClair)

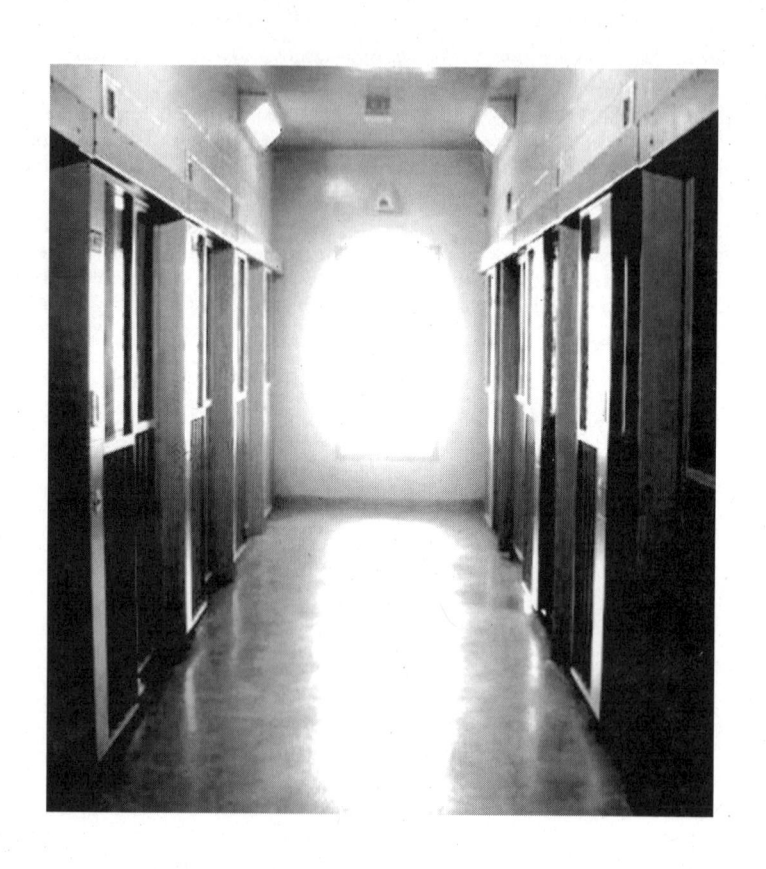

# 14

Dangerous Medicine: Social Control of the Mentally Ill and the Police Role

Gregory P. Brown
Department of Sociology, Criminal Justice & Social Welfare, Nipissing University

Ron Hoffman
Ontario Police College

INTRODUCTION

In February 2004 RCMP officers shot and killed Martin Ostopovich, 41, during a six hour long standoff at his Spruce Grove Alberta home. Police had been called to the home following a report that a vehicle parked in front of the home had been struck by a bullet. Upon arriving at the scene a panic-stricken woman ran from the home, warning officers that Ostopovich was very agitated, and armed. Ostopovich, who was mentally ill and had reported hearing voices telling him to kill police officers, was well-known to police.

The stand-off ended tragically when Ostopovich attempted to flee the home in his pick-up truck. Police rammed the vehicle as it backed out of the driveway. Exiting the vehicle with two rifles, Ostopovich fired at the officers, killing Corporal Jim Gallaway. Other officers returned fire, killing Ostopovich.

At the inquiry into the shootings, both Ostopovich's doctors and RCMP officers expressed frustration with laws and regulations that prevent them from intervening with mentally ill persons who are known to be at a high risk for committing a violent act. Ostopovich was diagnosed as a paranoid schizophrenic after suffering a brain injury in 1999 as the result of a truck crash. Doctors reported that Ostopovich believed police were 'out to get him' and that the RCMP had secretly implanted a transmitter in his neck. Ostopovich refused to remain in hospital for treatment, and only sporadically took the medications prescribed to treat his condition (Ryan Cormier, *Edmonton Journal*, January 26, 2006, p.A1; Ryan Cormier, *Windsor Star*, May 25, 2006, p.A7).

With increasing frequency, police are called to intervene in situations in which persons with a mental illness are at risk for violence toward others, as in the Ostopovich case above. Police are also often called to intervene in situations where the mentally ill person is at risk for violence against themselves, as in the case of suicide. Sometimes, as the ultimate authorities in legitimate use of violence, the police are called to assist others to exert control over persons with a mental illness, as in the case below.

> On April 12, 2006 Waterloo Regional Police were called to Grand River Hospital in Kitchener, Ontario to assist staff to subdue a 36 year-old male psychiatric patient who had become violent at the hospital. Police fired a Taser at the patient in an attempt to gain control of him.
>
> The Taser weapon fires two electrodes into the skin that deliver a high-voltage electric shock, temporarily immobilizing the subject.
>
> Unfortunately, use of the Taser weapon by the Waterloo Regional Police resulted in the patient suffering a near-fatal cardiac arrest. Ontario's Special Investigations Unit, a civilian agency that investigates police use of force, is looking into the incident (Frances Barrick, *Kitchener Record*, April 15, 2006, p.B1).

At still other times, police and other criminal justice officials are called upon to use their authority to maintain public order and protect property from the intrusion of those, like the homeless and the mentally ill, who are perceived to be a threat to other persons or property.

> Running for leadership of the Ontario Provincial Conservative party, leadership candidate Jim Flaherty proposed that the correctional centre in Guelph, Ontario about to be closed be used instead as a facility to house the homeless, including those with mental illness, prostitutes, drug addicts and alcoholics. By rounding up the homeless and placing them in the centre, Flaherty believed they could get the counseling, medical care and rehabilitation they require (Peggy O'Sullivan, *Kitchener Record*, March 4, 2004, p.A6).

Mr. Flaherty is now Minister of Finance in the federal Conservative government.

In a 2005 presentation to the Standing Senate Committee on Social Issues, Science and Technology, the Canadian Association of Chiefs of Police (CACP) called on the government to recognize that "the police should not be the de facto first line of support for most people with mental illnesses" and that "appropriate mental health services" must be put in place to permit officers to get individuals the help they need in a "timely manner" (CNCPMHL/CACP, 2005, p. 11). In similar fashion, the Ontario Association of Chiefs of Police (OACP) has called on the government to recognize the "inappropriateness of the enmeshing of the criminal justice system, and particularly police services, with health issues" and that the current state of affairs has resulted in "vulnerable individuals being at risk of increased contact with the police and increased involvement in the criminal justice system. This contact has resulted in the criminalization of behaviours associated to mental illness" (OACP, 2003, Resolution 03-03).

Confronted by rapid growth in calls to intervene with mentally ill persons, with consequently increased risks for arrests and possibly violence, police agencies across Canada are thus questioning the role that police should play in addressing the needs of mentally ill persons. For example, should the police be training to play the role of "psychiatrists in blue"? (Menzies, 1987; Cotton, 2003). Should we be asking the police to be the 'first line of support' in the mental health system, and what are the consequences of putting the police in this position? Alternatively, should practitioners and policy makers be looking elsewhere for the resources and supports needed by persons with a mental illness when in crisis?

THE EPIDEMIOLOGY OF POLICE CONTACT WITH MENTALLY ILL PERSONS IN CANADA

According to a 2002 Health Canada report, approximately 20% of Canadians will experience mental illness in any given year. A small proportion of these will come into contact with the police.

Estimating the number of persons with a mental illness who come into contact with the police is fraught with difficulty. Many contacts between police and members of the public, including those with a mental illness, are dealt with on an informal basis, and no official record is kept. Other contacts between the police and persons with a mental illness are in the form of a non-criminal or 'civil' commitment under mental health legislation, wherein a physician has ordered an individual to be apprehended by police and committed to a hospital for a period of psychiatric observation (Janus, 1998; Hiday, 2003; Vago and Nelson, 2004). Still other contacts between police and the mentally ill are in the form of an arrest for a criminal offence. Police agencies across Canada have reported substantial increases in all types of contacts with the mentally ill (Brown and Maywood, 2002; Heslop, Hartford, Rona, Stitt, and Schrecker, 2002).

Brown and Maywood (2003) analysed data from the Toronto Police Service on civil commitment apprehensions under the Ontario Mental Health Act. Between 1999 and 2002 apprehensions increased from 2,932 to 4,847, a growth of 65% in only 4 years. During the same period, persons charged with Criminal Code offences increased by only 3% (Brown and Maywood, 2003). Still, mental health act-related apprehensions represent only a small proportion of contacts between police and the mentally ill, and unfortunately very little information is recorded about individuals who are arrested for a criminal offence and who may also show evidence of a mental illness.

Most often, researchers have relied on tracking the arrests of psychiatric patients by police to establish a measure of contact. In their comprehensive review of the research, Schellenberg, Wasylenki, Webster, and Goering (1992) report that between one-third and one-half of psychiatric patients have been arrested at some time in their lives, and approximately 8% of patients will experience an arrest on an annual basis. Preliminary findings from an Ontario study of hospital and community psychiatric patients generally confirm these figures (Hoffman, Hirdes, and Montague, 2006). Still, some individuals who experience a mental illness will not seek treatment, and many more will not receive treatment in a formal 'psychiatric' setting (e.g., they will be treated by a family physician). Those treated in formal psychiatric settings are both more likely to suffer from more serious mental illness and to exhibit the severe symptoms that may bring them into contact with police (Lamb, Weinberger, and Gross, 2004).

Recent evidence (Arboleda-Florez, Holley, and Crisanti, 1996; Link, Monohan, Steuve, and Cullen, 1999; Swanson, Borum, Swartz, and Hiday, 1999; Markowitz, 2006) shows that, indeed, the police are more likely to come into contact with mentally ill persons who are severely mentally ill (e.g., psychotic, affective disorders including bi-polar) and who are also at a high risk for committing acts of violence or public disorder that will bring them to the attention of police. In large part, this increased contact with the severely mentally ill stems from the deinstitutionalization of hospitalized psychiatric patients that began in the 1960s (Lamb, Weinberger, and Gross, 2004). Thus, while it is estimated that between only 3% and 7% of the general public are thought to suffer from a severe mental illness (Broner, Lattimore, Cowell, and Schlenger, 2004), estimates of the proportion of offenders who come into contact with police and end up in jails, correctional centres, and prisons, and who are severely mentally ill, range from 10% to 15% (Lamb and Weinberger, 1998; Lamb et al., 2004; Laishes, 2006; Brown, Girard, and Mathias, 2006).

At the same time, those who are severely mentally ill, in particular those who also have a substance abuse problem, have been found to be significantly more likely to exhibit violent behaviours toward others (Arboleda-Florez, 1998; Marzuk, 1996; Arboleda-Florez et al., 1996; Mulvey, 1994). More than half of convicted offenders in jails, correctional centres, and prisons have a substance abuse problem, and nearly 50% of offenders with a diagnosed mental illness also have a substance abuse problem (Brown et al., 2006).

Thus, while it may be impossible to accurately estimate the proportion of persons with a mental illness who come into contact with the police, research shows that those who do come into contact with the police are more likely to be severely mentally ill and to be at a greater risk for exhibiting violent behaviour toward others. Given the role of the police, to enforce the law and protect the public through force if necessary, it is therefore not surprising that contacts between the police and persons with a mental illness have become a significant concern among key stakeholders including mentally ill persons, their families and friends, police, mental health professionals, media, government, and the general public. Consistently, calls are made for improved strategies and practices to address the problem (Mary-Jane Egan, *London Free Press*, August 26, 2003, n.p.).

Historical Notes on the Social Control of the Mentally Ill

Until the end of the European Middle Ages in the latter part of the 16th century, persons who were mentally ill, and who were defined normatively to be a 'problem' by other members of their social group, were understood in magical or religious terms as being somehow possessed by an evil spirit or the Devil that needed to be expelled or 'exorcised' (Szasz, 1961; Busfield, 1988). Not infrequently, the exorcism ceremonies involved physical torture or 'ordeals' that resulted in the death of the afflicted (Rosen, 1968).

With the onset of the Enlightenment in the 17th century, religious explanations gave way to scientific theories, including the causes (and cures) of human behaviour. Increasingly, 'lunacy,' or mental illness, was understood to be a medical illness, caused by some set of biological and environmental factors, including changes in the phases of the moon (lunar, hence lunacy and lunatic; *Oxford English Dictionary*, 1989; Torrey and Miller, 2001).

Now conceived as a medical condition, mental illness therefore obviously required care and treatment in an appropriate setting. Initially, the 'care' or custodial component was emphasized, and the mentally ill were housed in workhouses or boarded out in privately-run 'madhouses' (Parry-Jones, 1973). Violent or otherwise dangerous lunatics posed a unique problem. Often, the only facility capable of restraining them was the local gaol. The legal authority for confining lunatics in gaols stemmed from the English Vagrancy Act of 1714 (12 Anne.2.Cap.23), the first legislation to deal with dangerous lunatics. It empowered the magistrates to confine,

> *Persons of little or no Estates, who, by Lunacy, or otherwise, are furiously Mad, and dangerous to be permitted to go abroad, and to direct them to be kept safely locked up, and chained if necessary while the madness lasted* (Fessler, 1956, p. 902).

In the early 1800s, spurred on by sensational accounts of inhumane forms of treatment in the private madhouses and instances of wrongful detention of sane individuals, the English government established a series of parliamentary committees to investigate conditions in the madhouses (Bynum, 1964; Hoffman, 1985). Out of the deliberations of the committees arose the government-funded, publicly administered system of asylums and mental hospitals that persisted in one form or another in England until the 1960s.

The emergence of asylums in Canada generally followed the English experience. Public asylums were constructed in Saint John, New Brunswick (1835),

Toronto (1850), Quebec City (1850), Kingston (1856), St. John's, Newfoundland (1854), Halifax (1859), and Charlottetown (1879).

DEINSTITUTIONALIZATION AND GROWTH OF COMMUNITY MENTAL HEALTH

The era of the lunatic asylum in Britain, Canada, and other Western countries extended until the early 1960s, when psychiatric treatment in asylums and mental hospitals began to be replaced by treatment delivered in the community by community-based mental health agencies. Just as allegations of abuse, wrongful detention, and harsh treatment in the old private asylum system had contributed to the development of the public asylum system, similar sensational revelations had surfaced regarding the treatment of patients in public asylums and mental hospitals.

Beginning with Michel Foucault's *Madness and Civilization: A History of Insanity in the Age of Reason* (1965/1973) and followed by Szasz (1961), Rothman, (1971), Scull (1975, 1977, 1980), Horwitz (1982), and others, the role of asylums and mental hospitals in the social control of 'undesirables' in society, including homosexuals, political dissidents, the developmentally disabled, the homeless, and the mentally ill, came under scathing attack. The asylums were depicted as warehouses for otherwise non-criminal deviants in modern society (Scull, 1977). Author Ken Kesey's fictional account of life on a mental hospital ward titled *One Flew Over the Cuckoo's Nest* (1962) did much to galvanize public support to end the apparent cruelty of the asylum system, and by the end of the 1960s the deinstitutionalization movement was in full swing. At the same time, the development of an array of psychotropic medications to treat a variety of psychiatric conditions, including the psychoses, made the safe release of patients into the community truly possible (Markowitz, 2006).

Today, mental health professionals believe that the most effective and humane method of psychiatric treatment is to allow the individual to remain in the community, near family and friends. At the same time, the notion that the mental illness suffered by an individual must be *cured* through aggressive treatment has been replaced with the idea that successful management and *control* of the illness in the community, through use of psychotropic medications and family and social agencies support, should be the goal of treatment.

THE ROLE OF THE POLICE IN THE SOCIAL CONTROL OF THE MENTALLY ILL

The first police forces in Canada had little role in exerting control over persons with a mental illness. By the 1850s, the public asylum movement in Canada was already well under way, with its own core of 'asylum attendants' set aside for the purpose of apprehending and controlling persons with a mental illness. To remove a violent or dangerous mentally ill person to the asylum, a family member or public official could petition the local magistrate or Governor for an order for the mentally ill person to be apprehended. The phrase, "*watch out, or the men in white coats will come take you away!*" contained a good measure of truth in that asylum attendants were primarily responsible for apprehending and transporting the insane person to the asylum, rather than police (Sussman, 1998; Saving Lives, 2000).

Only with the onset of the deinstitutionalization movement in the 1960s were police called upon to intervene with the mentally ill. Without adequate funding in place to house and treat patients in the community, in particular those who were poor, recent immigrants, or minorities, police were thrust into the role of 'first point of contact' for dealing with mentally ill persons in crisis in the community (Lamb, Weinberger, and DeCuir, 2002; Lamb, Weinberger, and Gross, 2004).

Police contacts with the mentally ill have increased dramatically since deinstitutionalization. US research shows that the number of mental illness-related incidents handled by police increased over 200% between 1975 and 1979 after legislative changes made it easier to involuntarily commit people with mental illnesses (Bonovitz and Bonovitz, 1981). In Canada, increases of as much as 30% per year in mental health apprehensions have been reported (Shannon Black, *National Post*, August 19, 2000), and Brown and Maywood (2003) report a 65% increase in apprehensions by Toronto Police between 1999 and 2002. Increases in Canada in criminal offence arrests of persons with a mental illness are thought to be on the rise, though it is difficult to measure the exact extent of the increase. Newspaper accounts of police shootings of mentally ill persons are no longer a rare occurrence.

As a result of their increased contacts with persons with a mental illness, police are being called on to perform as "psychiatrists in blue" (Menzies, 1987; Cotton, 2003). Each of the Canadian provinces has legislation in place that permits a medical practitioner to issue an order of 'civil commitment' that an individual be apprehended by police and taken to a hospital or psychiatric facility for assessment of their mental health status (Vago and Nelson, 2004). Police can also be called upon to apprehend individuals who have violated a Community Treatment Order (CTO). A CTO may be issued by a psychiatric facility when an individual is discharged, and directs that the individual can live in the community so long as they attend required treatment and take any prescribed medications as directed. If the individual fails to abide by the conditions of the CTO, the police will be directed to apprehend the violator and return them to the facility (Meehan, 1995; Psychiatric Patient Advocate Office, 2003).

Police officers can also make apprehensions on their own initiative if they believe that an individual is suffering from a mental illness and is a danger to themselves or others (Ontario Ministry of Health and Long Term Care, 2006a).

In still other circumstances, police can be called to make an arrest of a person who has committed a criminal offence and who may also have a mental illness.

Whether or not first contact with the mentally ill in the community should or should not be the responsibility of the police, the reality is that police today have little choice and, in fact, are now *expected* to perform the function. On the other hand, police are much criticized for the way they perform this function, including the training they receive in dealing with the mentally ill, their use of discretion in making decisions about who is or is not mentally ill, and their choice to use informal means, apprehension, or arrest to resolve situations involving the mentally ill (Patch and Arrigo, 1999; Cotton, 2004).

POLICE RESPONSES TO DEALING WITH PERSONS WITH A MENTAL ILLNESS

Numerous studies (Abrahamson, 1972; Whitmer, 1980; Arrigo, 1993, 1996; Green, 1997; Laberge, Landerville, and Morin, 2000) have examined the process through which police officers come to decide on a course of action when dealing with emotionally disturbed persons, and the tendency for police officers to resort to laying criminal charges as the most expeditious means of resolving the situation has been reported frequently (Bittner, 1967; Menzies, 1987; Teplin and Pruett, 1992; Borum, 2000, Markowitz, 2006).

The increasingly important role of the police as 'gatekeepers' to mental health crisis intervention services, and the further tendency therefore to 'criminalize' the entire crisis intervention process, has been a focus of much additional research (Meehan, 1995; Panzarella and Alicea, 1997; Lamb and Weinberger, 1998). The results of this research show that, too often, police officers are confronted by a lack of accessible alternative services, or are unaware of such services, and so are forced to rely on their fundamental authorities as enforcers of the criminal law to address situations involving persons in crisis, including the emotionally disturbed (Janik, 1992; Lamb, Weinberger, and DeCuir, 2002).

Research in the area of community mental health tends to focus on the identification and evaluation of different organizational strategies and programs that can serve as alternatives to arresting, prosecuting, and incarcerating individuals who may be emotionally disturbed (Milestone, 1995; Cordner, 2000; Borum, 2000; Lamb, Weinberger, and DeCuir, 2002).

Police, community mental health agencies, and government policy makers have responded to the criticisms levelled against the police, and the results of research studies, by instituting a diverse array of training programs and crisis-response initiatives. Most police services in Canada now provide some training for police officers in recognizing and responding to persons who may have a mental illness. Assertive Community Treatment (ACT) programs that pair police officers with mental health professionals to address the needs of mentally ill persons in crisis are becoming increasingly common in larger centres (Bond, Drake, Mueser, and Latimer, 2001) with the result that a growing number of persons with a mental illness are being 'diverted' away from arrest and into the mental health care system, where their needs are better served (Cordner, 2000; Zealberg, Santos, and Fisher, 1993; Steadman, Deane, Borum, and Morrisey, 2000; Lamb, Weinberger, and Gross, 2004). Special courts designed to assess and, where appropriate, divert individuals with a mental illness from standing trial have been implemented in a number of larger centres in Canada, further reducing criminalization of the mentally ill (Lamb, Weinberger, and Gross, 1999; Steadman, Cocozza, and Veysey, 1999; Fisher, Packer, Grisso, McDermeit, and Brown, 2000; Watson, Hanrahan, Luchins, and Lurigo, 2001; Lattimore, Broner, Sherman, Frisman, and Shafer, 2003).

Nevertheless, critics continue to complain that investment in police training and joint crisis team initiatives begs the real question: should in fact the police be acting as the first line of response for mentally ill persons in crisis? As the ultimate authorities on the use of legitimate violence (Hoffman, Lawrence, and Brown, 2004), police carry guns and other weapons when responding to crisis situations, increasing the potential for serious harm or even death. Should we take this risk when responding to the needs of a mentally ill person in crisis? At the same time, chiefs of police across the country complain that a growing proportion of officers' time and police service budgets are being eaten up in responding to calls involving a person with a mental illness (CBC News, August 6, 2002; Scott Tracey, *Guelph Mercury*, May 23, 2003; Virginia McDonald, *Guelph Tribune*, August 2, 2005), and that too often mental health resources are not available when officers need them (Jeffrey Ougler, *Sudbury Star*, November 4, 2002; Mary-Jane Egan, *London Free Press*, August 26, 2003; Richard Dooley, *Halifax Daily News*, December 24, 2005).

RETHINKING THE POLICE ROLE IN RESPONDING TO MENTALLY ILL PERSONS IN CRISIS

As the extent of serious violence and crime has decreased in Western societies, reflected in police statistics showing a decline in calls to respond to criminal actions, there has been a concomitant increase in expectations for police to respond to non-criminal matters, ranging from a host of community policing initiatives, school liaison duties, and public education campaigns through to providing assistance and counselling to victims of crime, arbitrating verbal disputes, conducting environmental assessments to reduce crime risk, intervening and counselling youth and their parents who have come into contact with the law, enforcing CTO orders, and performing apprehensions of mentally ill persons (Shearing, 1984; Cordner, 1989; Brown and Seguin, 2002). According to Murphy (1993): "it remains an inescapable fact that on almost every measure of demand for police services, the trend is moving upwards" (p. 43).

As the front-line of response to almost any type of crisis in our society, as the voice at the end of the 911 call, police understand and accept the important role they play, and the need for training and programs that continuously improve their capacity to deal with crisis situations effectively (Teplin, 2000; Editorial, *Canadian Medical Association Journal,* March 4, 2001; Swaminath, Mendonca, Vidal, and Chapman, 2002; Cotton, 2004; Jonathan Kay, *National Post,* May 15, 2006). Rather, at issue for many in the police community is what follows after the crisis response, in terms of resources and other supports available to the police to get help for those in crisis, in particular those who have not committed a criminal offence (Brown and Maywood, 2003; Lamb, Weinberger, and DeCuir, 2004). Without the resources and supports available in community agencies or at the hospital to provide treatment and counselling for persons with a mental illness who come into contact with police, individuals are caught up in an inhumane cycle, therefore, of arrest, hospitalization, release, re-arrest, and so on (Lamb, Weinberger, and DeCuir, 2004; Hartford, Heslop, Stitt, and Hoch, 2005).

Is it reasonable to ask that police officers act as "psychiatrists in blue" (Menzies, 1987; Cotton, 2003)? The answer is a resounding 'no'—it is unlikely that officers will ever have the training and expertise to diagnose persons in crisis on-the-spot and determine the kinds of treatment and support they need. Rather, police officers require training and expertise to become better 'first responders' to mentally ill persons in crisis, to deal with the immediate threat to individuals themselves or to others around them, and to ensure that they are directed to the professional treatment and supports they need (Hoffman and Putnam, 2004). In fact, Brown and Maywood (2003) report that most Toronto police officers are generally accurate in their assessment of the types of situations they are likely to encounter in dealing with a mentally ill person in crisis, and their needs for counselling/support; what is lacking too often are the community and hospital supports necessary to get individuals the help that they require.

Governments are slowly starting to respond to calls for better funding for community mental health agencies and hospitals to address the needs of mentally ill persons living in the community. In 2005, Ottawa announced plans to establish a Canadian Mental Health Commission to promote cooperation and coordination 'to better address mental health and mental illness in Canada,' including fragmentation and gaps in services available to address the needs of mentally ill persons in crisis (Health Canada, 2005). In May, 2006 the Ontario government announced $68.5 million in funding for community mental health services, including $23 million targeted for ACT programs and other crisis response initiatives (Ontario Ministry of Health and Long-Term Care, 2006b).

Epilogue

On February 8, 2004 George Bell, Vivian McKay, Donald Evans and Joy Evans, all from Huntsville, Ontario died in a head-on crash outside of Orillia Ontario. Cynthia Oster, the driver of the car that slammed into their vehicle, also died in the crash.

Oster, who had a long history of psychiatric problems, had the day before been taken by police to hospital in Bracebridge after friends and others had reported that she had exhibited bizarre behaviour, including driving her car in circles around a parking lot, threatening an attendant at a gas bar and appearing angry and 'furious.'

Oster was released from the emergency room at the hospital by the doctor on duty. The community mental health worker on call was apparently not contacted, for reasons unknown.

The next day Oster drove the wrong way down the exit onto the northbound lanes of Highway 11. According to police, Oster drove for more than 10 kilometres against oncoming traffic before slamming into the sport utility vehicle, killing the four occupants and herself.

An inquest into the circumstances of the crash was called by the Ontario coroner. It is expected that among the recommendations will be yet another call for more resources and support to address the needs of mentally ill persons in crisis (*Barrie Examiner*, August 18, 2005; De La Vega, *Bracebridge Examiner*, September 22, 2005, p. 1; De La Vega, *Huntsville Forester*, April 5, 2006, p. A3).

References

Abrahamson, M.L. (1972). The criminalization of mentally disorder behavior: Possible side effects of a new mental health law. *Hospital and Community Psychiatry*, 23, 101-105.

Arboleda-Flórez, J., Holley, H.L., and Crisanti, A. (1996). *Mental illness and violence: Proof or stereotype?* Ottawa: Health Canada, Health Promotion and Programs Branch.

Arboleda-Flórez, J. (1998). Mental illness and violence: An epidemiological appraisal of the evidence, *Canadian Journal of Psychiatry*, 43, 989-996.

Arrigo, B. (1993). *Madness, language and the law*. Albany, NY: Harrow and Heston.

Arrigo, B. (1996). *The contours of psychiatric justice*. New York: Garland Publishing.

Barrick, F. (2006). Taser incident nearly fatal; Local psychiatric patient suffers cardiac arrest after being subdued. *Kitchener Record*, April 15, p.B1.

Barry Examiner (2005). News. August 18, np.

Black, S. (2000). The police and the mentally ill: Is there a better way? *National Post*, August 19, p.F1.FRO.

Bittner, E. (1967). Police discretion in emergency room apprehension of mentally ill persons. *Social Problems*, 14, 278-292.

Bond, G.R., Drake, R.E., Mueser, K.T., and Latimer, E. (2001). Assertive community treatment for people with severe mental illness: Critical ingredients and impact on patients. *Disease Management and Health Outcomes*, 9(3), 141-159.

Bonovitz, J.C., and Bonovitz, J.S. (1981). Diversion of the mentally ill into the criminal justice system: The police intervention perspective. *American Journal of Psychiatriatry Association*, 138, 973-976.

Borum, R. (2000). Improving high risk encounters between people with mental illness and the police. *Journal of the American Academy of Psychiatry and the Law*, 28, 332-337.

Broner, N., Lattimore, P.K., Cowell, A.J., and Schlenger, W.E. (2004). Effects of diversion on adults with co-occuring mental illness and substance abuse: Outcomes from a national multi-site study. *Behavioral Sciences and the Law*, 22, 519-541.

Brown, G., and Maywood, S. (2002). *Police response in situations involving emotionally disturbed persons: An analysis and update of data reported from the Toronto Police Service EDP report form*. Paper presented at the First National Conference on Police/Mental Health Liaison, Montreal, Canada.

Brown, G., and Seguin, R.C.J. (2002). *North Bay Police Service Patrol Workload Study: Final Report*. North Bay, ON: North Bay Police Service.

Brown, G., and Maywood, S. (2003). *Understanding interactions between the police and emotionally disturbed persons: An analysis of data from the Toronto Police Service EDP report form*. Unpublished paper.

Brown, G., Girard, L., and Mathias, K.(2006). *Identifying the psychiatric care needs of adult offenders in the Ontario Correctional System*. Presentation to the 20th Annual MHCP Forensic Conference, Penetanguishene, Ontario.

Canadian National Committee for Police/Mental Health Liaison/Canadian Association of Chiefs of Police (CNCPMHL/CACP) (2005). Presentation to the Senate Standing Senate Committee on Social Issues, Science and Technology. Ottawa: Senate of Canada.

Busfield, J. (1988). Mental illness as social product or social construct: A contradiction in feminists' arguments? *Sociology of Health and Illness*, 10(4), 521-542.

Bynum, W.F. (1964). Rationales for therapy in British psychiatry: 1780-1835. *Medical History*, 18, 323.

CBC News (2002). Alberta police deal increasingly with mentally ill people. Canadian Broadcasting Coroporation, August 6, *http://cbc.ca*.

Cordner, G.W. (1989). The police on patrol. In D.J. Kenny (Ed.), *Police and policing* (pp. 60-71). New York: Praeger Publishers.

Cordner, G.W. (2000). A community policing approach to persons with mental illness. *Journal of the American Academy of Psychiatry and the Law*, 28, 326-331.

Cormier, R. (2006). Mountie killer rejected treatment. *Edmonton Journal*, January 26, p.A1.

Cormier, R. (2006). Doctor felt helpless to stop officer's mentally ill killer. *Windsor Star*, May 25, p.A7.

Cotton, D. (2003). *Psychiatrists in Blue*. Annual Conference, Canadian National Committee for Police/Mental Health Liaison/Canadian Association of Chiefs of Police (CNCPMHL/CACP), Saskatoon, Saskatchewan, October, 2003.

Cotton, D. (2004). The attitudes of Canadian police officers toward the mentally ill. *International Journal of Law and Psychiatry*, 27, 135-146.

Davis, S. (1992). Assessing the criminalization of the mentally ill in Canada. *Canadian Journal of Psychiatry*, 37(October), 532-538.

De La Vega, T. (2005). Cynthia Oster led troubled life. *Bracebridge Examiner*, September 22, p. 1.

De La Vega, T. (2006). Agency suggests crisis worker could help with mental health patients in ER. *Huntsville Forester*, April 5, p. A3.

Dooley, R. (2005). Chief considers forming trained mental health unit. *Halifax Daily News*, December 24, p.5.

Editorial (2001). Mental illness in my backyard. *Canadian Medical Association Journal*, 164(7), 957.

Egan, M.J. (2003). Cops urge increase in mental health funding. *London Free Press*, August 26, n.p., www.ontario.cmha.ca.

Fessler, A. (1956). The management of lunacy in Seventeenth Century England. *Proceedings of the Royal Society of Medicine*, 49(11), 901-907.

Fisher, W.H., Packer, I.K., Grisso, T., McDermeit, M., and Brown, J.M. (2000). From case management to court clinic: Examining forensic system involvement of persons with severe mental illness. *Mental Health Services Research*, 2(1), 41-49.

Foucault, M. (1965). *Madness and civilization: A history of insanity in the Age of Reason*. New York: Pantheon Books.

Green, T.M. (1997). Police as frontline mental health workers: The decision to arrest or refer to mental health agencies. *International Journal of Law and Psychiatry*, 20(4), 469-486.

Hartford, K., Heslop, L., Stitt, L., and Hoch, J.S. (2005). Design of an algorithm to identify persons with mental illness in a police administrative database. *International Journal of Law and Psychiatry*, 28, 1-11.

Health Canada (2002). *A Report on Mental Illnesses in Canada*. Ottawa, Canada.

Health Canada (2005). Minister Dosanjh announced that the government of Canada will establish a Canadian Mental Health Commission. *News Release*, November 24.

Heslop, L., Hartford, K., Rona H., Stitt, L., and Schrecker, T. (2002). *Trends in police contact with persons with serious mental illnesses in London, Ontario*. Paper presented at the First National Conference on Police/Mental Health Liaison, Montreal, Canada.

Hiday, V.A. (2003). Civil commitment and arrests. *Current Opinion in Psychiatry*, 16(5), 575-580.

Hoffman, R.E. (1985). *Lunacy in Upper Canada: The viability of the social control theory*. Unpublished Masters Thesis. Psychology Department, Carleton University.

Hoffman, R.E., Lawrence, C., and Brown, G. (2004). Canada's national use-of-force framework for police officers. *The Police Chief*, 71(10), www.policechiefmagazine.net.

Hoffman, R.E., and Putnam, L. (2004). *Not just another call...Police response to persons with mental illnesses*. Sault Ste. Marie, ON: Ontario Association of Chiefs of Police.

Hoffman, R.E., Hirdes, J., and Montague, P. (2006). *Identifying characteristics of psychiatric patients involved in the criminal justice system in Ontario: Preliminary findings*. Presentation to the 2005 Canadian Psychiatric Association Conference, Vancouver, B.C.

Horwitz, A. (1982). *The social control of mental illness*. New York: Academic Press.

Janik, J. (1992). Dealing with mentally ill offenders. *FBI Law Enforcement Bulletin*, July, 22-26.

Janus, E. (1998). Hendricks and the moral terrain of police power civil commitment. *Psychology, Public Police and Law*, 4(2), 297-322.

Jones, J.E. (1924). *Pioneer crimes and punishments in Toronto and the Home District*. Toronto: George N. Morang.

Kay, J. (2006). Patients' rights vs. a father's anguish. *National Post*, May 15, p.A11.

Kesey, K. (1962). *One flew over the cuckoo's nest*. New York: New American Library.

Laberge, D., Landerville, P., and Morin, D. (2000). The criminalization of mental illness: A complex process of interpretation. In L.G. Beaman (Ed.), *New perspectives in deviance* (pp. 86-108). Scarborough, ON: Prentice-Hall.

Laishes, J. (2006). *The Correctional Service of Canada's Mental Health Strategy*. Mental Health Services: Correctional Service of Canada.

Lamb, H.R., and Weinberger, L.E. (1998). Persons with severe mental illness in jails and prisons: A review. *Psychiatric Services*, 49, 483-492.

Lamb, H.R., Weinberger, L.E., and Gross, B.H. (1999). Community treatment of severely mental ill offenders under the jurisdiction of the criminal justice system: A review. *Psychiatric Services*, 50(7), 907-914.

Lamb, H.R., Weinberger, L.E., and DeCuir, W.J. (2002). The police and mental health. *Psychiatric Services*, 53(10), 1266-1271.

Lamb, H.R., Weinberger, L.E., and Gross, B.H. (2004). Mentally ill persons in the criminal justice system: Some perspectives. *Psychiatric Quarterly*, 75(2), 107-126.

Lamb, H.R., Weinberger, L.E., and DeCuir, W.J. (2004). The police and mental health. *Psychiatric Services*, 53(10), 1266-1271.

Latimorre, P.K., Broner, N., Sherman, R., Frisman, L., and Shafer, M.S. (2003). A comparison of prebooking andf postbooking diversion programs for mentally ill substance-using individuals with justice involvement. *Journal of Contemporary Criminal Justice*, 19(1), 30-64.

Link, B.G., Monohan, J., Steuve, A., and Cullen, F.T. (1999). Real in their consequences: A sociological approach to understanding their association between psychotic symptoms and violence. *American Sociological Review*, 64, 316-332.

Markowitz, F.E. (2006). Psychiatric hospital capacity, homelessness and crime and arrest rates. *Criminology*, 44(1), 45-72.

Marzuk, P.M. (1996). Violence, crime and mental illness: How strong a link? *Archives of General Psychiatry*, 53(6), 481-486.

McDonald, V. (2005). Cops pick up mental health system's slack. *Guelph Tribune*, August 2, p.1.

Meehan, A.J. (1995). From conversion to coercion: The police role in medication compliance. *Psychiatric Quarterly*, 66(2), 163-184.

Menzies, R. (1987). Psychiatrists in blue: Police apprehension of mental disorder and dangerousness. *Criminology*, 25(3), 429-453.

Milestone, C. (1995). *The mentally ill and the criminal justice system*. Ottawa: Health Canada.

Mulvey, E.P. (1994). Assessing the evidence of a link between mental illness and violence. *Hospital and Community Psychiatry*, 45, 663-668.

Murphy, C. (1993). Thinking critically about police resources. In A.N. Doob (Ed.), *Thinking about police resources* (pp. 35-67). Toronto: Centre of Criminology, University of Toronto.

News (2005). Inquest will probe dealy collision. *Barrie Examiner*, August 18, p. A1.

Ontario Association of Chiefs of Police (2003). Annual Conference Proceedings; OACP Resolution 03-03.

Ontario Ministry of Health and Long-Term Care (2006a). *Brian's Law (Mnetal Helath Legislative Reform) 2000*. Toronto: Ontario: Ministry of Health and Long-Term Care. *www.health.gov.on*.

Ontario Ministry of Health and Long-Term Care (2006b). McGuinty government expanding community mental health services. *News Release*, May 19.

O'Sullivan, P. (2002). Rejig jail for homeless. *Kitchener Record*, March 4, p.A6.

Ougler, J. (2002). Mental health cuts lead to 'criminalization': Study. *Sudbury Star*, November 4, p.A2.

Oxford English Dictionary (1989). Online version. Oxford University Press, 2006.

Parry-Jones, W.L. (1973). English private madhouses in the Eighteenth and Nineteenth Centuries. *Proceedings of the Royal Society of Medicine*, 66, 659.

Patch, P.C., and Arrigo, B.A. (1999). Police officer attitudes and use of discretion in situations involving the mentally ill. *International Journal of Law and Psychiatry*, 22(1), 23-35.

Psychiatric Patient Advocate Office (2003). *Infoguide: Community Treatment Orders*. Toronto: Ontario Psychiatric Patient Advocate Office.

Rosen, G. (1968). *Madness in society: Chapters in the historical sociology of mental illness*. Chicago: University of Chicago Press.

Rothman, D.J. (1971). *The discovery of the asylum: Social order and disorder in the New Republic*. Boston: Little, Brown and Company.

Saving Lives: Alternatives to the Use of Lethal Force by Police. Report of a Conference held in Toronto (2000). June 23-24. Urban Alliance on Race Relations.

Schellenberg, E.G., Wasylenki, D., Webster, C.D., and Goering, P. (1992). A review of arrests among psychiatric patients. *International Journal of Law and Psychiaty*, 16, 251-264.

Scull, A. (1975). From madness to mental illness: Medical men as moral entrepreneurs. *European Journal of Sociology*, 16, 219-261.

Scull, A. (1977). Madness and segregative control: The rise of the insane asylum. *Social Problems*, 24, 337-351.

Scull, A. (1980). A convenient place to get rid of inconvenient people: The Victorian lunatic asylum. In A.D. King (Ed.), *Buildings and society* (pp. 37-60). London: Routledge and Kegan Paul.

Shearing, C.D. (1984). *Dial-a-cop: A study of police mobilization*. Toronto: Centre of Criminology, University of Toronto.

Steadman, H.J., Cocozza, J.J., and Veysey, B.M. (1999). Comparing outcomes for diverted and nondiverted jail detainees with mental illness. *Law and Human Behavior*, 23(6), 615-627.

Steadman, H.J., Deane, M.H., Borum, R., and Morrissey, J.P. (2000). Comparing outcomes of major models of police responses to mental health emergencies. *Psychiatric Services*, 51(5), 645-649.

Sussman, S. (1998). The first asylums in Canada: A response to neglectful community care and current trends. *Canadian Journal of Psychiatry*, 43, 260-264.

Szasz, T. (1961). *The myth of mental illness*. New York: Hoeber-Harper.

Swaminath, R.S., Mendonca, J.D., Vidal, C., and Chapman, P. (2002). Experiments in change: Pretrial diversion of offenders with mental illness. *Canadian Journal of Psychiatry*, 47(5), 450-458.

Swanson, J., Borum, R., Swartz, M., and Hiday, V. (1999). Violent behaviour preceding hospitalization among persons with a severe mental illness. *Law and Human Behavior*, 23(2), 185-204.

Teplin, L.A. (2000). Keeping the peace: Police discretion and mentally ill persons. *National Institute of Justice Journal*, 244, 8-15.

Torrey, E.F., and Miller, J. (2001). *The invisible plague: The rise of mental Illness from 1750 to the Present*. Piscataway, NJ: Rutgers University Press.

Tracey, S. (2003). Handling mental illness calls boosts police overtime claims. *Guelph Mercury*, May 23, p.A4.

Vago, S., and Nelson, A. (2004). *Law and society*. Toronto: Pearson Education.

Watson, A., Hanrahan, P., Lucins, D., and Lurigio, A. (2001). Mental health courts and the complex issue of mentally ill offenders. *Psychiatric Services*, 52(4), 477-481.

Whitmer, G. (1980). From hospitals to jails: The fate of California's deinstitutionalized mentally ill. *American Journal of Orthopsychiatry*, 50, 65-75.

Zealberg, J.J., Santos, A.B., and Fisher, R.K. (1993). Benefits of mobile crisis programs. *Hospital and Community Psychiatry*, 44(1) 16-17.

Plate 10 "Meaning" (Ferruccio Sardella)

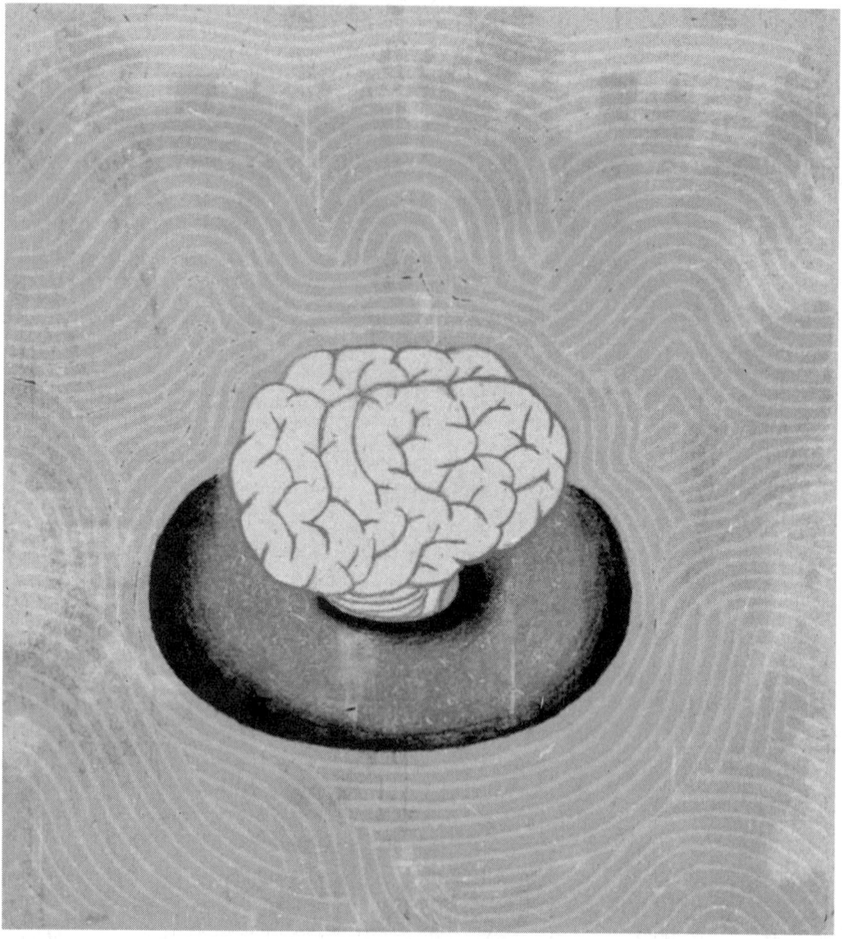

Integration of Mind: How Superstition Amplifies Discrimination and Blocks Empowerment

15

Tim King
Upper Grand District School Board, Ontario

INTRODUCTION

In my undergraduate-level course on mental health, the social stigma attached to mental illness was an issue raised repeatedly. The detrimental effects of this are readily seen: children with attention deficit disorder/attention deficit hyperactivity disorder (ADD/ADHD) are often seen as 'trouble makers,' or as merely incapable of completing curriculum requirements. Adults with clinical depression are considered 'defective,' and risk abandonment by their friends. Duncan McKinlay, a psychologist from Toronto who is also dealing with Tourette's syndrome (*www.lifesatwitch.com*), contemplates taking his own life because his 'defect' has rendered him terrified of publicly showing his illness. The debilitating effects of mental illness are commonly seen in society.

In my own considerations of the issues surrounding the stigma of mental health problems, I have come to believe that this stigmatization can be clearly described in terms of public perceptions of mind, body, and soul. Ideas concerning the mind-body-soul connection have evolved over time, and my hope is that changes in attitudes—most notably a change in our superstitious conceptualizations of the mind-body-soul connection—will eventually produce a vast reduction in the stigma associated with mental illness. Encouraging this change is vital to the well-being and overall quality of life for the people afflicted with mental illnesses.

THE MIND AS MYTH

A number of years ago, I was listening to an interview on CBC radio with a Halifax neurologist (his name and affiliation escape me) who was conducting leading edge research on the brain. His conceptualization of the brain left me rather stunned, listening in silence as I tried to grapple with the implications of his way of thinking. When asked what he thought of the idea that the mind was the centre of consciousness, he suggested that there was no such thing as a mind. When the interviewer questioned his approach, and offered that it simply did not fit with how most people saw things, he asserted that most people were grossly ignorant of how the brain functioned, and that if people could get over this ridiculous concept of 'mind,' we could overcome our superstition and deal with ourselves in a more realistic manner.

It seems that this neuroscientist was fighting the age-old idea that the mind somehow exists outside of physical reality. Having worked on brain research exhaustively for years, he had a very clear idea of how the brain worked, and had concluded that the 'mind' as a separate entity unto itself simply did not exist. His understanding of thought processes and complex structures such as memory, imagination, and intelligence were all based on a very real biology rather than the spurious notion of a mind that exists metaphysically beyond the material world. This kind of thinking challenged some of my basic assumptions about human consciousness and put me on a quest to find out more about other, alternative ways that human cognition could be understood.

PHILOSOPHY OF THE MIND

The notion of brain function versus the metaphysical mind is further elucidated in Bertand Russell's philosophical thesis, *Analysis of Mind* (Russell,1995). Although Russell's argument is complex, he essentially asserts that there is no mental/physical duality. The mental world and the physical world are not in conflict, because the distinction of a mental world is meaningless. Russell's book was a progression of thought that began with the idea of physical body and spiritual soul, and evolved into Rene Descartes' theory of mind/body duality.

In fairness to Descartes, his distinction overturned millennia of religious doctrine and prompted a movement toward a more rational enquiry of human thought by considering people in terms of empirically provable criteria as opposed to religious or mystical doctrine. Prehistoric humans had no social distinction between medicine, magic, and religion (Goshen, 1967). Magic was eventually seen as completely spurious and religious beliefs were used to explain phenomena such as mental illness.

By making the distinction of a mind/body duality instead of a body/soul symbiosis, Descartes had removed a spiritual definition from the equation. While still speculation, Descartes' ghostly mind was at least something that existed without a supernatural explanation. Descartes' notion of a 'ghost in the machine' was still going strong in the mid-20th century, embraced in works such as Gilbert Ryle's (1949) *Concept of Mind*.

The duality between mind and body is still strongly supported in today's thinking, with over 80% (Harris, 1998) of people expressing their belief in a non-physical component to their being. If that leading edge researcher of brains was right, then a vast majority of us are deluding ourselves as to our true nature.

So, what does all this have to do with mental health?

RATIONAL ENQUIRY MAKES FOR LESS STIGMA

Through the remainder of this chapter, I hope to show that scientific thought is nudging public perception away from a mind-body duality, and toward a more methodical, empirical understanding of the human mind. This push stands to produce some decidedly positive effects on how mental health and mental illness are understood by the public. Much of the stigma associated with mental health problems may be related to our oft-expressed reverence for and supernatural view of the mind/soul.

Physical abnormalities have, for the most part, lost the stigmatization to which they were often subject in the past. This is likely a reflection of the fact that physical abnormalities are quantifiable, examinable, and understandable; they lend themselves to scientific analysis. Mental abnormalities, on the other hand, are often invisible and hidden in a superstitiously shrouded, ego-focused seat of power: the human self image.

Our minds are our most coveted attribute. While any biologist will tell you that we are not the fastest, strongest or most agile animal on the planet, we do have a large and decidedly complex brain which, as far as we know, makes us the smartest. When something goes wrong with one of our 'lesser' physical components, we may not think so much of it. When something goes wrong with the one thing that makes us so special—and in a way that we cannot easily explain—we revert to historically-biased beliefs that wallow in ego-inspired superstition.

THE BRIEF HISTORY OF MENTAL ILLNESS: OUR PREJUDICES SHOW

A thousand years ago, someone with mental illness was considered supernaturally afflicted, under the influence of the devil, or suffering from failures in past lives—all depending on who was doing the explaining (Buchanan, 1999). Just a century ago, depression or 'nervous breakdown' was described in gender-based terms such as 'domestic illness' (Glossary of Old Names, nd). This kind of approach reveals significant differences between physical and mental irregularities, and says more about the society of the time than it does about the illness in question. A shift from witch trials to domestic illness could certainly be considered a good step toward rational explanation, but far from accurately understanding how our minds work. Until we achieve an accurate understanding without false notions, perceptions of mental illness will continue to be coloured by ignorance and superstition.

Previously, mental illness was considered to be found in the soul (later to be understood as the mind of the individual), and could only be explained (or cured) through supernatural and then psychological means (William, 1957). The shift to mind from soul was significant, and although an entire branch of research sprang up around it, little else changed. Psychology continued its evolutionary "process of alternate progress and retrogression" (Turner, 1957, p. 446), always dodging around an honest answer to the mind/body duality. Shrouded in the idea that the mind exists beyond the physical realm, early psychology focused on explaining mental illness in terms of a patient's own experience and thoughts—hence terms like 'domestic illness.' In this context, those with an obsessive-compulsive disorder are acting out against a lonely childhood, or a person suffering from depression is thus because they have no close friends. Psychology, like the religions before it, tried to explain mental illness in terms of its own understandings.

Today, research is slowly uncovering the complexities of the brain, and in doing so it is starting to consider thought processes from an empirical rather than fanciful basis. If this kind of thinking continues, people may begin to see mental illness as a quantifiable, physical issue rather than an abstract, superstitious defect that somehow reflects on the value of the afflicted person. The stigma of mental illness may be ingrained as it is in public consciousness because it is fixed to these historical, superstitious ideas. A person with an 'abnormal' mind is tied to this idea of metaphysical value. In short, mental illness carries with it spiritual connotations from previous religious and psychological ideas of mind and soul. Those suffering from a mental illness are not viewed as sick or injured; rather, they are seen as no longer possessing those attributes which make humans spiritually superior.

THE NEGATIVE CYCLE

Ironically, the power of the brain in the brain/body system has often been overlooked by medicine simply because it is not an easily understood and analysed connection. By integrating the concept of mind back into the brain, and the brain back into the body, a very complex but essential understanding might be realized.

Approaching mental wellness is a vital part of overcoming any kind of physical imbalance, from breaking an ankle to developing depression (Brewer and Petipas, 2006). By appreciating mental/physical oneness we are able to deal with a situation rationally and completely without stigma sneaking in to weaken the work of healing. I am a good example of this. Currently labouring under the agony of a 3-month-old back injury, I am in anguish whenever I sit down. I have been injured in this manner before, and have recovered much more quickly, but the stress of being away from my family and working 60-plus hours per week on my studies while not producing income and worrying about finances has greatly aggravated it, just as any rough physical activity would have. I am so tired and mentally stressed that I am unable to find the time to relax and laugh. As a consequence, I am denying myself important, natural support mechanisms. Happiness and laughter produce chemicals similar to those released by cocaine or amphetamines.

Imagining a person with a depressive disorder in this circumstance produces some dark possibilities. If a mechanism in the brain is not working properly, and as a result one finds that they are depressed, it would seem almost impossible to get the positive chemical reward that the brain delivers from laughter. Considering the negative external stimuli that further create a downward tailspin (social stigma), it is little wonder that depression can be such a devastating illness. Clear, biological explanations for some forms of depression are becoming evident. Serotonin and norepinephrine (HealthyPlace.com, nd) are both hormones that have been linked with sleeplessness, irritability, and anxiety. Prior to this biological connection, depression was assessed psychologically (you're sad because of your childhood, for example), and before that, spiritually (the devil's got you!). This cycle of negativity is chemical and internal, but the detrimental effects of mental illness produce far more negative results than just the chemical cycle described.

A mentally ill person also faces the social pressures previously mentioned. Not only are they dealing with their chemical imbalances, they are also dealing with their own fear of the mental health system, born of the historical stigma still so prevalent in society (Surgeon General, 1999). Mental health issues are more than an illness in the public mind—recall the spiritual association. Fear of the unknown keeps stereotypical, superstitious ideas about mental illness alive, and creates a patina of fear around the entire profession. And while social support is vital to people in successfully dealing with their mental illness (Hafen, Karren, Frandsen, and Smith, 1996), the lack of such support can become the 'final straw' for many people; without their social network, they fall further and more quickly than their condition alone could accomplish.

The Positive Cycle

So how can this work to heal rather than hurt? Positive support can have a tremendous impact on the deleterious effects of mental illness. Beginning at home, an educated, understanding family can assist an adolescent in coming to terms with a newly discovered mental illness, assist an adult in modifying their lifestyle to cope with their illness, or provide an elderly patient with a loving, safe environment. This is to say nothing about the preventative effects of a robust, understanding family. Many people who might be at risk for illness may never have it manifest because they are never put into a negative cycle that prompts the imbalance. Understanding just what the mental illness is without all the negative stereotyping and mysticism that surrounds it can free both the patient and the family from the guilt that often accompanies mental illness. The empirical, scientific approach mentioned at the beginning of this chapter can assist in this as it clears away the historical baggage and allows supporters to see the problem with greater clarity.

Dealing with mental illness is not like dealing with the majority of physical illnesses. In most cases, physical injuries can repair themselves quite quickly. The vast majority of mental illnesses are related to deeper concerns and a happy, quick conclusion to the imbalance is often unlikely. Those imbalances are often hidden, being genetic or developmental, and solutions are, at best, 'guessed at.' Psychiatrists specialize in both general medicine and a range of psychological and pharmaceutical options in order to try to 'cover the bases' in this rather complex exercise in speculation (Birecree and Cutler, 1998). Keeping this complexity in mind is the key to realizing the truth of mental illness and how best to come to terms with it.

By surrounding patients with positive support and open, unprejudiced minds willing to learn the truth of the issue, potential stressors related to societal dysfunction and personal abhorrence are mitigated. Such supportive experiences serve to prompt positive chemical responses and enhance recovery.

Conclusion

As noted elsewhere in this volume, mental health issues are among the most significant of social problems in contemporary society. The hidden nature of this infirmity and its historical connotations still 'creep up' to confound the best intentions of the agents of social change. The majority of the population still holds misconceptions about human thought and the illnesses associated with it. I have suggested that an empirical, scientific understanding of the brain and the chemical processes within it would go a long way toward resolving these social fallacies, but these beliefs are tied up in metaphysical and spiritual concepts that are fundamentally connected with how people see themselves. Many people still chafe at the idea of being conceptualized as an animal; they continue to cling to the idea of mind and soul, and have the need for a connection to the metaphysical. Being a wonderfully complex, intelligent, dexterous animal is, seemingly, not enough. Does seeing the mind as an illusion and thought as physical process make us any less wonderful? Did finally accepting the fact that the Earth is not the centre of the universe detract that much from who we are?

I suspect that mental illness will lose much of its stigma when we finally let go of the 500-year-old idea that we are Descartes' ghost in a machine. The mind-body/soul-body duality is an old fantasy that should be put in the dustbin of history. Not only would stigma born of ignorance vanish, but we would finally begin to mould the mind to something functionally accurate and empowering. Accurately engineered mind support could amplify the positive effects of the workings of the brain—such as the effects of laughter—in powerful, more efficient ways. Just as with any science, we *can* make great strides forward if we get our historical prejudices out of the way first.

REFERENCES

Andersen, M.B. (2005). *Sports psychology in practice*. Campaign, IL: Human Kinetics. p.93.

Birecree, E., and Cutler, D.L. (1998). What makes a community psychiatrist? *Community Mental Health Journal*, 34(4), 433-435.

Brendan Malley, P. (1999). Legal and ethical dimensions for mental health professionals. Bridgeport, NJ: George H. Buchanan Co.

Brewer, B.W., and Petipas, A.J. (2006). Returning to self: The anxieties of coming back after injury. In M.B. Andersen (Ed.), *Sports psychology in practice* (pp. 93-108). Champaign, IL: Human Kinetics.

Brown, M., Ralph, S., and Brember, I. (2002). Change-linked work-related stress in British teachers. *Journal of Research in Education*, 67, 1-12.

Glossary of Old Names (nd). Retrieved December 21, 2006 from http://www.bignell.uk.com/glossary_of_old_names.htm.

Goshen, C.E. (1967). *Documentary history of psychiatry: A source book on historical principles*. New York: Vision Press,

Hafen, B.Q., Karren, K.J., Frandsen, K.J., and Smith, N.L. (1996). *Mind/body health: The effects of attitudes, emotions, and relationships*. Boston: Allyn & Bacon.

HealthyPlace.com (nd). Depression community: Causes of depression. Retrieved December 21, 2006 from http://www.healthyplace.com/communities/depression/causes.asp.

Røysamb, E., Tambs, K., Reichborn-Kjennerud, T., Neale, M.C., and Harris, J.R. (2003). Happiness and health: Environmental and genetic contributions to the relationship between subjective well-being, perceived health, and somatic illness. *Journal of Personality and Social Psychology*, 85(6), 1136-1146.

Russell, B.A. (1995). *Analysis of mind*. New York: Routledge.

Ryle, G. (1949). *The concept of mind*. University of Chicago Press.

Surgeon General (1999). Mental health: A report of the Surgeon General. Retrieved December 21, 2006 from http://www.surgeongeneral.gov/library/mentalhealth/home.html.

Taylor, H. (1998). Large majority of people believe they will go to heaven; only one in fifty thinks they will go to hell. A paradox: Many Christians and non-Christians believe in astrology, ghosts and reincarnation. Retrieved December 21, 2006 from http://www.harrisinteractive.com/harris_poll/index.asp?PID=167 #41.

Turner, W. (1957). *History of philosophy*. New York: Ginn & Company.

Plate 11 "Labyrinth" (J. LeClair)

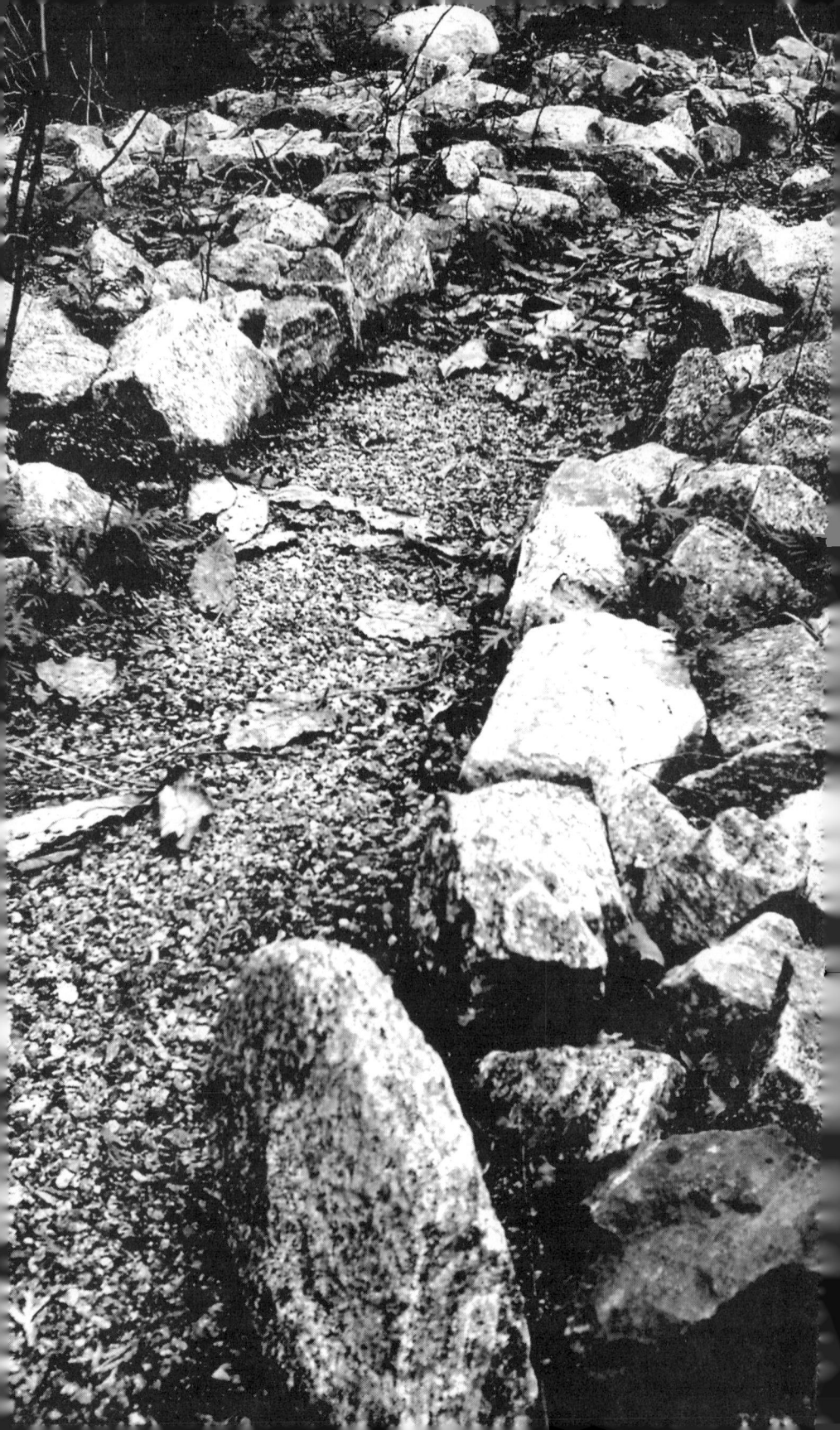